Biological Efficacy of Natural and Chemically Modified Products against Oral Inflammatory Lesions

Biological Efficacy of Natural and Chemically Modified Products against Oral Inflammatory Lesions

Special Issue Editor

Hiroshi Sakagami

MDPI • Basel • Beijing • Wuhan • Barcelona • Belgrade

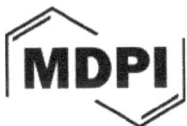

MDPI

Special Issue Editor
Hiroshi Sakagami
Meikai University Research Institute of Odontology (M-RIO)
Japan

Editorial Office
MDPI
St. Alban-Anlage 66
4052 Basel, Switzerland

This is a reprint of articles from the Special Issue published online in the open access journal *Medicines* (ISSN 2305-6320) from 2018 to 2019 (available at: https://www.mdpi.com/journal/medicines/special_issues/natural_products_stomatitis).

For citation purposes, cite each article independently as indicated on the article page online and as indicated below:

LastName, A.A.; LastName, B.B.; LastName, C.C. Article Title. *Journal Name* **Year**, *Article Number, Page Range.*

ISBN 978-3-03897-992-0 (Pbk)
ISBN 978-3-03897-993-7 (PDF)

Cover image courtesy of Hiroshi Sakagami.

Contents

About the Special Issue Editor

Hiroshi Sakagami was born in Tokyo (1952) and obtained his Ph.D. from the Faculty of Pharmaceutical Sciences, University of Tokyo (1980). He worked for 17 years in the Department of Biochemistry, School of Medicine, Showa University, Tokyo, with a three-year stay as a visiting researcher in Roswell Park Memorial Institute, Buffalo, NY. He became a professor in the Division of Pharmacology, Meikai University School of Dentistry (1997) and the director of Meikai Pharmaco-Medical Laboratory (MPL) (1999). He also worked as a professor at Meikai University Research Institute of Odontology (M-RIO) (2017). His research interests include the biological function of lignin–carbohydrate complexes, the application of plant extracts to oral diseases, the exploration of anticancer drugs that have the least keratinocyte toxicity and the creation of new fields of research by international collaboration. He was the principal investigator for seven Grants-in-Aid from the Ministry of Education, Science, Sports and Culture of Japan. He is also the director of the board of the trustees for both Meikai and Asahi Universities

Preface to "Biological Efficacy of Natural and Chemically Modified Products against Oral Inflammatory Lesions"

Stomatitis is not life-threatening, but its occasional recurrence significantly reduces our quality of life. It is unclear to what extent prolonged stomatitis is involved in life span and cancer development. Among natural products, Kampo is the most popular to treat stomatitis, possibly due to its high therapeutic effect. Kampo is the mixture of at least two different constitutional plant extracts. The choice of which plant combination to use depends on the diagnostic power and experience of the physician. From plant extracts, various bioactive substances have been isolated and manufactured into gel-entrapped and oral care products. There are still many unknown compounds in nature. By introducing substituents into a basic framework, compounds with higher activity and lower side effects can be produced. Finally, by combining selected compounds, a treatment that is more clinically effective than the existing Kampo prescriptions can be explored. The present Special Issue, entitled "Biological Efficacy of Natural and Chemically Modified Products against Oral Inflammatory Lesions", is a collection of 11 articles written by virologists, bacteriologists, immunologists, molecular biologists, pharmacologists and clinical doctors. The editorial serves to introduce and summarize the included topics, as well as to survey the publication incidence rates for each age group, etiology and treatment of stomatitis. This Special Issue, written by specialists from a wide range of fields, will interest and enlighted readers. It will be useful not only for researchers, but also for beginners such as students. I hope that this book can contribute to the treatment of stomatitis.

Hiroshi Sakagami
Special Issue Editor

medicines

MDPI

Editorial

Introduction to the Special Issue "Biological Efficacy of Natural and Chemically Modified Products against Oral Inflammatory Lesions"

Hiroshi Sakagami

Meikai University Research Institute of Odontology (M-RIO), 1-1 Keyakidai, Sakado, Saitama 350-0283, Japan; sakagami@dent.meikai.ac.jp; Tel.: +81-49-279-2758 (office); +81-49-279-2787 (M-RIO) (dial-in)

Received: 23 April 2019; Accepted: 25 April 2019; Published: 28 April 2019

Abstract: This editorial is a brief introduction to the Special Issue of "Biological Efficacy of Natural and Chemically Modified Products against Oral Inflammatory Lesions". From the natural resources and chemical modifications of the backbone structures of natural products, various attractive substances with new biological functions were excavated. Best fit combination of these materials may contribute in the treatment of oral diseases.

Keywords: Kampo medicine; constituent plant extract; stomatitis; oral inflammation; quantitative structure-activity relationship (QSAR) analysis; metabolomics

---

Stomatitis is a sore and often recurrent inflammatory condition of the oral mucosa. Approximately 28,542 published papers of stomatitis were found by the recent PubMed search (Survey 1, Table 1). When searched by keyword A (stomatitis) and keyword B (patient's age), 7695, 10,241, 1142, 2990 and 920 publications were found in elders, adults, young, child and pediatrics, respectively. This indicates that the citing number of older populations in the papers of stomatitis (6695 + 10,241/2 = 8968) were approximately 5.3 times higher than that of younger populations (1142 + 2990 + 929/3 = 1684). Similar trends were found in the papers of herpes stomatitis, aphthous stomatitis, oral inflammation, periodontitis and gingivitis. This may reflect the age-related increase in the incidence of stomatitis.

Oral inflammation is triggered or aggravated by various factors, but how much is each factor involved in the generation of stomatitis? To address this question, the numbers of publications of each factor was searched (Survey 2, Table 1). The most frequently cited factor was virus infection, followed by bacterial infection and radiotherapy. Surprisingly, fungal infection, autoimmune diseases, immune suppression, stress, nutritional deficiency, genetic background, reactive oxygen species (ROS), cigarette and dental prosthetics were cited much less frequently.

The most popular therapeutic agents for stomatitis was searched next (Survey 3, Table 1). Antiviral agents seem to be the most popular for the treatment of stomatitis and herpes stomatitis, followed by antibacterial agents. On the other hand, antibacterial and anti-inflammatory agents appeared to be most often used for the treatment of aphthous stomatitis, oral inflammation, periodontitis and gingivitis. It is surprising that the citation numbers of Traditional Chinese Medicine (TCM) and Kampo medicines were much less, only one tenth that of natural products.

This Special Issue picks up 11 articles, that are listed in four separate sections: Section 1 (Antiviral and antibacterial agents [1,2]); Section 2 (Kampo medicine and constitutive plant extracts [3–6]); Section 3 (Protection mechanism, [7,8]; (Application of metabolomics and quantitative structure-activity relationship (QSAR) [9–11]).

Table 1. Survey of publications of stomatitis and related oral inflammations, narrowed down by age-difference, etiology and treatment (based on PubMed search, 13 April 2019).

Keyword B	Number of Cited References					
	Keyword B	Keyword A				
	Stomatitis	Herpes Stomatitis	Aphthous Stomatitis	Oral Inflammation	Periodontitis	Gingivitis
Total	28,542 (100)	1935 (100)	3781 (100)	35,354 (100)	37,596 (100)	13,902 (100)
Survey 1: Age-related citation rate						
Elderly	7695 (27)	349 (18)	1081 (29)	8677 (25)	12,603 (34)	3833 (28)
Adult	10,241 (36)	599 (31)	1712 (45)	12,122 (34)	17,833 (47)	6092 (44)
Young	1142 (4)	88 (5)	243 (6)	2413 (7)	2603 (7)	1026 (7)
Child	2990 (10)	434 (22)	655 (17)	2708 (8)	2339 (6)	2239 (16)
Pediatric	920 (3)	83 (4)	235 (6)	1449 (4)	660 (2)	403 (3)
Survey 2: Etiology						
Virus infection	6267 (22)	1582 (82)	670 (18)	1437 (4)	689 (2)	650 (5)
Bacterial infection	1658 (6)	174 (9)	267 (7)	4529 (13)	3852 (10)	1711 (12)
Radiotherapy	1521 (5)	46 (2)	54 (1)	352 (1.0)	210 (0.6)	57 (0.4)
Inflammation	1181 (4)	53 (3)	164 (4)	N.D.	5989 (16)	2669 (19)
Autoimmune diseases	941 (3)	82 (4)	248 (7)	1885 (5)	709 (2)	370 (3)
Drug-induced	546 (1.9)	8 (0.4)	22 (0.6)	265 (0.7)	53 (0.1)	485 (3)
Fungal infection	1048 (4)	186 (10)	164 (4)	735 (2)	198 (0.5)	214 (2)
Immune suppression	428 (1.5)	55 (3)	40 (1.1)	603 (2)	131 (0.4)	98 (0.7)
Stress	267 (0.9)	13 (0.7)	92 (2)	2361 (7)	997 (3)	227 (1.6)
Nutritional deficiencies	250 (0.9)	9 (0.5)	90 (2)	1243 (4)	110 (0.3)	162 (1.2)
Genetic background	202 (0.7)	4 (0.2)	40 (1.1)	240 (0.7)	450 (1.2)	47 (0.3)
Reactive oxygen species	119 (0.4)	0 (0)	19 (0.5)	902 (3)	24 (0.06)	150 (1.1)
Vitamin B deficiency	107 (0.4)	0 (0)	52 (1.4)	26 (0.1)	2 (0.01)	14 (0.1)
Cigarette	60 (0.2)	9 (0.5)	18 (0.5)	250 (0.7)	323 (0.9)	82 (0.6)
Dental prosthetics	18 (0.06)	0 (0)	1 (0.03)	19 (0.05)	42 (0.1)	14 (0.1)

Table 1. *Cont.*

Keyword B	Number of Cited References					
	Keyword A					
	Stomatitis	Herpes Stomatitis	Aphthous Stomatitis	Oral Inflammation	Periodontitis	Gingivitis
Survey 3: Treatment						
Antiviral agent	3716 (13)	579 (30)	116 (3)	1028 (3)	321 (0.9)	102 (0.7)
Antibacterial agent	2333 (8)	86 (4)	324 (9)	3036 (9)	2907 (8)	660 (5)
Anti-inflammatory agent	1492 (5)	66 (3)	357 (9)	4975 (14)	1036 (3)	474 (3)
Steroid	1234 (4)	59 (3)	319 (8)	2761 (8)	583 (2)	342 (2)
Natural product	1105 (4)	85 (4)	120 (3)	2063 (6)	640 (2)	314 (2)
Trad. Chinese Med.	54 (0.2)	2 (0.1)	24 (0.6)	349 (1.0)	45 (0.1)	3 (0.02)
Kampo medicine	14 (0.05)	0 (0)	1 (0.03)	27 (0.1)	4 (0.01)	2 (0.01)
Anti-fungal agent	1029 (4)	48 (2)	55 (1.5)	674 (2)	128 (0.3)	37 (0.3)
Immunopotentiator	359 (1.2)	40 (2)	127 (3)	723 (2)	128 (0.3)	37 (0.3)

The top 2 keywords B with high citation rate for each item of Keyword A is highlighted in blue.

1. Antiviral and Antibacterial Agents

Herpes simplex virus (HSV) infects mainly around the mouth and lips. Epstein–Barr virus (EBV) can manifest in the oral cavity and/or head and neck region. Human papilloma virus (HPV) is often found in oral lesions, including oral hairy leukoplakia (OHL) and/or cancers. Common or notable human immunodeficiency virus (HIV)-related oral conditions include xerostomia (dry mouth), candidiasis, OHL, periodontal diseases, Kaposi sarcoma (KS), HPV-associated warts and ulcerative conditions. Asai and Nakashima stated that among natural sources, the red algal protein GRFT and the algae-derived polysaccharide carrageenan (CG) showed excellent antiviral effects on HIV, HSV-2 and HPV, whereas lignin-carbohydrate (LCC) and sulfated polysaccharide showed the highest anti-HIV activity among natural polyphenols and polysaccharides, by non-specific inhibition of virus adsorption [1].

The human oral cavity is assumed to be a reservoir for the pathogens of many systemic infective diseases. Kanamoto et al. investigated seven *Abiotrophia defectiva*, 17 *Granulicatella adiacens* and six *Granulicatella elegans*, isolated from human oral microbiota for their susceptibility to 15 antimicrobial agents. They found that these bacteria were most sensitive to imipenem and amoxicillin, and there was species-related differences with respect to susceptibilities to ciprofloxacin and minocycline [2].

2. Kampo Medicine and Constitutive Plant Extracts

Kampo consists of natural herbs—roots and barks—and has more than 3000 years of history. Watanabe et al. manufactured a Kampo gargle and mastic gel dentifrice for the treatment of peri-implant and severe periodontitis. They found that Kampo reduced the oral bacteria number in vitro, inhibited the bacteria-induced alveolar bone loss and the osteoclast differentiation in vivo, and improved the inflammatory response in the periodontal tissues of patients [3].

Sunagawa et al. reviewed the clinical effect of Hangeshashinto (HST) on cancer patients with chemotherapy-induced mucositis. HST significantly decreased the mean Common Terminology Criteria for Adverse Events grade in the patients and inhibited the growth of Gram-negative bacteria, and the production of PGE_2 and the expression of COX-2 protein. Its constitutive plant extracts (*Glycyrrhizae* Radix, *Pinelliae* Tuber, *Coptidis* Rhizoma and *Ginseng* Radix) enhanced immunity and increased the activity of natural killer cells in mice [4].

Hara et al. showed that among 18 Kampo medicines, HST is most frequently used in Japan, possibly due to the presence of *glycyrrhiza* that contains anti-inflammatory glycyrrhizin. It was surprising that HST had not been used in China [5]. Traditional medicines have been prescribed to elders and adults rather than children, but inclusion of sweet licorice as an ingredient will make it easier for children to take [5].

Ara et al. reviewed the anti-inflammatory action of various natural products [6]. HST inhibited arachidonic acid cascade at multiple points (both COX-1 and COX-2 activities; cPLA2 and COX-2 expressions; ERK phosphorylation). Gingerols and shogaols, the major ingredients in ginger, suppressed NF-κB activation directly or indirectly, leading to the inhibition of COX-2 expression. Recently, β-cryptoxanthin, naringenin, ellagic acid and (-)-epigallocatechin-3-gallate have been reported to show anti-osteoclast characteristics. Since rheumatoid arthritis (RA) is a disease associated with inflammation and bone destruction, and RA prevalence is increased in patients with periodontitis, these natural products may be applicable to treat the periodontitis.

3. Protection and Regeneration Mechanism

Quercetin is a dietary flavonoid found in red wine, tea, many fruits and onions, and well known for its radical scavenging, anti-diabetic, antiviral, anti-pollinosis and anti-allergic activity in vitro and animal models. Edo et al. demonstrated that oral administration of quercetin significantly elevated thioredoxin (TRX) levels in nasal lavage fluids and reduced nasal sneezes and nasal rubbing behaviors.

Quercetin's ability to increase TRX production may account, at least in part, for its clinical efficacy toward allergic rhinitis [7].

Moritani et al. provided a new standpoint of action mechanism of fluocinolone acetonide (synthetic glucocorticoid having 6α,9α-difluoro- and 16,17-acetonide structure) and harmine (one of the β-carboline alkaloids). These compounds strongly induced Cellular Communication Network Factor 2 (CNN2), which encodes protein that is critical in wound healing. Since CNN2 potentiated TGF-β-associated chondrogenesis of bone marrow mesenchymal stem/progenitor cells, harmine may effective to treat stomatitis [8].

4. Application of Metabolomics and QSAR

In dentistry, zinc oxide-eugenol formulations have been used for many years as the preferred material for root canal fillings. However, zinc oxide-eugenol released cytotoxic concentrations of eugenol, and induced chronic inflammation. Sakagami et al. demonstrated by metabolomics analysis that Eugenol rapidly induced the vacuolization and suppressed the TCA cycle in human gingival fibroblast, periodontal ligament fibroblast and pulp cells. Similarly, sodium fluoride, that is included in several dentifrices, and benzaldehyde, anticancer principle of figs, blocked the TCA cycle of human oral squamous cell carcinoma cell lines. It is crucial to pursue the biological significance of the inhibition of the TCA cycle in each case for the safe and effective clinical application of these substances [9].

Sakagami et al. reported that among three major natural polyphenols, lignin-carbohydrate complexes (LCC) showed the highest anti-HIV activity, while chemically-modified chromone derivatives (backbone structure of flavonoids) showed much higher anti-tumor activity than most of tannins and flavonoids. QSAR (quantitative structure-activity relationship) analysis suggests a possible link between their tumor-specificity and three-dimensional molecular shape [10]. Although the anti-periodontitis activity of synthetic angiotensin II blockers has been suggested in many papers, natural angiotensin II blockers have not yet been tested for their possible anti-periodontitis activity. Basic structures of the dental plaque is produced from sucrose by glucosyltransferase enzymes (GTFs). Various tannins were found to be excellent inhibitors of GTFs, leading to the manufacture of the gel-entrapped catechin. QASR analysis can be used to explore more selective GTFs and angiotensin II receptor blockers (ARB).

Nagai et al. analyzed the merged data of cytotoxic activities and chemical structures of a total of 494 compounds, and found that the structure-toxicity relationship prediction model showed higher prediction accuracy than the tumor selectivity prediction model. This was mainly due to the fact that descriptors with a high contribution differed for tumor and normal cells. Construction of the tumor selective toxicity prediction model with a higher predictive accuracy may contribute to the screening of candidate compounds for new anticancer drugs [11].

Natural resources provide numerous useful compounds for treating stomatitis. We can modify their backbone structure to synthesize more active compounds, using QSAR analysis. We can change the combination of candidate components, measure their determined biological activity, and repeat this process until the best combination is determined. Accumulation of such data may lead us to manufacture the best Kampo medicine (Figure 1).

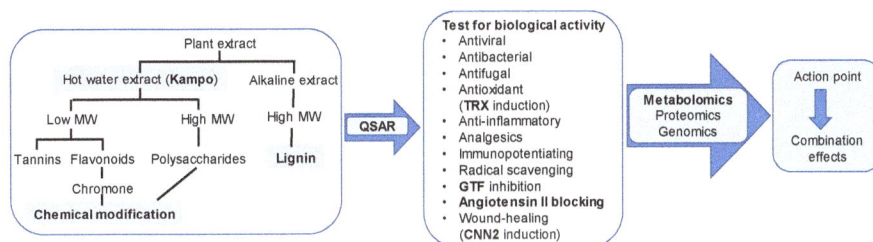

Figure 1. Flow chart to select the best combination of Kampo ingredients.

References

1. Asai, D.; Nakashima, H. Pathogenic Viruses Commonly Present in the Oral Cavity and Relevant Antiviral Compounds Derived from Natural Products. *Medicines* **2018**, *5*, 120. [CrossRef] [PubMed]
2. Kanamoto, T.; Terakubo, S.; Nakashima, H. Antimicrobial Susceptibilities of Oral Isolates of Abiotrophia and Granulicatella According to the Consensus Guidelines for Fastidious Bacteria. *Medicines* **2018**, *5*, 129. [CrossRef] [PubMed]
3. Shuji Watanabe, S.; Toyama, T.; Sato, T.; Suzuki, M.; Morozumi, A.; Sakagami, H.; Hamada, N. Kampo Therapies and the Use of Herbal Medicines in the Dentistry in Japan. *Medicines* **2019**, *6*, 34. [CrossRef] [PubMed]
4. Sunagawa, M.; Yamaguchi, K.; Tsukada, M.; Ebihara, N.; Ikemoto, H.; Hisamitsu, T. Kampo (Traditional Japanese Herbal) Formulae for Treatment of Stomatitis and Oral Mucositis. *Medicines* **2018**, *5*, 130. [CrossRef] [PubMed]
5. Hara, Y.; Shiratuchi, H.; Kaneko, T.; Sakagami, H. Search for Drugs Used in Hospitals to Treat Stomatitis. *Medicines* **2019**, *6*, 19. [CrossRef] [PubMed]
6. Ara, T.; Nakatani, S.; Kobata, K.; Sogawa, N.; Sogawa, C. The Biological Efficacy of Natural Products against Acute and Chronic Inflammatory Diseases in the Oral Region. *Medicines* **2018**, *5*, 122. [CrossRef] [PubMed]
7. Edo, Y.; Otaki, A.; Asano, K. Quercetin Enhances the Thioredoxin Production of Nasal Epithelial Cells In Vitro and In Vivo. *Medicines* **2018**, *5*, 124. [CrossRef] [PubMed]
8. Moritani, N.H.; Hara, E.S.; Kubota, S. New Functions of Classical Compounds against Orofacial Inflammatory Lesions. *Medicines* **2018**, *5*, 118. [CrossRef] [PubMed]
9. Sakagami, H.; Sugimoto, M.; Kanda, Y.; Murakami, Y.; Amano, O.; Saitoh, J.; Kochi, A. Changes in Metabolic Profiles of Human Oral Cells by Benzylidene Ascorbates and Eugenol. *Medicines* **2018**, *5*, 116. [CrossRef] [PubMed]
10. Sakagami, H.; Watanabe, T.; Hoshino, T.; Suda, N.; Mori, K.; Yasui, T.; Yamauchi, N.; Kashiwagi, H.; Gomi, T.; Oizumi, T.; et al. Recent Progress of Basic Studies of Natural Products and Their Dental Application. *Medicines* **2019**, *6*, 4. [CrossRef] [PubMed]
11. Nagai, J.; Imamura, M.; Sakagami, H.; Uesawa, Y. QSAR Prediction Model to Search for Compounds with Selective Cytotoxicity Against Oral Cell Cancer. *Medicines* **2019**, *6*, 45. [CrossRef] [PubMed]

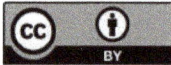

medicines MDPI

Review

Pathogenic Viruses Commonly Present in the Oral Cavity and Relevant Antiviral Compounds Derived from Natural Products

Daisuke Asai and **Hideki Nakashima** *

Department of Microbiology, St. Marianna University School of Medicine, Kawasaki 216-8511, Japan
* Correspondence: nakahide@marianna-u.ac.jp; Tel.: +81-44-977-8111

Received: 24 October 2018; Accepted: 7 November 2018; Published: 12 November 2018

Abstract: Many viruses, such as human herpesviruses, may be present in the human oral cavity, but most are usually asymptomatic. However, if individuals become immunocompromised by age, illness, or as a side effect of therapy, these dormant viruses can be activated and produce a variety of pathological changes in the oral mucosa. Unfortunately, available treatments for viral infectious diseases are limited, because (1) there are diseases for which no treatment is available; (2) drug-resistant strains of virus may appear; (3) incomplete eradication of virus may lead to recurrence. Rational design strategies are widely used to optimize the potency and selectivity of drug candidates, but discovery of leads for new antiviral agents, especially leads with novel structures, still relies mostly on large-scale screening programs, and many hits are found among natural products, such as extracts of marine sponges, sea algae, plants, and arthropods. Here, we review representative viruses found in the human oral cavity and their effects, together with relevant antiviral compounds derived from natural products. We also highlight some recent emerging pharmaceutical technologies with potential to deliver antivirals more effectively for disease prevention and therapy.

Keywords: anti-human immunodeficiency virus (HIV); antiviral; natural product; human virus

1. Introduction

The human oral cavity is home to a rich microbial flora, including bacteria, fungi, and viruses. Oral tissues are constantly exposed to these microbes, which form a complex ecological community that influences oral and systemic health [1]. Discussion of the microbiological aspects of oral disease traditionally focuses on bacteria and fungi, but viruses are attracting increasing attention as pathogens. Viruses are generally more difficult to detect among pathogenic microbes, at least with traditional methods such as in vitro cultivation; however, the development of sophisticated molecular tools, including monoclonal antibodies and viral genome sequencing, have greatly advanced the field of virology over the past decade or so. A number of viruses have been found in the oral cavity, of which many are thought to be involved in the development of various types of oral ulcers, oral tumors, classical oral infectious diseases, and periodontitis. For example, herpes simplex virus 1 (HSV-1) causes gingivostomatitis, and the virus can subsequently enter a dormant state in the trigeminal ganglion. Blood-borne viruses such as human immunodeficiency virus (HIV) can enter the mouth via gingival crevicular fluid, and viruses causing upper respiratory tract infections are also found in the mouth [2]. Similarly, the mumps virus is known to infect the salivary glands and can be found in saliva of affected individuals. Human papillomavirus (HPV) is responsible for several oral conditions, including papilloma, condylomas, and focal epithelial hyperplasia, and has also been implicated in head and neck squamous cell carcinoma.

The field of antiviral research acquired new urgency since the 1980s, owing to the global spread of HIV, which causes acquired immune deficiency syndrome (AIDS). HIV is a member of the RNA retroviruses, which contain a reverse transcriptase (RT) enzyme that transcribes RNA into DNA in infected cells, leading to integration of the retroviral genomic information into chromosomal DNA of the host cell. Antiretroviral drugs (ARVs) often target RT, but are always given in combination with other ARVs for antiretroviral therapy (ART) in order to increase efficacy and reduce the development of resistance. The anti-HIV agent zidovudine (AZT) is a representative ARV, and was the first to be approved in the United States in 1986; however, recently, many new classes of drugs have been introduced [3], together with new formulations such as long-acting depot-type anti-HIV drugs and easy-to-use gel formulations for preventing rectal HIV infection [4].

The enormous research effort directed at the treatment of HIV has led to important advances in basic science and many therapeutic breakthroughs, including the development of inhibitors targeting a range of human viruses. Nevertheless, large-scale screening of natural products, such as extracts of marine sponges, sea algae, plants, and arthropods, remains an important source of leads for new antiviral agents, whose potency and selectivity can then be optimized with the aid of rational design strategies, including computational approaches. Thus, the aim of this review is to provide a personal viewpoint on natural-product-derived antiviral agents that are available for the treatment of pathogenic viruses, especially HIV, that may cause symptoms in the oral cavity, considered from a historic perspective. As major candidates for viruses involved in oral diseases, we focus on (1) HSV-1 and HSV-2; (2) Epstein–Barr virus (EBV); (3) Kaposi sarcoma-associated herpesvirus (KSHV); (4) human papilloma virus (HPV); and (5) HIV.

2. Viruses Associated with Oral Diseases of Humans

Members of the human herpesvirus (HHV) family cause common primary viral infections of the oral mucous membrane, and may also play a role in periodontitis. There are eight members of the HHV family, which are among the largest and most complex human viruses. We focus here on HSV-1, HSV-2, EBV, and KSHV; the others are varicella-zoster virus (VZV), human cytomegalovirus (HCMV), HHV-6, and HHV-7 (Table 1). HPV is a diverse family of viruses, which can cause a variety of pathologies, including oral squamous cell carcinoma, and chronic infection of the skin or mucosal epithelium. Furthermore, the retrovirus HIV causes a decline in immunocompetence, which can lead to various cutaneous manifestations [5]. In this section, we present a brief overview of these viruses.

Table 1. Human herpesviruses (HHVs) and their associated diseases.

Type	Target	Oral Manifestations	Other Pathology
1. HSV-1	Mucoepithelial	Herpes ulcers	Genital ulcers
2. HSV-2	Mucoepithelial	Herpes ulcers	Genital ulcers
3. VZV	Mucoepithelial	Possible oral manifestations of chicken pox and herpes zoster	Chicken pox and herpes zoster
4. EVB	B cells and epithelial cells	Hairy leukoplakia, Periodontitis (nasopharyngeal carcinoma)	Mononucleosis and lymphoma
5. HCMV	Monocytes, lymphocytes, and epithelial cells	Periodontitis	
6. HHV-6	Monocytes and macrophages		Roseola in infants
7. HHV-7	T cells and possibly others		Roseola in infants
8. KSHV	B cells and possibly others		Kaposi sarcoma (in AIDS patients)

HSV-1, herpes simplex virus 1; HSV-2, herpes simplex virus 2; VZV, varicella-zoster virus; EBV, Epstein–Barr virus; HCMV, human cytomegalovirus; HHV-6, human herpesvirus 6; HHV-7, human herpesvirus 7; KSHV, Kaposi sarcoma-associated herpesvirus; AIDS, acquired immune deficiency syndrome.

2.1. HSV-1 and HSV-2

HSVs are relatively large, enveloped, double-stranded DNA viruses with icosahedral symmetry. Infections by HSV-1 are referred to as upper body infections to distinguish them from the genital infection caused by HSV-2. The formal designations of these viruses are human herpesvirus 1 (HHV-1) and 2 (HHV-2). Oral herpes is a viral infection mainly around the mouth and lips caused by herpes simplex viruses. HSV-1 causes painful sores on the upper and lower lips, gums, tongue, roof of the mouth, inside the cheeks or nose, and sometimes on the face, chin, and neck. In addition, HSV-1 can cause symptoms such as swollen lymph nodes, fever, and muscle aches. HSV-2 is primarily associated with the genitals and most often causes genital herpes. However, it may spread to the mouth during oral sex, causing oral herpes. HSVs characteristically establish latent infection in sensory nerve ganglia, and, in this case, signs appear only when the virus is reactivated. Following recovery from primary oropharyngeal infection, the individual retains HSV DNA in the trigeminal ganglion, but the virus becomes dormant. Infected individuals have at least a 50% chance of suffering sporadic recurrent attacks of herpes labialis (otherwise known as facial herpes, herpes simplex, fever blisters, or cold sores) from time to time throughout the remainder of their life.

At present, the drug of choice for the treatment of HSV infections is acyclovir (ACV; 9-(2-hydroxyethoxymethyl)guanine). Its unique advantage over earlier nucleoside derivatives is that HSV-encoded thymidine kinase (TK), which has broader specificity than cellular TK, phosphorylates ACV to ACV-monophosphate (ACV-P). A cellular guanosine monophosphate (GMP) kinase then completes the phosphorylation to generate the active agent, ACV-triphosphate (ACV-PPP). ACV-PPP acts as both an inhibitor and a substrate of the viral enzyme, competing with guanosine triphosphate (GTP) for incorporation into DNA; this results in chain termination, because ACV lacks the 3′-hydroxyl group required for chain elongation. Before ACV was introduced, vidarabine (Ara-A) which was the first nucleoside analog antiviral to be systemically administered, was used. Ara-A is also sequentially phosphorylated by kinases to afford the triphosphate ara-ATP, which competitively inhibits deoxyATP (dATP). However, the mechanism of Ara-A is different in that all three phosphorylations are mediated by host adenosine kinases, resulting in a lack of specificity. Indeed, Ara-A is more toxic and less metabolically stable than ACV, although it is still employed against ACV-resistant strains. In addition, valaciclovir (VACV), an ester of ACV, is a prodrug that has greater oral bioavailability than ACV. VACV provides high plasma levels of the parent compound and offers greater efficacy, as well as decreased dosing frequency. Additionally, guanosine analog famciclovir (FCV) is another choice for the treatment of HSV infections.

2.2. EBV

EBV, formally human herpesvirus 4 (HHV-4), has a small DNA genome, and its main host cells are B lymphocytes and epithelial cells. EBV replicates in epithelial cells of the nasopharynx and salivary glands, especially the parotid, lysing them and releasing infectious virions into saliva. EBV attaches to B lymphocytes via binding of the viral glycoprotein gp350/EBV to CD21 receptors on the lymphocyte. The major characteristic of infected B lymphocytes is transformation. When this occurs, only a small amount of the viral DNA integrates into the host chromosome, and most of the viral DNA stays in a separate circular episome form. The B lymphocytes infiltrating the lymphatic tissue of the infected oropharyngeal mucosa may, in turn, become infected, but are generally not permissive for virus production. EBV is transmitted only after repeated contact with infected individuals. It can manifest in the oral cavity and/or head and neck region, e.g., as Burkitt's lymphoma (BL), mononucleosis, or oral hairy leukoplakia (OHL), and the prevalence and disease severity are increased in individuals co-infected with HIV. Mononucleosis is common, irrespective of HIV infection status, and is associated with a primary EBV infection during adolescence and young adulthood. OHL is an oral mucosal lesion that is associated with EBV infection and is often asymptomatic, commonly presenting as non-removable white patches on the lateral borders of the tongue. OHL is now an established phenomenon in a range of conditions affecting immune competence, e.g., in immunosuppressed patients with HIV infection or bone marrow transplant recipients [6]. EBV-positive Hodgkin's and non-Hodgkin's lymphomas may manifest in the head and neck. Nasopharyngeal carcinoma (NPC) is also a head and neck cancer associated with EBV infection. No effective anti-EBV drugs have yet been developed. EBV is sensitive to ACV in vitro, but systemic administration of this drug has little effect on clinical illness.

2.3. KSHV

The formal designation of human herpesvirus 8 (HHV-8) was proposed for KSHV, in keeping with the systematic nomenclature adopted for all human herpesviruses. KSHV is the causative virus of Kaposi sarcoma (KS), multicentric Castleman's disease, and primary effusion lymphoma. Humans are thought to be the natural host for KSHV, which is primarily transmitted via saliva. Infection occurs during childhood and increases with age. KSHV is detected in endothelial and spindle cells of Kaposi sarcoma lesions, as well as in circulating endothelial cells, primary effusion lymphoma cells, B lymphocytes, macrophages, dendritic cells, oropharynx and prostatic glandular epithelium, and keratinocytes. Epidemiological studies indicate that there are four clinical variants of KS: (1) classic; (2) endemic (African); (3) iatrogenic (transplant-associated); and (4) HIV/AIDS-associated (epidemic) (HIV-KS). It is well known that KS is an AIDS-defining illness and the most frequent AIDS-associated neoplasm. HIV-KS commonly affects the oral cavity, with the oral mucosa being the initial site of clinical disease in 20% of patients [7]. ART has successfully decreased the prevalence and incidence of HIV-KS. A liposome-encapsulated form of doxorubicin (Doxil) is often used primarily for the treatment of AIDS-related KS.

2.4. HPV

HPV is a small, non-enveloped, double-stranded DNA virus with icosahedral symmetry. There is wide genetic diversity among HPVs, and more than 70 genotypes of HPVs have been identified so far. Some of them are associated with a variety of benign papillomatous lesions of the skin and squamous mucosa. The mechanism of malignant transformation is not fully understood and is difficult to study because HPV is difficult to grow in culture. It is thought that the viral DNA remains episomal in benign lesions, whereas it is integrated into host chromosomal DNA in malignant cells, e.g., cervical carcinoma. Oral papillomas of the conventional kind can be caused by sexually transmitted HPV types 6, 11, and 16. Common warts are most frequently caused by type 2 [8].

HPVs induce benign tumors of the epithelium in their natural host. The discovery of the role of HPV in cervical cancer has led to the widespread use of HPV vaccines for young women, but it is still uncertain whether HPV actually plays an essential role [9]. Based on their putative role in cervical carcinoma, the viruses are classified as having either high (primarily 16 and 18) or low (primarily 6 and 11) oncogenic potential. HPVs are often found in oral samples from healthy mouths, such as brush samples of mucosa, but their prevalence is typically reported to be higher in biopsies from oral lesions, including leukoplakia and/or cancers. The association with oncogenic HPVs is less obvious in the case of leukoplakia, while there are many reports of HPVs in malignant cancers. The observed prevalence in oral cancers is considerably lower than that in cervical cancers, but the case for a role of HPVs is still reasonably strong [2]. When generations who have received papillomavirus vaccines grow up, we should find out whether the prevalence of oral carcinomas declines along with the expected decline in cervical cancer. Imiquimod is used as a patient-applied cream to treat genital warts. Imiquimod is a Toll-like receptor 7 (TLR7) agonist, promoting the secretion of inflammatory cytokines. Traditional treatments consist of locally destructive techniques, such as cautery, surgical excision, and cryotherapy using liquid nitrogen.

2.5. HIV

HIV is an enveloped retrovirus that is transmitted through sexual contact or by contact with infected body fluids. Retroviral RT allows the virus to integrate its genetic information into the host chromosome. HIV targets CD4-positive T-helper cells, and the resulting development of immunodeficiency leads to AIDS. Viral infections are a significant cause of morbidity and mortality in immunosuppressed patients. In general, diseases or medical treatments that have cytostatic or cytotoxic effects on lymphocytes increase the risk of viral infections, and the viral infection rate depends on the nature and degree of immunosuppression. The reactivation of latent virus is the most important determinant of the type of viral infection, and this occurs most commonly in immunosuppressed patients. Skin and mucous membrane manifestations of HIV infection may result from opportunistic disorders secondary to the decline in immunocompetence caused by the infection. HIV-related oral conditions occur in a large proportion of patients, and frequently are misdiagnosed or inadequately treated. Dental expertise is necessary for appropriate management of oral manifestations of HIV infection; however, in practice, many patients do not receive adequate dental care. Common or notable HIV-related oral conditions include the following symptoms: xerostomia (dry mouth), candidiasis, OHL, periodontal diseases such as linear gingival erythema and necrotizing ulcerative periodontitis, KS, HPV-associated warts, ulcerative conditions including HSV lesions, recurrent aphthous ulcers, and neutropenic ulcers. In 1993, consensus was reached on the classification of the oral manifestations of HIV, so-called the 1993 EC-Clearinghouse classification. It classifies oral lesions associated with HIV (HIV-OLs) into three groups: (1) lesions strongly associated with HIV infection; (2) those less commonly associated with HIV infection; and (3) lesions seen in HIV infection [10]. The sequence of events associated with HIV infection, from the cellular level of infection to oral manifestations in HIV-infected patients, is illustrated in Figure 1, together with the classification of HIV-OLs.

HIV is one of the best-studied viruses and, thus, anti-HIV agents show the widest range of structural variation among antiviral agents. Since the introduction of combination therapy (ART) for patients, HIV infection has been transformed into a long-term and manageable disorder; indeed, ART can reduce plasma virus titers to below detectable levels for more than one year and slow the disease progression. The major classes of drugs used in ART regimens include entry inhibitors (EI), nucleoside reverse-transcriptase inhibitors (NRTI), non-nucleoside reverse-transcriptase inhibitors (NNRTI), protease inhibitors (PI), and integrase strand-transfer inhibitors (INSTI).

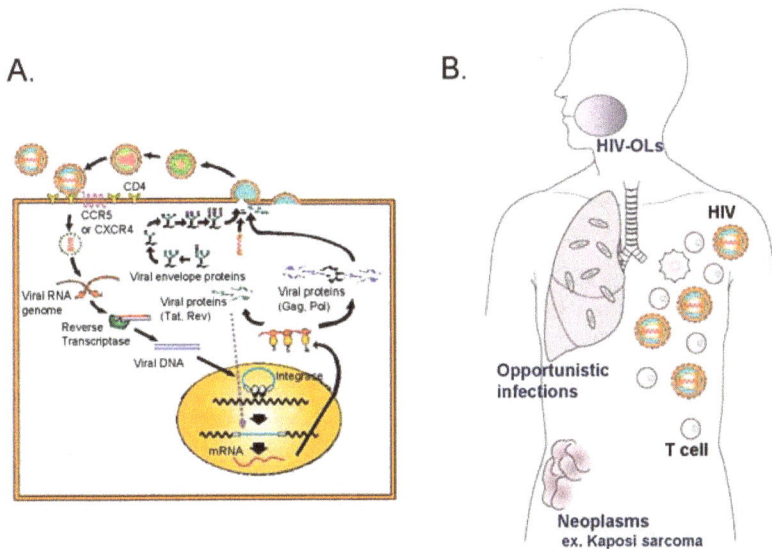

Figure 1. *Cont.*

C.

HIV-OLs

(1) Lesions strongly associated with HIV infection

- Candidiasis
  - Erythematous
  - Pseudomembranous
- Hairy leukoplakia
- Kaposi sarcoma

- Non Hodgkin's lymphoma
- Periodontal disease
  - Linear gingival erythema
  - Necrotizing (ulcerative) gingivitis
  - Necrotizing (ulcerative) periodontitis

(2) Lesions less commonly associated with HIV infection

- Bacterial infections
  - Mycobacterium avium-intracellulare
  - Mycobacterium tuberculosis
- Melanotic hyperpigmentation
- Necrotizing (ulcerative) stomatitis
- Salivary gland disease
  - Dry mouth due to decreased salivary flow rate
- Unilateral or bilateral swelling of the major salivary glands
- Thrombocytopenic purpura
- Ulceration NOS (not otherwise specified)

- Viral infections
  - Herpes simplex virus
  - Human papillomavirus (wart like lesions)
  - Condyloma acuminatum
  - Focal epithelial hyperplasia
  - Verruca vulgaris
  - Varicella zoster virus
  - Herpes zoster
  - Varicella

(3) Lesions seen in HIV infection

- Bacterial infections
  - Actinomyces Israel
  - Escherichia coli
  - Klebsiella pneumoniae
- Cat scratch disease
- Drug reactions
  (ulcerative, erythema multiforme, lichenoid, toxic epidermolysis)
- Epithelioid (bacillary) angiomatosis
- Neurologic disturbances
  - Facial palsy
  - Trigeminal neuralgia

- Fungal infection other than candidiasis
  - Cryptococcus neoformans
  - Geotrichum candidum
  - Histoplasma capsulatum
  - Mucoraceae (mucormycosis/zygomycosis)
  - Aspergillus flavus
- Recurrent aphthous stomatitis
- Viral infections
  - Cytomegalovirus
  - Molluscum contagiosum

Kaposi's sarcoma

Hairy Leukoplakia

Oral Candidiasis

Herpes simplex virus

Dry mouth (Xerostomia)

Herpes zoster

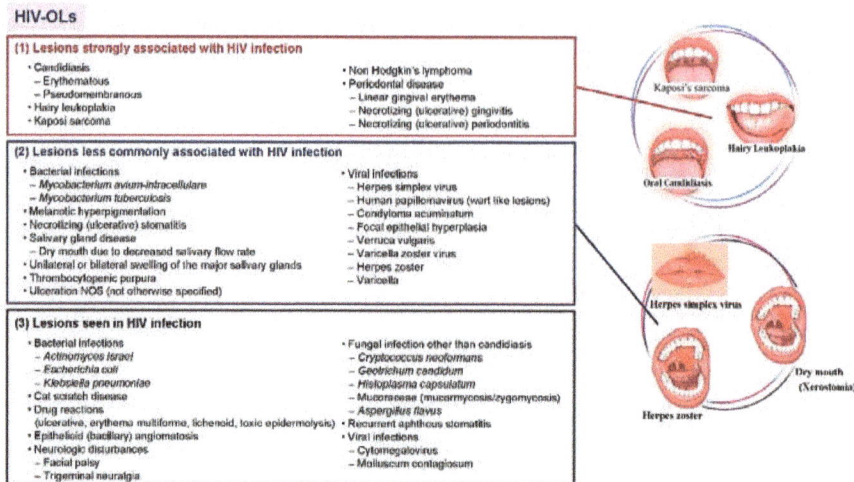

Figure 1. Life cycle and effects of human immunodeficiency virus (HIV). (**A**) The HIV infection of cells begins when the envelope glycoprotein of a viral particle binds to both cluster of differentiation 4 (CD4) and a co-receptor that is a member of the chemokine receptor family. Once inside the cells, the viral genome is reverse-transcribed into DNA and incorporated into the cellular genome. Viral gene transcription and viral reproduction are stimulated by signals that normally activate the host cell. Production of the virus is accompanied by cell death. (**B**) Infection with HIV induces immunosuppression, which in turn enables many kinds of bacteria, fungi, and viruses to grow in the oral cavity. HIV-infected individuals usually exhibit immune dysfunction prior to depletion of their CD4-positive T-helper cells. The progressive immune deficiency is accompanied by a wide range of opportunistic infections and neoplasms, such as candidiasis, Kaposi sarcoma, and hairy leukoplakia, in the oral cavity. (**C**) The 1993 EC-Clearinghouse classification for oral lesions associated with HIV (HIV-OLs) is still globally used, despite some controversy as to its current relevance to periodontal diseases.

3. Natural Products as Antiviral Agents

3.1. Early History of Antivirals

Extracts of natural materials, such as herbs, spices, roots, tree barks, leaves, etc., have a long anecdotal, as well as proven history of use in treating human ailments. Indeed, many drugs now in clinical use have their origins in plants, marine organisms, bacteria, and fungi that were traditionally believed to have desirable pharmacological activities. However, it is difficult to isolate pure active compounds from a complex array of substances, some of which may be cytotoxic, present in natural materials. Nevertheless, the discoveries of antiviral-active nucleosides, spongothymidine and spongouridine, more than half a century ago made scientists aware of the potential value of antivirals from natural sources (Figure 2) [11].

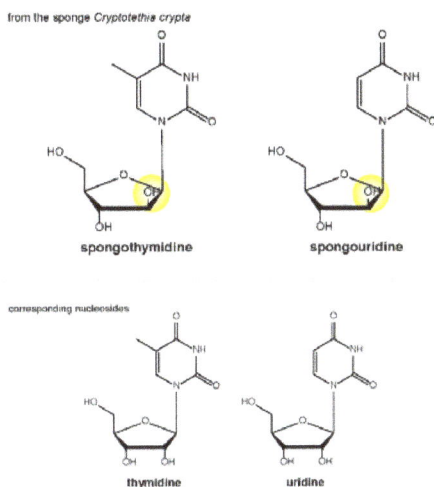

Figure 2. Chemical structures of arabinosyl nucleosides from the sponge *Cryptotethia crypta*, together with the corresponding human nucleosides. The key structural features are highlighted in yellow. Arabinosyl nucleosides contain arabinofuranose instead of β-D-ribofuranose.

3.2. Antivirals in the Latter Half of the 20th Century

Since the early work on marine-derived antivirals, thousands of novel compounds with antiviral activities have been isolated from natural sources, and some have been successfully developed for clinical use. Perhaps the most important contribution was the isolation and characterization of arabinosyl nucleosides from a Caribbean sponge (phylum Porifera) called *Tethya crypta* (Tethylidae), which provided the basis for drug design of nucleoside analogs used in medicine today. In this context, the most important antivirals that have come onto the market so far are acyclovir (ACV) [12], vidarabine (Ara-A) [13], and azidothymidine (zidovudine) (AZT) [14] (Figure 3). ACV and Ara-A are nucleic acid analogs that competitively inhibit herpes viral DNA polymerases, preventing further viral DNA synthesis. As for AZT, the active intracellular metabolite, AZT-triphosphate, is an HIV RT inhibitor, and is a key constituent of standard ART regimens. Our group investigated the inhibition of HIV replication by AZT and its cytopathic effect by means of time-of-addition experiments using HIV-bearing MT-4 cells [15], confirming and extending previous work [16].

Given the history of marine organism-based drug discovery, attention subsequently turned to marine sponges, which proved to be a rich source of compounds with antiviral properties (Table 2). Cytarabine (Ara-C) is a structural analog of cytosine arabinoside and is currently used in the routine treatment of patients with leukemia and lymphoma [13]. Avarol blocks the synthesis of glutamine transfer RNA (tRNA), which is crucial for a viral protein synthesis [17]. Manzamine A is an alkaloid with a diverse range of bioactivity, including anti-HIV activity [18]. Mycalamide A was found to inhibit HSV-1 replication by blocking viral protein synthesis [19]. Papuamide A inhibits viral entry into host cells independently of the CD4-gp120/HIV and C–C chemokine receptor type 5 (CCR5)-gp41/HIV interactions [20].

Synthetic derivatives of arabinosyl nucleosides from sponge, *Tethya cripta*

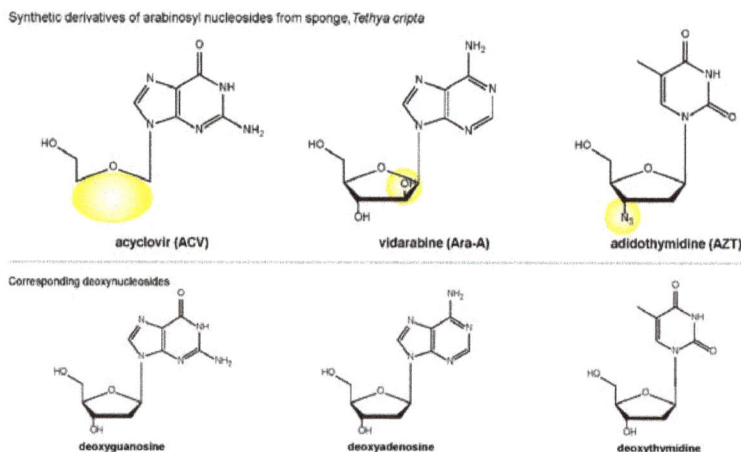

acyclovir (ACV)   vidarabine (Ara-A)   adidothymidine (AZT)

Corresponding deoxynucleosides

deoxyguanosine   deoxyadenosine   deoxythymidine

Figure 3. Chemical structures of nucleic acid analogs clinically used as key antivirals today, together with those of analogous competitors. Acyclovir (ACV) is used for the treatment of herpes simplex virus infections, chickenpox, and shingles. ACV inhibits viral DNA polymerase activity in a deoxyguanosine triphosphate (dGTP)-competitive manner. Vidarabine (Ara-A) is active against herpes simplex and varicella zoster viruses. Ara-A inhibits viral DNA polymerase activity in a deoxyadenosine triphosphate (dATP)-competitive manner. Azidothymidine, also called zidovudine (AZT), is the most common drug prescribed for individuals who have acquired immune deficiency syndrome (AIDS). AZT inhibits viral reverse transcriptase (RT) activity in a deoxythymidine triphosphate (dTTP)-competitive manner. The key structural features are highlighted in yellow.

Table 2. Sponge-derived antivirals reported in the latter part of the twentieth century. Compounds below the horizontal dotted line are more recent medicines. HIV—human immunodeficiency virus.

Compound	Organism	Target Virus	Reference
Acyclovir	*Tethya cripta*	HSV, VZV	Elion et al., 1977 [12]
Cytarabine	*Tethya cripta*	HSV [*1]	Privat and de Rudder, 1964 [13]
Vidarabine	*Tethya cripta*	HSV	Privat and de Rudder, 1964 [13]
Zidovudine	*Tethya cripta*	HIV	Horwitz et al., 1964 [14]
Avarol	*Disidea avara*	HIV	Muller et al., 1987 [17]
Manzamine A	*Haliclona* sp.	HIV	Sakai et al., 1986 [18]
Mycalamide A	*Mycale*	HSV	Perry et al., 1988 [19]
Papuamide A	*Theonella mirabilis*		Ford et al., 1999 [20]

[*1]: presently used as an anti-tumor agent.

Compounds extracted from algae have activity against a wide range of viruses, including HIV and HSV [21]. For example, galactan sulfate, which is a polysaccharide isolated from the red seaweed *Agardhiella tenera*, shows potent HIV replication-inhibitory activity [22]. A citrate buffer extract of the marine red alga *Schizymenia pacifca* inhibited RT of avian myeloblastosis virus and Rauscher murine leukemia virus [23], and the main component of this "sea algal extract" (SAE) was characterized as a member of the λ-carrageenan family, being a sulfated polysaccharide composed of galactose (73%), sulfonate (20%), and 3,6-anhydrogalactose (0.65%) with a molecular weight of approximately 2000 kDa [24]. SAE was demonstrated to be a specific inhibitor of HIV RT and HIV replication in vitro, and its sulfate residues were hypothesized to play a key role in the inhibition. Various types of sulfated polysaccharides such as dextran sulfate have been reported as potent inhibitors of HIV infection by researchers from around the world, including our group [25–34]. However, these observations did not generate much interest because the antiviral actions of these compounds were considered to be largely nonspecific [35]. Subsequent studies revealed that the target of sulfated polysaccharides is the binding of gp120/HIV to the cell-surface protein CD4 on naive cells [36–38].

Various plant-derived natural products have also been reported as potential lead compounds for anti-HIV agents. Lignin extracted from pine cones is a natural polyphenolic material generated by oxidative polymerization of phenylpropanoid monomers. Sakagami and co-workers have reported on the anti-HIV activity of lignin toward cultured cells [39,40]. Lignin was suggested to suppress the absorption of HIV onto the surface of cultured cells, although the details are unclear. Mitsuhashi et al. proposed that low-molecular-weight lignin inhibits HIV replication through suppression of HIV transcription from long terminal repeats (LTRs), including activation via nuclear factor kappa B (NF-κB) [41]. Betulinic acid (triterpenoid), isolated from the leaves of *Syzigium claviflorum*, inhibited HIV replication in a mechanism-blind screening [42]. The activity-directed derivatization of betulinic acid contributed to the creation of bevirimat, which disrupts core condensation by targeting a late step in Gag/HIV processing [43–45].

Cationic host-defense peptides, tachyplesins and polyphemusins, which were isolated from the hemocytes of horseshoe crabs (*Tachypleus tridentatus* and *Limulus polyphemus*), were reported to possess anti-HIV activity by Iwanaga's group [46,47]. These peptides consist of 17 or 18 amino-acid residues with two intramolecular disulfide bridges. We investigated the structure–anti-HIV activity relationship (SAR) of these peptides and found that [Tyr-5,12, Lys-7]polyphemusin II (named T22) showed strong anti-HIV activity and low cytotoxicity [48,49]. Our continuing studies led to shortened polyphemusin analogs comprising 14 amino-acid residues, T134 [50] and T140 [51], as potent anti-HIV peptides. Moreover, FC131, which has a lower molecular weight than T134/T140, was found in a library of cyclic pentapeptides designed by means of a pharmacophore-guided approach based on SAR studies [52]. These peptides include a potent C–X–C chemokine receptor type 4 (CXCR4; HIV co-receptor) antagonist that strongly blocks X4-HIV-1 entry through competitive binding to CXCR4 [53–55]. Development of polyphemusin-derived CXCR4 antagonists from natural sources is a good example of a success story from natural product screening supported by fine synthetic technology using peptide chemistry (Figure 4). Currently, the biostable T140 analog BKT-140 (BioLineRx Ltd.) is a phase II drug candidate for the treatment of acute myeloid leukemia (AML) [56].

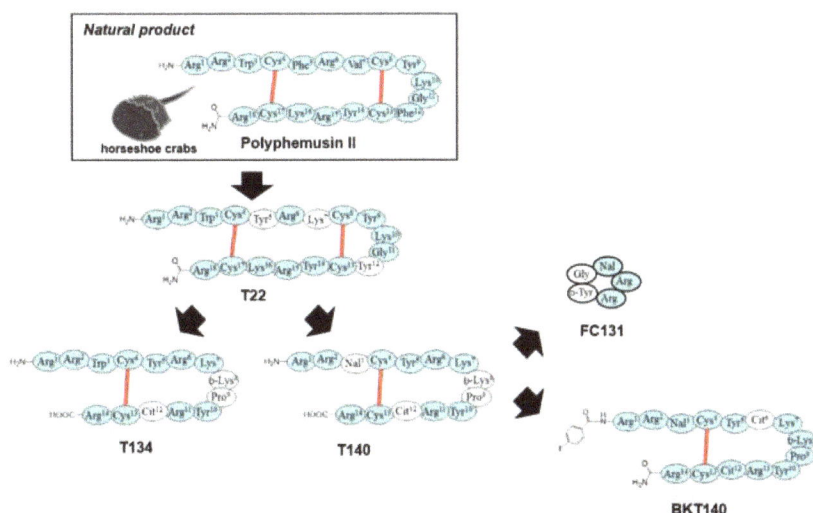

Figure 4. Discovery and development of C–X–C chemokine receptor type 4 (CXCR4) antagonists with potent anti-HIV activity from host-defense peptide of horseshoe crabs. Substitutions are highlighted in white. Red lines indicate intramolecular disulfide bond formation. Cit, L-citrulline; Nal, L-3-(2-naphthyl)alanine.

3.3. Antivirals in the 21st century

3.3.1. Status of Anti-HIV Natural Products

The mainstream of antiviral discovery from natural sources continues to be directed against HIV and HSV. In the past decade, some unique compounds with anti-HIV activity have been reported from sponges, algae, and also from natural product libraries. Ma et al. reported the isolation of phenylspirodrimane, named stachybotrin D, from the marine sponge-associated fungus *Stachybotrys chartarum* MXH-X73, as a novel NNRTI [57]. Vidal et al. reported that daphnane diterpenes (daphnetoxin) extracted from the aerial parts of *Daphne gnidium* L. (Thymelaeaceae) with dichloromethane possessed anti-HIV inhibitory activity, interfering directly with the expression of the two main HIV co-receptors, CCR5 and CXCR4 [58]. Ixoratannin A-2 (doubly linked, A-type proanthrocyanidin trimer) and boldine (aporphine alkaloid) were identified as novel viral protein U (Vpu)/HIV-interacting anti-HIV inhibitors from the pan-African Natural Product Library (p-ANAPL), which is the largest collection of medicinal plant-derived pure compounds on the African continent [59]. The activities of these compounds require further characterization. The red algal protein griffithsin (GRFT) comprising 121 amino-acid residues shows promising potent anti-HIV inhibitory activity without cellular toxicity [60]. The potent HIV entry inhibitor GRFT was found to be a lectin that targets high-mannose N-linked glycans displayed on the surface of HIV envelope glycoproteins, and is of interest because unique technology has been developed for its large-scale production by genetic engineering using *Nicotiana benthamiana* plants transduced with a tobacco mosaic virus (TMV)-based vector expressing GRFT [61]. Recently, gnidimacrin, a daphnane-type diterpenoid extracted from the roots of *Stellera chamaejasme* (Thymelaeaceae), was reported to reduce latent HIV-1 DNA and the frequency of HIV-1-infected cells through activation of protein kinase C beta 1 and 2 (PKCβI and βII) in peripheral blood mononuclear cells (PBMC) from patients [62]. Persistent HIV infection is currently incurable owing to the presence of latent viral reservoirs of long-lived memory T cells, so targeting of latent viruses is an attractive strategy for complete HIV eradication, especially for ART-interrupted patients.

3.3.2. Status of Anti-HSV Natural Products

The second most advanced antiviral development program after anti-HIV is anti-HSV. Anti-herpes drugs were the first antivirals targeting human pathogenic viruses and, thus, HSV infections are considered to be manageable, even though the available drugs have only limited therapeutic efficacy. It should be noted that chronic HSV infections of HIV-positive individuals, or solid organ transplant recipients, or patients with cancer may require prolonged antiviral treatment. In particular, HSV encephalitis is highly lethal. Unfortunately, prolonged therapies with available anti-herpes drugs may result in undesirable side effects, and can also induce the emergence of drug-resistant strains. Therefore, the discovery of novel anti-herpesvirus agents is still necessary.

There are many reports of compounds derived from various plant species as potential antiherpetic agents. Hassan et al. recently published a comprehensive review about bioactive natural products with anti-HSV properties, including nucleosides, polysaccharides, proteins, peptides, terpenes, phenolic compounds, and alkaloids [63]. Here, we focus on some of the materials currently considered most promising. Based on the successful development of ACV and Ara-A, marine organisms are anticipated to be a key source of novel anti-HSV drugs [64]. Mandal et al. showed that the polysaccharide xylan isolated from red algae *Scinaia hatei* exhibits activity against HSVs [65]. In addition, some sulfated polysaccharides, such as sulfated galactan, were reported to have antiviral activity for HSV [66,67], as well as HIV. These compounds may inhibit virus adsorption on cells. In 2005, a methanol extract of algae *Sargassum latiuscula* (Rhodomelaceae) collected in Korea was reported to display antiviral activities against not only wild-type HSV-1, but also ACV-resistant and/or thymidine kinase-deficient HSV-1 strains in vitro without apparent cytotoxicity, and it was also effective in a mouse HSV-1 infection model without noticeable toxic effects [68]. Fractionation of this extract afforded the active components 2,3,6-tribromo-4,5-dihydroxybenzyl methyl ether (TDB) and TDB alcohol. Meliacine isolated from *Melia azedarach* is a plant-derived glycopeptide exhibiting a therapeutic effect on HSV-induced ocular disease and genital herpetic infection in mice, possibly by inhibiting viral protein synthesis [69,70]. Various other natural products have yielded candidate anti-HSVs, including diterpenes from *Scoparia dulcis* L. (a medicinal plant) [71], a sulfated polysaccharide called calcium spirulan (Ca-SP) from *Spirulina platensis* (cyanobacteria) [72], fucoidan from *Undaria pinnatifida* (edible seaweed) [73], and nostoflan from *Nostoc flagelliforme* (terrestrial cyanobacterium) [74].

3.3.3. Status of Natural Products with Activity against Other Viruses

Although HIV and HSVs have been the mainstream of attention, screening for and testing of natural compounds for activity against other viruses has also been progressing. For example, resveratrol (trans-3,4′,5 trihydroxystilbene) has in vitro antiviral activities against several members of the HHV family, including varicella-zoster virus (VZV) [75], EBV [76], human cytomegalovirus (HCMV) [77], and KSHV [78]. The compound appears to act on cellular pathways that affect viral replication, though the details are unclear. Anti-EBV peptide, an N-myristoylated peptide containing six amino acids, was isolated from hemolymph (blood) of larvae of tobacco budworm, *Heliothis virescens* [79]. This peptide has antiviral activity against several viruses, and Ourth proposed that the "myristate plus basic" motif in this peptide may prevent assembly and/or budding of viruses from the host cell. These two compounds are of interest, because there are no effective antiviral drugs or vaccines in clinical use for diseases caused by EBV and KSHV. Curcumin, a natural polyphenol derived from the rhizome of the medical plant *Curcuma longa Linn*, was reported to have anti-HPV activity due to downregulation of HPV18 transcription via inhibition of activator protein 1 (AP-1) [80]. This seems noteworthy, because curcumin is readily available and inexpensive. Slater et al. reported that indolocarbazoles derived from the natural product arcyriafavin A (an alkaloid) are potent and selective inhibitors of replication of HCMV [81]. Arcyriafavin A is a potent cyclin-dependent kinase 4 (CDK4)/cyclin D1 and Ca^{2+}/calmodulin-dependent (CaM) kinase II inhibitor, and seems to be a promising candidate for further development.

At present, the most promising next-generation antiviral agents from natural sources may be the red algal protein GRFT and the algae-derived polysaccharide carrageenan (CG). GRFT is a potent anti-HIV agent, and also inhibits infection with other sexually transmitted infectious viruses, including HSV by targeting viral entry and cell-to-cell transmission [82], HPV by mediating receptor internalization [83], and HCV by targeting cell entry [84]. CG blocks the binding of HPV to cells [85,86], and is well established as a thickening agent in various foods and cosmetic products, including some brands of sexual lubricant [87]. It has, therefore, the advantage of being recognized as safe by the Food and Drug Administration (FDA), and a microbicide gel formulation for vaginal application has been developed, taking advantage of its gel-forming property. Recently, the combination of GRFT and CG was reported to show broad antiviral activity against HSV-2 and HPV in murine models [83]. The combination of GRFT and CG seems promising, and we discuss it further below in connection with new pharmaceutical formulation technologies.

4. Formulation of Natural-Product-Derived Antivirals Using New Pharmaceutical Technologies

Recently, innovations in drug formulation technology have attracted great interest as a means of improving clinical outcomes. Drug delivery systems (DDS) such as nano- and microparticles, targeted carriers, prodrugs, polyethylene glycol (PEG)ylation, hydrogel depots, and so on are attractive technologies to enable a drug to act at the right time, at the right site, and at the required concentration. The objectives of these systems include controlled drug release, prolongation of drug lifetime, acceleration of drug permeation and absorption, and drug targeting. For example, a prodrug modification of ACV is the L-valyl ester (VACV), which shows increased cell-membrane permeability, enabling a reduction in the frequency of administration and reduced side effects. Some formulations of natural products themselves have been reported to serve as topical microbicides. Cellulose sulfate, an HIV entry inhibitor in vitro, was investigated for use as a sulfated polysaccharide vaginal gel formulation [88,89]. Unfortunately, however, no significant effect of cellulose sulfate on the risk of HIV acquisition was found, compared with the placebo [90]. In an alternative approach, sodium carboxymethylcellulose (Na CMC) has been used as a gelling agent together with maraviroc and tenofovir (both of which are in clinical use) for prevention of rectal acquisition of HIV [4]. In a macaque model, these drugs were detectable in plasma at 30 minutes after gel application and remained in rectal fluids at more than 95%-inhibitory concentrations for 24 h. The algae-derived anti-HPV polysaccharide CG (see Section 3.3.3) is a macromolecular gel, and the CG-based gel formulation Carraguard is now a phase III drug candidate as a sexual lubricant with anti-HPV properties. More recently, the combination of the red algal protein GRFT and CG in a novel formulation called a freeze-dried fast-dissolving insert (FDI) was reported to protect rhesus macaques from vaginal simian–human immunodeficiency virus (SHIV) challenge, as well as mice from vaginal HSV-2 and HPV pseudovirus challenge, and current phase I trials are looking at the anti-HPV properties of a GRFT/CG combination gel as a sexual lubricant [91]. Thus, formulations with good retention at invasion sites using natural products acting outside infected cells, e.g., entry and/or budding inhibitors for host cells, seem promising, especially for pre-exposure prophylaxis (PrEP).

Some drug formulation studies of curcumin, an anti-HPV natural product from medical plants, were recently reported. Curcumin inspired considerable interest based on its extensive physiological activities; however, poor bioavailability restricts its clinical translation. Treatment of cervical cancer with a curcumin nanoparticle formulation in poly(lactic-*co*-glycolic acid) (PGLA) was investigated in an orthotopic mouse model [92,93]. Various hydrogel formulations for curcumin have also been proposed [94,95]. The results of these pre-clinical experiments suggested that suitably formulated curcumin could be an effective therapeutic modality for HPV-induced cervical cancer.

5. Prospects

Most viral infections of the oral cavity involve HHVs, especially in HIV-infected individuals. As described in Section 2, HSV type 1 (HHV-1) and 2 (HHV-2) produce shallow, small, painful ulcers which may coalesce. The development of antiviral agents with their delivery systems that successfully stop the recurrence of oral ulceration (recurrent aphthous stomatitis (RAS)) is anticipated [96]. VZV (HHV-3) is responsible for chickenpox upon primary infection, and shingles in its reactivated form. EBV (HHV-4) causes infectious mononucleosis and/or glandular fever. HCMV (HHV-5) can cause large, painful ulceration on any oral surface. EBV and HCMV were also reported to associate with periodontitis [97]; therefore, the discovery of new antiviral agents is necessary, especially for chronic periodontitis. HHV-6 and -7 are associated with facial rashes in babies and oral ulceration. Also, reactivated HHV-6 can cause encephalitis in patients after transplantation [98]. KSHV (HHV-8) is associated with KS in AIDS patients. In HIV-infected individuals, herpes infections often persist for long period of time. In addition, HPV infections are also found in AIDS patients, and may give rise to exophytic warts, often at the corners of the mouth. In patients with AIDS, there is a danger that viremias may spread to life-threatening sites, and early treatment of oral herpetic infections is essential.

Recent developments in anti-HIV drugs has mainly been focused on creating novel formulations to improve medication compliance, such as mixed formulations including drugs with different mechanisms of action in a single tablet. For example, Complera® is a once-a-day medication, consisting of a single tablet containing rilpivirine (NNRTI), emtricitabine (NRTI), and tenofovir (NRTI). Prezcobix® utilizes a pharmacokinetic (PK) booster strategy, with a single tablet containing darunavir (PI) and a cytochrome P450 3A (CYP3A) inhibitor to prolong the blood half-life of darunavir. We have reported a depot strategy for the peptide drug Fuzeon®, which is used for the treatment of HIV-infected individuals and AIDS patients with multidrug-resistant HIV infections [99]. Natural-product-derived peptides with anti-viral activity may be candidates for PrEP and post-exposure therapy if appropriate pharmaceutical technology is employed. Also, there is still an enormous range of natural resources (plants, etc.) that remain to be explored for new antiviral candidates. Thus, discovery and development of new drugs in combination with improved pharmaceutical formulation technologies offers great promise for the future treatment of viral infections.

Author Contributions: D.A. wrote the first draft of the manuscript and reviewed it under research supervision by H.N. H.N. reviewed and edited the manuscript.

Funding: This work was supported by Grant-in-Aid for Scientific Research (C) (15K01319 and 17K08254) of Japan.

Acknowledgments: We thank the members of the Department of Microbiology, St. Marianna University School of Medicine, and the Department of Microbiology and Immunology, Kagoshima University Dental School, for much helpful discussion and technical support. We also thank Dr. Nobutaka Fujii (Kyoto University), Dr. Hiroshi Sakagami (Meikai University), and Dr. Naoki Yamamoto (Tokyo Medical and Dental University) for collaboration in our research on anti-HIV compounds.

Conflicts of Interest: The authors declare no conflicts of interest.

References

1. Aas, J.A.; Paster, B.J.; Stokes, L.N.; Olsen, I.; Dewhirst, F.E. Defining the normal bacterial flora of the oral cavity. *J. Clin. Microbiol.* **2005**, *43*, 5721–5732. [CrossRef] [PubMed]
2. Grinde, B.; Olsen, I. The role of viruses in oral disease. *J. Oral Microbiol.* **2010**, *2*. [CrossRef] [PubMed]
3. Caplan, M.R.; Daar, E.S.; Corado, K.C. Next generation fixed dose combination pharmacotherapies for treating HIV. *Expert Opin. Pharmacother.* **2018**, *19*, 589–596. [CrossRef] [PubMed]
4. Dobard, C.W.; Taylor, A.; Sharma, S.; Anderson, P.L.; Bushman, L.R.; Chuong, D.; Pau, C.P.; Hanson, D.; Wang, L.; Garcia-Lerma, J.G.; et al. Protection Against Rectal Chimeric Simian/Human Immunodeficiency Virus Transmission in Macaques by Rectal-Specific Gel Formulations of Maraviroc and Tenofovir. *J. Infect. Dis.* **2015**, *212*, 1988–1995. [CrossRef] [PubMed]
5. Cedeno-Laurent, F.; Gomez-Flores, M.; Mendez, N.; Ancer-Rodriguez, J.; Bryant, J.L.; Gaspari, A.A.; Trujillo, J.R. New insights into HIV-1-primary skin disorders. *J. Int. AIDS Soc.* **2011**, *14*, 5. [CrossRef] [PubMed]
6. Khammissa, R.A.; Fourie, J.; Chandran, R.; Lemmer, J.; Feller, L. Epstein-Barr Virus and Its Association with Oral Hairy Leukoplakia: A Short Review. *Int. J. Dent.* **2016**, *2016*, 4941783. [CrossRef] [PubMed]
7. Khammissa, R.A.; Pantanowitz, L.; Feller, L. Oral HIV-Associated Kaposi Sarcoma: A Clinical Study from the Ga-Rankuwa Area, South Africa. *AIDS Res. Treat.* **2012**, *2012*, 873171. [CrossRef] [PubMed]
8. Cubie, H.A. Diseases associated with human papillomavirus infection. *Virology* **2013**, *445*, 21–34. [CrossRef] [PubMed]
9. Giuliano, A.R.; Tortolero-Luna, G.; Ferrer, E.; Burchell, A.N.; de Sanjose, S.; Kjaer, S.K.; Munoz, N.; Schiffman, M.; Bosch, F.X. Epidemiology of human papillomavirus infection in men, cancers other than cervical and benign conditions. *Vaccine* **2008**, *26* (Suppl. 10), K17–K28. [CrossRef] [PubMed]
10. Classification and Diagnostic Criteria for Oral Lesions in HIV Infection. EC-Clearinghouse on Oral Problems Related to HIV Infection and WHO Collaborating Centre on Oral Manifestations of the Immunodeficiency Virus. *J. Oral Pathol. Med.* **1993**, *22*, 289–291. [CrossRef]
11. Bergmann, W.; Feeney, R.J. Contributions to the study of marine products. XXXII. The nucleosides of sponges. I. *J. Org. Chem.* **1951**, *16*, 981–987. [CrossRef]
12. Elion, G.B.; Furman, P.A.; Fyfe, J.A.; de Miranda, P.; Beauchamp, L.; Schaeffer, H.J. Selectivity of action of an antiherpetic agent, 9-(2-hydroxyethoxymethyl) guanine. *Proc. Natl. Acad. Sci. USA* **1977**, *74*, 5716–5720. [CrossRef] [PubMed]
13. Privat de Garilhe, M.; de Rudder, J. Effect of 2 arabinose nucleosides on the multiplication of herpes virus and vaccine in cell culture. *C. R. Hebd. Seances Acad. Sci.* **1964**, *259*, 2725–2728.
14. Horwitz, J.P.; Chua, J.; Noel, M. Nucleosides. V. The Monomesylates of 1-(2′-Deoxy-β-D-lyxofuranosyl)thymine[1,2]. *J. Org. Chem.* **1964**, *29*, 2076–2078. [CrossRef]
15. Nakashima, H.; Matsui, T.; Harada, S.; Kobayashi, N.; Matsuda, A.; Ueda, T.; Yamamoto, N. Inhibition of replication and cytopathic effect of human T cell lymphotropic virus type III/lymphadenopathy-associated virus by 3′-azido-3′-deoxythymidine in vitro. *Antimicrob. Agents Chemother.* **1986**, *30*, 933–937. [CrossRef] [PubMed]

16. Mitsuya, H.; Weinhold, K.J.; Furman, P.A.; St Clair, M.H.; Lehrman, S.N.; Gallo, R.C.; Bolognesi, D.; Barry, D.W.; Broder, S. 3′-Azido-3′-deoxythymidine (BW A509U): An antiviral agent that inhibits the infectivity and cytopathic effect of human T-lymphotropic virus type III/lymphadenopathy-associated virus in vitro. *Proc. Natl. Acad. Sci. USA* **1985**, *82*, 7096–7100. [CrossRef] [PubMed]

17. Muller, W.E.; Sobel, C.; Diehl-Seifert, B.; Maidhof, A.; Schroder, H.C. Influence of the antileukemic and anti-human immunodeficiency virus agent avarol on selected immune responses in vitro and in vivo. *Biochem. Pharmacol.* **1987**, *36*, 1489–1494. [CrossRef]

18. Sakai, R.; Higa, T.; Jefford, C.W.; Bernardinelli, G. Manzamine A, a novel antitumor alkaloid from a sponge. *J. Am. Chem. Soc.* **1986**, *108*, 6404–6405. [CrossRef]

19. Perry, N.B.; Blunt, J.W.; Munro, M.H.G.; Pannell, L.K. Mycalamide A, an antiviral compound from a New Zealand sponge of the genus Mycale. *J. Am. Chem. Soc.* **1988**, *110*, 4850–4851. [CrossRef]

20. Ford, P.W.; Gustafson, K.R.; McKee, T.C.; Shigematsu, N.; Maurizi, L.K.; Pannell, L.K.; Williams, D.E.; de Silva, E.D.; Lassota, P.; Allen, T.M.; et al. Papuamides A−D, HIV-inhibitory and cytotoxic depsipeptides from the sponges *Theonella mirabilis* and *Theonella swinhoei* collected in Papua New Guinea. *J. Am. Chem. Soc.* **1999**, *121*, 5899–5909. [CrossRef]

21. Yasuhara-Bell, J.; Lu, Y. Marine compounds and their antiviral activities. *Antivir. Res.* **2010**, *86*, 231–240. [CrossRef] [PubMed]

22. Witvrouw, M.; Este, J.A.; Mateu, M.Q.; Reymen, D.; Andrei, G.; Snoeck, R.; Ikeda, S.; Pauwels, R.; Bianchini, N.V.; Desmyter, J.; et al. Activity of a sulfated polysaccharide extracted from the red seaweed *Aghardhiella tenera* against human immunodeficiency virus and other enveloped viruses. *Antivir. Chem. Chemother.* **1994**, *5*, 297–303. [CrossRef]

23. Nakashima, H.; Kido, Y.; Kobayashi, N.; Motoki, Y.; Neushul, M.; Yamamoto, N. Antiretroviral activity in a marine red alga: Reverse transcriptase inhibition by an aqueous extract of *Schizymenia pacifica*. *J. Cancer Res. Clin. Oncol.* **1987**, *113*, 413–416. [CrossRef] [PubMed]

24. Nakashima, H.; Kido, Y.; Kobayashi, N.; Motoki, Y.; Neushul, M.; Yamamoto, N. Purification and characterization of an avian myeloblastosis and human immunodeficiency virus reverse transcriptase inhibitor, sulfated polysaccharides extracted from sea algae. *Antivir. Chem. Chemother.* **1987**, *31*, 1524–1528. [CrossRef]

25. Mitsuya, H.; Looney, D.J.; Kuno, S.; Ueno, R.; Wong-Staal, F.; Broder, S. Dextran sulfate suppression of viruses in the HIV family: Inhibition of virion binding to CD4$^+$ cells. *Science* **1988**, *240*, 646–649. [CrossRef] [PubMed]

26. Nakashima, H.; Yoshida, O.; Baba, M.; De Clercq, E.; Yamamoto, N. Anti-HIV activity of dextran sulphate as determined under different experimental conditions. *Antivir. Res.* **1989**, *11*, 233–246. [CrossRef]

27. Busso, M.E.; Resnick, L. Anti-human immunodeficiency virus effects of dextran sulfate are strain dependent and synergistic or antagonistic when dextran sulfate is given in combination with dideoxynucleosides. *Antimicrob. Agents Chemother.* **1990**, *34*, 1991–1995. [CrossRef] [PubMed]

28. Yoshida, T.; Nakashima, H.; Yamamoto, N.; Uryu, T. Anti-AIDS virus activity in vitro of dextran sulfates obtained by sulfation of synthetic and natural dextrans. *Polym. J.* **1993**, *25*, 1069–1077. [CrossRef]

29. Yoshida, O.; Nakashima, H.; Yoshida, T.; Kaneko, Y.; Yamamoto, I.; Matsuzaki, K.; Uryu, T.; Yamamoto, N. Sulfation of the immunomodulating polysaccharide lentinan: A novel strategy for antivirals to human immunodeficiency virus (HIV). *Biochem. Pharmacol.* **1988**, *37*, 2887–2891. [CrossRef]

30. Kaneko, Y.; Yoshida, O.; Nakagawa, R.; Yoshida, T.; Date, M.; Ogihara, S.; Shioya, S.; Matsuzawa, Y.; Nagashima, N.; Irie, Y.; et al. Inhibition of HIV-1 infectivity with curdlan sulfate in vitro. *Biochem. Pharmacol.* **1990**, *39*, 793–797. [CrossRef] [PubMed]

31. Gao, Y.; Fukuda, A.; Katsuraya, K.; Kaneko, Y.; Mimura, T.; Nakashima, H.; Uryu, T. Synthesis of regioselective substituted curdlan sulfates with medium molecular weights and their specific anti-HIV-1 activities. *Macromolecules* **1997**, *30*, 3224–3228. [CrossRef]

32. Yamamoto, I.; Takayama, K.; Gonda, T.; Matsuzaki, K.; Hatanaka, K.; Yoshida, T.; Uryu, T.; Yoshida, O.; Nakashima, H.; Yamamoto, N.; et al. Synthesis, structure and antiviral activity of sulfates of curdlan and its branched derivatives. *Br. Polym. J.* **1990**, *23*, 245–250. [CrossRef]

33. Koizumi, N.; Sakagami, H.; Utsumi, A.; Fujinaga, S.; Takeda, M.; Asano, K.; Sugawara, I.; Ichikawa, S.; Kondo, H.; Mori, S.; et al. Anti-HIV (human immunodeficiency virus) activity of sulfated paramylon. *Antivir. Res.* **1993**, *21*, 1–14. [CrossRef]

34. Nakashima, H.; Inazawa, K.; Ichiyama, K.; Ito, M.; Ikushima, N.; Shoji, T.; Katsuraya, K.; Uryu, T.; Yamamoto, N.; Juodawlkis, A.S.; et al. Sulfated alkyl oligosaccharides inhibit human immunodeficiency virus in vitro and provide sustained drug levels in mammals. *Antivir. Chem. Chemother.* **1995**, *6*, 271–280. [CrossRef]

35. Witvrouw, M.; De Clercq, E. Sulfated polysaccharides extracted from sea algae as potential antiviral drugs. *Gen. Pharmacol.* **1997**, *29*, 497–511. [CrossRef]

36. Batinic, D.; Robey, F.A. The V3 region of the envelope glycoprotein of human immunodeficiency virus type 1 binds sulfated polysaccharides and CD4-derived synthetic peptides. *J. Biol. Chem.* **1992**, *267*, 6664–6671. [PubMed]

37. Callahan, L.N.; Phelan, M.; Mallinson, M.; Norcross, M.A. Dextran sulfate blocks antibody binding to the principal neutralizing domain of human immunodeficiency virus type 1 without interfering with gp120-CD4 interactions. *J. Virol.* **1991**, *65*, 1543–1550. [PubMed]

38. Mbemba, E.; Chams, V.; Gluckman, J.C.; Klatzmann, D.; Gattegno, L. Molecular interaction between HIV-1 major envelope glycoprotein and dextran sulfate. *Biochim. Biophys. Acta* **1992**, *1138*, 62–67. [CrossRef]

39. Lai, P.K.; Donovan, J.; Takayama, H.; Sakagami, H.; Tanaka, A.; Konno, K.; Nonoyama, M. Modification of human immunodeficiency viral replication by pine cone extracts. *AIDS Res. Hum. Retrovir.* **1990**, *6*, 205–217. [CrossRef] [PubMed]

40. Nakashima, H.; Murakami, T.; Yamamoto, N.; Naoe, T.; Kawazoe, Y.; Konno, K.; Sakagami, H. Lignified materials as medicinal resources. V. Anti-HIV (human immunodeficiency virus) activity of some synthetic lignins. *Chem. Pharm. Bull.* **1992**, *40*, 2102–2105. [CrossRef] [PubMed]

41. Mitsuhashi, S.; Kishimoto, T.; Uraki, Y.; Okamoto, T.; Ubukata, M. Low molecular weight lignin suppresses activation of NF-κB and HIV-1 promoter. *Bioorg. Med. Chem.* **2008**, *16*, 2645–2650. [CrossRef] [PubMed]

42. Fujioka, T.; Kashiwada, Y.; Kilkuskie, R.E.; Cosentino, L.M.; Ballas, L.M.; Jiang, J.B.; Janzen, W.P.; Chen, I.S.; Lee, K.H. Anti-AIDS agents, 11. Betulinic acid and platanic acid as anti-HIV principles from *Syzigium claviflorum*, and the anti-HIV activity of structurally related triterpenoids. *J. Nat. Prod.* **1994**, *57*, 243–247. [CrossRef] [PubMed]

43. Kashiwada, Y.; Hashimoto, F.; Cosentino, L.M.; Chen, C.H.; Garrett, P.E.; Lee, K.H. Betulinic acid and dihydrobetulinic acid derivatives as potent anti-HIV agents. *J. Med. Chem.* **1996**, *39*, 1016–1017. [CrossRef] [PubMed]

44. Kanamoto, T.; Kashiwada, Y.; Kanbara, K.; Gotoh, K.; Yoshimori, M.; Goto, T.; Sano, K.; Nakashima, H. Anti-human immunodeficiency virus activity of YK-FH312 (a betulinic acid derivative), a novel compound blocking viral maturation. *Antimicrob. Agents Chemother.* **2001**, *45*, 1225–1230. [CrossRef] [PubMed]

45. Li, F.; Goila-Gaur, R.; Salzwedel, K.; Kilgore, N.R.; Reddick, M.; Matallana, C.; Castillo, A.; Zoumplis, D.; Martin, D.E.; Orenstein, J.M.; et al. PA-457: A potent HIV inhibitor that disrupts core condensation by targeting a late step in Gag processing. *Proc. Natl. Acad. Sci. USA* **2003**, *100*, 13555–13560. [CrossRef] [PubMed]

46. Morimoto, M.; Mori, H.; Otake, T.; Ueba, N.; Kunita, N.; Niwa, M.; Murakami, T.; Iwanaga, S. Inhibitory effect of tachyplesin I on the proliferation of human immunodeficiency virus in vitro. *Chemotherapy* **1991**, *37*, 206–211. [CrossRef] [PubMed]

47. Murakami, T.; Niwa, M.; Tokunaga, F.; Miyata, T.; Iwanaga, S. Direct virus inactivation of tachyplesin I and its isopeptides from horseshoe crab hemocytes. *Chemotherapy* **1991**, *37*, 327–334. [CrossRef] [PubMed]

48. Nakashima, H.; Masuda, M.; Murakami, T.; Koyanagi, Y.; Matsumoto, A.; Fujii, N.; Yamamoto, N. Anti-human immunodeficiency virus activity of a novel synthetic peptide, T22 ([Tyr-5,12, Lys-7]polyphemusin II): A possible inhibitor of virus-cell fusion. *Antimicrob. Agents Chemother.* **1992**, *36*, 1249–1255. [CrossRef] [PubMed]

49. Masuda, M.; Nakashima, H.; Ueda, T.; Naba, H.; Ikoma, R.; Otaka, A.; Terakawa, Y.; Tamamura, H.; Ibuka, T.; Murakami, T.; et al. A novel anti-HIV synthetic peptide, T-22 ([Tyr5,12,Lys7]-polyphemusin II). *Biochem. Biophys. Res. Commun.* **1992**, *189*, 845–850. [CrossRef]

50. Arakaki, R.; Tamamura, H.; Premanathan, M.; Kanbara, K.; Ramanan, S.; Mochizuki, K.; Baba, M.; Fujii, N.; Nakashima, H. T134, a small-molecule CXCR4 inhibitor, has no cross-drug resistance with AMD3100, a CXCR4 antagonist with a different structure. *J. Virol.* **1999**, *73*, 1719–1723. [PubMed]

51. Tamamura, H.; Xu, Y.; Hattori, T.; Zhang, X.; Arakaki, R.; Kanbara, K.; Omagari, A.; Otaka, A.; Ibuka, T.; Yamamoto, N.; et al. A low-molecular-weight inhibitor against the chemokine receptor CXCR4: A strong anti-HIV peptide T140. *Biochem. Biophys. Res. Commun.* **1998**, *253*, 877–882. [CrossRef] [PubMed]

52. Fujii, N.; Oishi, S.; Hiramatsu, K.; Araki, T.; Ueda, S.; Tamamura, H.; Otaka, A.; Kusano, S.; Terakubo, S.; Nakashima, H.; et al. Molecular-size reduction of a potent CXCR4-chemokine antagonist using orthogonal combination of conformation- and sequence-based libraries. *Angew. Chem. Int. Ed. Engl.* **2003**, *42*, 3251–3253. [CrossRef] [PubMed]

53. Murakami, T.; Nakajima, T.; Koyanagi, Y.; Tachibana, K.; Fujii, N.; Tamamura, H.; Yoshida, N.; Waki, M.; Matsumoto, A.; Yoshie, O.; et al. A small molecule CXCR4 inhibitor that blocks T cell line-tropic HIV-1 infection. *J. Exp. Med.* **1997**, *186*, 1389–1393. [CrossRef] [PubMed]

54. Xu, Y.; Tamamura, H.; Arakaki, R.; Nakashima, H.; Zhang, X.; Fujii, N.; Uchiyama, T.; Hattori, T. Marked increase in anti-HIV activity, as well as inhibitory activity against HIV entry mediated by CXCR4, linked to enhancement of the binding ability of tachyplesin analogs to CXCR4. *AIDS Res. Hum. Retrovir.* **1999**, *15*, 419–427. [CrossRef] [PubMed]

55. Murakami, T.; Zhang, T.Y.; Koyanagi, Y.; Tanaka, Y.; Kim, J.; Suzuki, Y.; Minoguchi, S.; Tamamura, H.; Waki, M.; Matsumoto, A.; et al. Inhibitory mechanism of the CXCR4 antagonist T22 against human immunodeficiency virus type 1 infection. *J. Virol.* **1999**, *73*, 7489–7496. [CrossRef] [PubMed]

56. Ohashi, N.; Tamamura, H. Peptide-derived mid-sized anti-HIV agents. *Amino Acids Pept. Proteins* **2017**, *41*, 1–29. [CrossRef]

57. Ma, X.; Li, L.; Zhu, T.; Ba, M.; Li, G.; Gu, Q.; Guo, Y.; Li, D. Phenylspirodrimanes with anti-HIV activity from the sponge-derived fungus *Stachybotrys chartarum* MXH-X73. *J. Nat. Prod.* **2013**, *76*, 2298–2306. [CrossRef] [PubMed]

58. Vidal, V.; Potterat, O.; Louvel, S.; Hamy, F.; Mojarrab, M.; Sanglier, J.J.; Klimkait, T.; Hamburger, M. Library-based discovery and characterization of daphnane diterpenes as potent and selective HIV inhibitors in *Daphne gnidium*. *J. Nat. Prod.* **2012**, *75*, 414–419. [CrossRef] [PubMed]

59. Tietjen, I.; Ntie-Kang, F.; Mwimanzi, P.; Onguene, P.A.; Scull, M.A.; Idowu, T.O.; Ogundaini, A.O.; Meva'a, L.M.; Abegaz, B.M.; Rice, C.M.; et al. Screening of the Pan-African natural product library identifies ixoratannin A-2 and boldine as novel HIV-1 inhibitors. *PLoS ONE* **2015**, *10*, e0121099. [CrossRef] [PubMed]

60. Mori, T.; O'Keefe, B.R.; Sowder, R.C., 2nd; Bringans, S.; Gardella, R.; Berg, S.; Cochran, P.; Turpin, J.A.; Buckheit, R.W., Jr.; McMahon, J.B.; et al. Isolation and characterization of griffithsin, a novel HIV-inactivating protein, from the red alga *Griffithsia* sp. *J. Biol. Chem.* **2005**, *280*, 9345–9353. [CrossRef] [PubMed]

61. O'Keefe, B.R.; Vojdani, F.; Buffa, V.; Shattock, R.J.; Montefiori, D.C.; Bakke, J.; Mirsalis, J.; d'Andrea, A.L.; Hume, S.D.; Bratcher, B.; et al. Scaleable manufacture of HIV-1 entry inhibitor griffithsin and validation of its safety and efficacy as a topical microbicide component. *Proc. Natl. Acad. Sci. USA* **2009**, *106*, 6099–6104. [CrossRef] [PubMed]

62. Lai, W.; Huang, L.; Zhu, L.; Ferrari, G.; Chan, C.; Li, W.; Lee, K.H.; Chen, C.H. Gnidimacrin, a Potent Anti-HIV Diterpene, Can Eliminate Latent HIV-1 Ex Vivo by Activation of Protein Kinase C beta. *J. Med. Chem.* **2015**, *58*, 8638–8646. [CrossRef] [PubMed]

63. Hassan, S.T.; Masarcikova, R.; Berchova, K. Bioactive natural products with anti-herpes simplex virus properties. *J. Pharm. Pharmacol.* **2015**, *67*, 1325–1336. [CrossRef] [PubMed]

64. Vo, T.S.; Ngo, D.H.; Ta, Q.V.; Kim, S.K. Marine organisms as a therapeutic source against herpes simplex virus infection. *Eur. J. Pharm. Sci.* **2011**, *44*, 11–20. [CrossRef] [PubMed]

65. Mandal, P.; Pujol, C.A.; Damonte, E.B.; Ghosh, T.; Ray, B. Xylans from *Scinaia hatei*: Structural features, sulfation and anti-HSV activity. *Int. J. Biol. Macromol.* **2010**, *46*, 173–178. [CrossRef] [PubMed]

66. Duarte, M.E.; Noseda, D.G.; Noseda, M.D.; Tulio, S.; Pujol, C.A.; Damonte, E.B. Inhibitory effect of sulfated galactans from the marine alga *Bostrychia montagnei* on herpes simplex virus replication in vitro. *Phytomedicine* **2001**, *8*, 53–58. [CrossRef] [PubMed]

67. Talarico, L.B.; Zibetti, R.G.; Faria, P.C.; Scolaro, L.A.; Duarte, M.E.; Noseda, M.D.; Pujol, C.A.; Damonte, E.B. Anti-herpes simplex virus activity of sulfated galactans from the red seaweeds *Gymnogongrus griffithsiae* and *Cryptonemia crenulata*. *Int. J. Biol. Macromol.* **2004**, *34*, 63–71. [CrossRef] [PubMed]

68. Park, H.J.; Kurokawa, M.; Shiraki, K.; Nakamura, N.; Choi, J.S.; Hattori, M. Antiviral activity of the marine alga *Symphyocladia latiuscula* against herpes simplex virus (HSV-1) in vitro and its therapeutic efficacy against HSV-1 infection in mice. *Biol. Pharm. Bull.* **2005**, *28*, 2258–2262. [CrossRef] [PubMed]

69. Pifarre, M.P.; Berra, A.; Coto, C.E.; Alche, L.E. Therapeutic action of meliacine, a plant-derived antiviral, on HSV-induced ocular disease in mice. *Exp. Eye Res.* **2002**, *75*, 327–334. [CrossRef] [PubMed]

70. Petrera, E.; Coto, C.E. Therapeutic effect of meliacine, an antiviral derived from *Melia azedarach* L., in mice genital herpetic infection. *Phytother. Res.* **2009**, *23*, 1771–1777. [CrossRef] [PubMed]
71. Hayashi, T.; Kawasaki, M.; Miwa, Y.; Taga, T.; Morita, N. Antiviral agents of plant origin. III. Scopadulin, a novel tetracyclic diterpene from *Scoparia dulcis* L. *Chem. Pharm. Bull.* **1990**, *38*, 945–947. [CrossRef] [PubMed]
72. Hayashi, T.; Hayashi, K.; Maeda, M.; Kojima, I. Calcium spirulan, an inhibitor of enveloped virus replication, from a blue-green alga *Spirulina platensis*. *J. Nat. Prod.* **1996**, *59*, 83–87. [CrossRef] [PubMed]
73. Lee, J.B.; Hayashi, K.; Hashimoto, M.; Nakano, T.; Hayashi, T. Novel antiviral fucoidan from sporophyll of *Undaria pinnatifida* (Mekabu). *Chem. Pharm. Bull.* **2004**, *52*, 1091–1094. [CrossRef] [PubMed]
74. Kanekiyo, K.; Lee, J.B.; Hayashi, K.; Takenaka, H.; Hayakawa, Y.; Endo, S.; Hayashi, T. Isolation of an antiviral polysaccharide, nostoflan, from a terrestrial cyanobacterium, *Nostoc flagelliforme*. *J. Nat. Prod.* **2005**, *68*, 1037–1041. [CrossRef] [PubMed]
75. Docherty, J.J.; Sweet, T.J.; Bailey, E.; Faith, S.A.; Booth, T. Resveratrol inhibition of varicella-zoster virus replication in vitro. *Antivir. Res.* **2006**, *72*, 171–177. [CrossRef] [PubMed]
76. De Leo, A.; Arena, G.; Lacanna, E.; Oliviero, G.; Colavita, F.; Mattia, E. Resveratrol inhibits Epstein Barr Virus lytic cycle in Burkitt's lymphoma cells by affecting multiple molecular targets. *Antivir. Res.* **2012**, *96*, 196–202. [CrossRef] [PubMed]
77. Evers, D.L.; Wang, X.; Huong, S.M.; Huang, D.Y.; Huang, E.S. 3,4′,5-Trihydroxy-trans-stilbene (resveratrol) inhibits human cytomegalovirus replication and virus-induced cellular signaling. *Antivir. Res.* **2004**, *63*, 85–95. [CrossRef] [PubMed]
78. Dyson, O.F.; Walker, L.R.; Whitehouse, A.; Cook, P.P.; Akula, S.M. Resveratrol inhibits KSHV reactivation by lowering the levels of cellular EGR-1. *PLoS ONE* **2012**, *7*, e33364. [CrossRef] [PubMed]
79. Ourth, D.D. Susceptibility in vitro of Epstein-Barr Virus to myristoylated-peptide. *Peptides* **2010**, *31*, 1409–1411. [CrossRef] [PubMed]
80. Prusty, B.K.; Das, B.C. Constitutive activation of transcription factor AP-1 in cervical cancer and suppression of human papillomavirus (HPV) transcription and AP-1 activity in HeLa cells by curcumin. *Int. J. Cancer* **2005**, *113*, 951–960. [CrossRef] [PubMed]
81. Slater, M.J.; Cockerill, S.; Baxter, R.; Bonser, R.W.; Gohil, K.; Gowrie, C.; Robinson, J.E.; Littler, E.; Parry, N.; Randall, R.; et al. Indolocarbazoles: Potent, selective inhibitors of human cytomegalovirus replication. *Bioorg. Med. Chem.* **1999**, *7*, 1067–1074. [CrossRef]
82. Nixon, B.; Stefanidou, M.; Mesquita, P.M.; Fakioglu, E.; Segarra, T.; Rohan, L.; Halford, W.; Palmer, K.E.; Herold, B.C. Griffithsin protects mice from genital herpes by preventing cell-to-cell spread. *J. Virol.* **2013**, *87*, 6257–6269. [CrossRef] [PubMed]
83. Levendosky, K.; Mizenina, O.; Martinelli, E.; Jean-Pierre, N.; Kizima, L.; Rodriguez, A.; Kleinbeck, K.; Bonnaire, T.; Robbiani, M.; Zydowsky, T.M.; et al. Griffithsin and Carrageenan Combination To Target Herpes Simplex Virus 2 and Human Papillomavirus. *Antimicrob. Agents Chemother.* **2015**, *59*, 7290–7298. [CrossRef] [PubMed]
84. Takebe, Y.; Saucedo, C.J.; Lund, G.; Uenishi, R.; Hase, S.; Tsuchiura, T.; Kneteman, N.; Ramessar, K.; Tyrrell, D.L.; Shirakura, M.; et al. Antiviral lectins from red and blue-green algae show potent in vitro and in vivo activity against hepatitis C virus. *PLoS ONE* **2013**, *8*, e64449. [CrossRef] [PubMed]
85. Buck, C.B.; Thompson, C.D.; Roberts, J.N.; Muller, M.; Lowy, D.R.; Schiller, J.T. Carrageenan is a potent inhibitor of papillomavirus infection. *PLoS Pathog.* **2006**, *2*, e69. [CrossRef] [PubMed]
86. Roberts, J.N.; Buck, C.B.; Thompson, C.D.; Kines, R.; Bernardo, M.; Choyke, P.L.; Lowy, D.R.; Schiller, J.T. Genital transmission of HPV in a mouse model is potentiated by nonoxynol-9 and inhibited by carrageenan. *Nat. Med.* **2007**, *13*, 857–861. [CrossRef] [PubMed]
87. Marais, D.; Gawarecki, D.; Allan, B.; Ahmed, K.; Altini, L.; Cassim, N.; Gopolang, F.; Hoffman, M.; Ramjee, G.; Williamson, A.L. The effectiveness of Carraguard, a vaginal microbicide, in protecting women against high-risk human papillomavirus infection. *Antivir. Ther.* **2011**, *16*, 1219–1226. [CrossRef] [PubMed]
88. Malonza, I.M.; Mirembe, F.; Nakabiito, C.; Odusoga, L.O.; Osinupebi, O.A.; Hazari, K.; Chitlange, S.; Ali, M.M.; Callahan, M.; Van Damme, L. Expanded Phase I safety and acceptability study of 6% cellulose sulfate vaginal gel. *AIDS* **2005**, *19*, 2157–2163. [CrossRef] [PubMed]
89. El-Sadr, W.M.; Mayer, K.H.; Maslankowski, L.; Hoesley, C.; Justman, J.; Gai, F.; Mauck, C.; Absalon, J.; Morrow, K.; Masse, B.; et al. Safety and acceptability of cellulose sulfate as a vaginal microbicide in HIV-infected women. *AIDS* **2006**, *20*, 1109–1116. [CrossRef] [PubMed]

90. Van Damme, L.; Govinden, R.; Mirembe, F.M.; Guedou, F.; Solomon, S.; Becker, M.L.; Pradeep, B.S.; Krishnan, A.K.; Alary, M.; Pande, B.; et al. Lack of effectiveness of cellulose sulfate gel for the prevention of vaginal HIV transmission. *N. Engl. J. Med.* **2008**, *359*, 463–472. [CrossRef] [PubMed]

91. Derby, N.; Lal, M.; Aravantinou, M.; Kizima, L.; Barnable, P.; Rodriguez, A.; Lai, M.; Wesenberg, A.; Ugaonkar, S.; Levendosky, K.; et al. Griffithsin carrageenan fast dissolving inserts prevent SHIV HSV-2 and HPV infections in vivo. *Nat. Commun.* **2018**, *9*, 3881. [CrossRef] [PubMed]

92. Punfa, W.; Yodkeeree, S.; Pitchakarn, P.; Ampasavate, C.; Limtrakul, P. Enhancement of cellular uptake and cytotoxicity of curcumin-loaded PLGA nanoparticles by conjugation with anti-P-glycoprotein in drug resistance cancer cells. *Acta Pharmacol. Sin.* **2012**, *33*, 823–831. [CrossRef] [PubMed]

93. Zaman, M.S.; Chauhan, N.; Yallapu, M.M.; Gara, R.K.; Maher, D.M.; Kumari, S.; Sikander, M.; Khan, S.; Zafar, N.; Jaggi, M.; et al. Curcumin Nanoformulation for Cervical Cancer Treatment. *Sci. Rep.* **2016**, *6*, 20051. [CrossRef] [PubMed]

94. Gong, C.; Wu, Q.; Wang, Y.; Zhang, D.; Luo, F.; Zhao, X.; Wei, Y.; Qian, Z. A biodegradable hydrogel system containing curcumin encapsulated in micelles for cutaneous wound healing. *Biomaterials* **2013**, *34*, 6377–6387. [CrossRef] [PubMed]

95. Chen, G.; Li, J.; Cai, Y.; Zhan, J.; Gao, J.; Song, M.; Shi, Y.; Yang, Z. A Glycyrrhetinic Acid-Modified Curcumin Supramolecular Hydrogel for liver tumor targeting therapy. *Sci. Rep.* **2017**, *7*, 44210. [CrossRef] [PubMed]

96. Porter, S.R.; Al-Johani, K.; Fedele, S.; Moles, D.R. Randomised controlled trial of the efficacy of HybenX in the symptomatic treatment of recurrent aphthous stomatitis. *Oral Dis.* **2009**, *15*, 155–161. [CrossRef] [PubMed]

97. Nibali, L.; Atkinson, C.; Griffiths, P.; Darbar, U.; Rakmanee, T.; Suvan, J.; Donos, N. Low prevalence of subgingival viruses in periodontitis patients. *J. Clin. Periodontol.* **2009**, *36*, 928–932. [CrossRef] [PubMed]

98. Agut, H.; Bonnafous, P.; Gautheret-Dejean, A. Laboratory and clinical aspects of human herpesvirus 6 infections. *Clin. Microbiol. Rev.* **2015**, *28*, 313–335. [CrossRef] [PubMed]

99. Asai, D.; Kanamoto, T.; Takenaga, M.; Nakashima, H. In situ depot formation of anti-HIV fusion-inhibitor peptide in recombinant protein polymer hydrogel. *Acta Biomater.* **2017**, *64*, 116–125. [CrossRef] [PubMed]

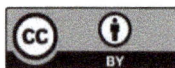

medicines

MDPI

Article

Antimicrobial Susceptibilities of Oral Isolates of *Abiotrophia* and *Granulicatella* According to the Consensus Guidelines for Fastidious Bacteria

Taisei Kanamoto [1,2,*], Shigemi Terakubo [2] and Hideki Nakashima [2]

[1] Laboratory of Microbiology, Showa Pharmaceutical University, Machida, Tokyo 194-8543, Japan

[2] Department of Microbiology, St. Marianna University School of Medicine, Kawasaki, Kanagawa 216-8511, Japan; biseibutsu-001@marianna-u.ac.jp (S.T.); nakahide@marianna-u.ac.jp (H.N.)

* Correspondence: kanamoto@ac.shoyaku.ac.jp; Tel.: +81-42-721-1551; Fax: +81-42-721-1552

Received: 7 November 2018; Accepted: 29 November 2018; Published: 3 December 2018

Abstract: Background: The genera *Abiotrophia* and *Granulicatella*, previously known as nutritionally variant streptococci (NVS), are fastidious bacteria requiring vitamin B_6 analogs for growth. They are members of human normal oral microbiota, and are supposed to be one of the important pathogens for so-called "culture-negative" endocarditis. **Methods:** The type strains and oral isolates identified, by using both phenotypic profiles and the DNA–DNA hybridization method, were examined for susceptibilities to 15 antimicrobial agents including penicillin (benzylpenicillin, ampicillin, amoxicillin, and piperacillin), cephem (cefazolin, ceftazidime, ceftriaxone, and cefaclor), carbapenem (imipenem), aminoglycoside (gentamicin), macrolide (erythromycin), quinolone (ciprofloxacin), tetracycline (minocycline), glycopeptide (vancomycin), and trimethoprim-sulfamethoxazole complex. The minimum inhibitory concentration and susceptibility criterion were determined, according to the consensus guideline from the Clinical and Laboratory Standards Institute. **Results:** Isolates of *Abiotrophia defectiva* were susceptible to ampicillin, amoxicillin ceftriaxone, cefaclor, imipenem, ciprofloxacin, and vancomycin. Isolates of *Granulicatella adiacens* were mostly susceptible to benzylpenicillin, ampicillin, amoxicillin, cefazolin, ceftriaxone, imipenem, minocycline, and vancomycin. The susceptibility profile of *Granulicatella elegans* was similar to that of *G. adiacens*, and the susceptibility rate was higher than that of *G. adiacens*. **Conclusions:** Although *Abiotrophia* and *Granulicatella* strains are hardly distinguishable by their phenotypic characteristics, their susceptibility profiles to the antimicrobial agents were different among the species. Species-related differences in susceptibility of antibiotics should be considered in the clinical treatment for NVS related infections.

Keywords: nutritionally variant streptococci; antimicrobial susceptibilities; oral microbiota; infective endocarditis

---

1. Introduction

The bacteria formerly known as nutritionally variant streptococci (NVS) are characterized by their growth as small satellite colonies supported by helper bacteria such as *Staphylococcus aureus* [1]. The NVS strains require vitamin B_6 analogs for growth and produce bacteriolytic enzymes, pyrrolidonyl arylamidase and chromophore in common and were supposed to be auxotrophic variants of viridans group streptococci [2]. After several taxonomic alterations, they were finally transferred into two new genera, *Abiotrophia* and *Granulicatella*, on the basis of 16S rRNA gene sequence homology analysis [3,4]. They have been estimated as one of the important pathogens of so-called 'culture-negative endocarditis' [2,5,6]; however, because of their fastidiousness in growth, difficulty in identification, and complication in taxonomic position, the clinical importance of these bacteria has been underestimated by clinicians [7].

Although there have been several studies on the antimicrobial susceptibility of NVS, most of the previous studies dealt with a small number of strains, and methods and results were variable [2]. Furthermore, the taxonomic backgrounds of the tested isolates were uncertain. Commercial identification systems, based on the phenotypic characteristics of cultured bacteria, have often misidentified the clinical isolates of *Granulicatella* as *Gemella morbillorum*, and cannot distinguish *Granulicatella adiacens* and *Granulicatella elegans* [8–10]. To distinguish the two species of *Granulicatella*, molecular genetic analysis is required [11]. We previously isolated 91 strains of NVS from the human oral microbiota and classified them based on the phenotypic characteristics [9]. Among the oral isolates, 37 isolates confirmed their taxonomic identification by using DNA–DNA hybridization homology analysis, and we reported genetic heterogeneities in genus *Granulicatella* [10].

The Clinical and Laboratory Standards Institute (CLSI) published a laboratory guideline of antimicrobial susceptibility testing of infrequently encountered or fastidious bacteria, not covered in previous CLSI publications [12]. In this study, we determined the minimum inhibitory concentrations (MICs) of the taxonomically confirmed strains of *Abiotrophia* and *Granulicatella*, according to the consensus guideline provided by CLSI.

2. Materials and Methods

2.1. Bacterial Strains

Seven *Abiotrophia defectiva*, 17 *Granulicatella adiacens*, and six *Granulicatella elegans* (including type strains and oral isolates) were examined (see Tables 1 and 2). All isolates were identified using the rapid ID32 STREP system (Bio Mérieux SA, Marcy-l'Etoile, France) and DNA-DNA hybridization homology analysis [10]. The reference strains, *A. defectiva* ATCC 49176^T, NVS-47, and PE7, *G. adiacens* ATCC 49175^T, and *G. elegans* DSM11693^T, were from patients with endocarditis or bacteremia [13–15], and the other 25 isolates were derived from the oral cavity of healthy volunteers [9]. The strain *Streptococcus pneumoniae* ATCC 49619 was included in the assay to monitor accuracy of the MIC tests. The ATCC strains were obtained from American Type Culture Collection (Manassas, VA, USA), the DSM strain was obtained from Deutsche Sammlung von Mikroorganismen und Zellkulturen GmbH (Braunschweig, Germany), and the other strains were from the stock culture collection in our laboratory.

Table 1. MICs (µg/mL) of 15 antibiotics against *Abiotrophia* isolates.

Strains	PEN	AMP	AMX	PIP	CFZ	CAZ	CRO	CEC	IPM	GEN	ERY	CIP	MIN	VAN	SXT
A. defectiva															
ATCC49176[T]	0.125	0.016	0.016	1	1	16	1	0.125	0.125	32	0.5	1	0.063	0.25	256/4864
NVS-47	0.125	0.032	0.016	1	2	16	1	0.125	0.125	32	0.5	1	0.032	0.25	256/4864
PE7	0.032	0.016	0.016	4	1	8	1	0.125	0.125	32	0.5	1	0.063	0.25	256/4864
YTS2	0.063	0.016	0.063	1	4	8	0.5	0.5	0.125	32	0.5	1	0.063	0.25	256/4864
C8-3	0.25	0.125	0.063	1	2	8	0.5	0.5	0.125	16	0.25	0.5	4	0.25	0.016/0.3
C1-2	2	0.5	0.25	4	16	16	1	32	0.25	16	128	1	8	0.25	128/2432
YK-3	0.25	0.125	0.125	2	16	16	1	1	0.25	64	4	1	16	0.25	128/2432
range	0.032	0.016	0.016	1	1	8	0.5	0.125	0.125	16	0.25	0.5	0.032	0.25	0.016/0.3
	– 2	– 0.5	– 0.25	– 4	– 16	– 16	– 1	– 32	– 0.25	– 64	– 128	– 1	– 16	–	– 256/4864

Type strain and strains NVS-47 and PE7 were derived from blood cultures with endocarditis and the others were oral isolates from healthy volunteers. MIC: minimum inhibitory concentration, PEN: benzylpenicillin, AMP: ampicillin, AMX: amoxicillin, PIP: piperacillin, CFZ: cefazolin, CAZ: ceftazidime, CRO: ceftriaxone, CEC: cefaclor, IPM: imipenem, GEN: gentamicin, ERY: erythromycin, CIP: ciprofloxacin, MIN: minocycline, VAN: vancomycin, SXT: sulfamethoxazole-trimethoprim complex.

Table 2. MICs (µg/mL) of 15 antibiotics against *Granulicatella* isolates.

Strains	PEN	AMP	AMX	PIP	CFZ	CAZ	CRO	CEC	IPM	GEN	ERY	CIP	MIN	VAN	SXT
G. adiacens															
ATCC49175[T]	0.032	0.032	0.016	0.5	0.125	16	0.25	0.5	0.016	32	0.5	2	0.063	0.5	128/2432
HHC3	0.125	0.063	0.032	1	2	32	0.5	2	0.032	32	0.25	4	8	0.5	64/1216
HHP1	0.063	0.032	0.016	0.25	0.25	4	0.25	1	0.016	32	0.5	2	0.063	0.5	256/4864
P6-1	0.063	0.032	0.016	0.25	0.25	4	0.25	2	0.016	64	0.25	1	0.063	0.5	64/1216
YTC1	0.125	0.063	0.032	0.5	1	32	0.5	2	0.016	16	0.5	2	0.032	0.5	256/4864
S961-2	0.032	0.032	0.016	0.25	0.25	4	2	0.25	0.016	32	0.5	1	0.016	0.5	32/608
S1058-2	0.125	0.032	0.032	0.25	0.25	2	0.25	1	0.016	32	0.25	2	0.032	0.5	32/608
TK-T1	0.032	0.032	0.032	0.25	0.25	4	1	0.5	0.016	32	0.5	2	0.125	0.5	64/1216
HKT1-4	0.25	0.125	0.063	0.5	1	8	1	4	0.032	32	0.5	2	0.125	0.5	32/608
HKT2-2	0.125	0.125	0.063	0.5	1	8	0.25	4	0.032	32	0.125	2	0.016	0.25	32/608
C4-3	0.016	0.008	0.008	0.063	0.125	4	1	0.5	0.016	16	0.25	4	0.016	0.5	256/4864

Table 2. Cont.

Strains	PEN	AMP	AMX	PIP	CFZ	CAZ	CRO	CEC	IPM	GEN	ERY	CIP	MIN	VAN	SXT
HKT1-1	0.25	0.125	0.063	0.5	1	16	2	4	0.032	32	0.125	1	0.016	0.25	64/1216
NMP2	0.125	0.125	0.063	0.5	1	4	1	2	0.032	32	0.25	2	0.032	0.5	64/1216
P74	0.5	0.25	0.125	0.5	2	4	4	4	0.016	32	0.25	2	0.016	0.5	16/304
S49-2	0.032	0.032	0.032	0.25	0.25	4	8	0.5	0.016	32	0.25	2	0.063	0.5	128/2432
YTT3	0.063	0.032	0.032	0.25	0.25	64	0.25	1	0.032	16	0.25	2	0.125	0.5	64/1216
TK-T2	0.063	0.063	0.063	0.25	0.5	16	1	1	0.016	32	0.5	2	0.125	0.5	256/4864
range	0.016	0.008	0.008	0.063	0.125	2	0.25	0.25	0.016	16	0.125	1	0.016	0.25	16/304
	–	–	–	–	–	–	–	–	–	–	–	–	–	–	–
	0.5	0.25	0.125	1	2	64	8	4	0.032	64	0.5	4	8	0.5	256/4864
G. elegans															
DSM11693^T	0.016	0.063	0.125	0.125	0.125	2	0.5	0.5	0.016	16	8	1	0.25	4	0.5/9.5
NMP3	0.032	0.032	0.016	0.125	0.25	1	0.008	0.5	0.016	16	0.5	2	0.032	0.5	1/19
S1052-1	0.016	0.016	0.016	0.25	0.5	2	0.008	0.5	0.032	16	1	2	0.063	0.5	2/38
YTM1	0.032	0.032	0.016	0.25	0.25	1	0.016	0.5	0.016	16	0.5	4	0.063	0.5	512/9728
HHC5	0.032	0.032	0.016	0.25	0.5	2	0.032	0.5	0.032	8	0.5	2	0.016	0.5	2/38
C9-2	0.063	0.063	0.063	0.25	0.5	1	0.032	2	0.063	16	32	4	2	0.5	1/19
range	0.016	0.016	0.016	0.125	0.125	1	0.08	0.5	0.016	8	0.5	1	0.016	0.5	0.5/9.5
	–	–	–	–	–	–	–	–	–	–	–	–	–	–	–
	0.063	0.63	0.125	0.25	0.5	2	0.5	2	0.63	16	32	4	2	4	512/9728

Type strains were derived from blood cultures with endocarditis and the others were oral isolates from healthy volunteers. MIC: minimum inhibitory concentration, PEN: benzylpenicillin, AMP: ampicillin, AMX: amoxicillin, PIP: piperacillin, CFZ: cefazolin, CAZ: ceftazidime, CRO: ceftriaxone, CBC: cefaclor, IPM: imipenem, GEN: gentamicin, ERY: erythromycin, CIP: ciprofloxacin, MIN: minocycline, VAN: vancomycin, SXT: sulfamethoxazole-trimethoprim complex.

2.2. Antimicrobial Agents

Fifteen antimicrobial agents including penicillin, cephem, carbapenem, aminoglycoside, macrolide, tetracycline, quinolone, glycopeptide, and sulfonamide were used for this study (see Table 3). The following agents were purchased from Wako Pure Chemical Industries, Ltd. (Osaka, Japan): benzylpenicillin, cefazolin, piperacillin, ciprofloxacin, minocycline, and trimethoprim-sulfamethoxazole complex. Ampicillin, ceftazidime, ceftriaxone, cefaclor, gentamicin, erythromycin, and vancomycin were obtained from Sigma Chemical Co. (St. Louis, MO, USA). Amoxicillin was purchased from Fluka Biochemika (Bucks, Switzerland). Imipenem was kindly supplied by the Banyu Pharmaceutical Co., Ltd. (Tokyo, Japan).

Table 3. Percentage of susceptible isolates of *Abiotrophia* and *Granulicatella* against antimicrobial agents.

Antimicrobial Agent	% of Susceptible Isolates		
	A. defectiva (n = 7)	G. adiacens (n = 17)	G. elegans (n = 6)
Penicillin			
Benzylpenicillin	57.1	82.4	100
Ampicillin	85.7	100	100
Amoxicillin [a]	100	100	100
Piperacillin [a]	0	52.9	100
Cephem			
Cefazolin [b]	28.6	88.2	100
Ceftazidime [b]	0	0	50
Ceftriaxone	100	76.4	100
Cefaclor [b]	85.7	52.9	83.3
Carbapenem			
Imipenem	100	100	100
Aminoglycoside			
Gentamicin [c]	0	0	0
Macrolide			
Erythromycin	14.3	58.8	0
Quinolone			
Ciprofloxacin	100	17.6	16.7
Tetracycline			
Minocycline [d]	57.1	94.1	100
Glycopeptide			
Vancomycin	100	100	83.3
Other			
Sulfamethoxazole-trimethoprim [e]	14.3	0	16.7

Susceptibilities of the strains to the antimicrobial agents were determined according to the CLSI guideline M45-A2 for *Abiotrophia* spp. and *Granulicatella* spp. Susceptibilities to the antimicrobial agents unlisted in the guideline were determined as below; [a,b] Determined according to the guideline for ampicillin and cephems, respectively; [c] Determined according to the CLSI guideline M100-S18 for *S. aureus*; [d] Determined according to the CLSI guideline M100-S18 for tetracycline for *Streptococcus* spp. Viridans group; [e] Determined by the MIC values under 2/38 µg/mL.

2.3. MIC Testing

For preparation of inoculum, tested isolates were cultured anaerobically at 37 °C for 20 to 24 h with Mueller-Hinton broth (MHB; Difco Becton Dickinson and company, Sparks, MD, USA) containing 0.001% pyridoxal hydrochloride (Wako) and the bacterial cell suspensions were adjusted to yield about 5×10^5 CFU/mL. MICs for the *Abiotrophia* and *Granulicatella* strains were determined using the microdilution broth method with MHB containing 2.5% lysed horse blood (Strepto hemo supplement 'Eiken', Eiken Chemical Co., Ltd., Tokyo, Japan) and 0.001% pyridoxal hydrochloride, according to the consensus guideline from the CLSI for fastidious bacteria [12]. Briefly, the antimicrobial agents (100 µL/well) were diluted on 96-well round bottom plates (Sumilon, Sumitomo Bakelite Co., Ltd.,

Tokyo, Japan) in serial two-fold with the supplemented MHB, and 5 μL of the bacterial inoculum was added to each well. The plates were incubated at 35 °C in anaerobic condition for 20 h. The MIC values were defined as the lowest concentrations of antimicrobial agents that completely inhibited the bacterial growth in the microdilution wells, detected by unaided eyes. The strain of *S. pneumoniae* ATCC 49619 was used for quality control testing, and all MIC values for the strain were within the acceptable limits.

2.4. Susceptibility Criteria

The MIC values for bacterial isolates to the antimicrobial agents benzylpenicillin, ampicillin, ceftriaxone imipenem, erythromycin, ciprofloxacin, and vancomycin were interpreted into 3 categories: Susceptible, intermediate, and resistant, according to the CLSI guideline for *Abiotrophia* spp. and *Granulicatella* spp.

The MIC values for amoxicillin and piperacillin, and those for cefazolin, ceftazidime, and cefaclor were interpreted using criteria for ampicillin and cephems in the guideline for *Abiotrophia* and *Granulicatella*, respectively [16]. The MIC values for gentamicin and minocycline were interpreted using criteria in the CLSI guideline for *S. aureus* and for *Streptococcus* spp. Viridans group, respectively. The MIC values under 2/38 μg/mL for trimethoprim-sulfamethoxazole were interpreted as susceptible [17].

3. Results

The susceptibility percentage of the NVS isolates for 15 antimicrobial agents was summarized in Table 3. Although the phenotypic characteristics of the NVS isolates were similar, the profiles of susceptibility were unique among the species. The NVS isolates were susceptible to ampicillin (96.7%), amoxicillin (100%), imipenem (100%), and vancomycin (96.7%). In addition, *A. defectiva* strains were susceptible to ceftriaxone (100%), cefaclor (85.7%), and ciprofloxacin (100%); and *G. adiacens* strains were susceptible to benzylpenicillin (82.7%), cefazolin (88.2%), ceftriaxone (76.4%), and minocycline (94.1%). The susceptibility profile of *G. elegans* was similar to that of *G. adiacens*, and the susceptibility percentages of *G. elegans* to beta-lactams were higher than that of *G. adiacens*. On the other hand, no NVS strains were susceptible to gentamicin, and 93.3% of the strains were not susceptible to trimethoprim/sulfamethoxazole. Piperacillin susceptibility rate of *A. defectiva* was 0%, while that of *G. adiacens* and *G. elegans* were 52.9% and 100%, respectively. All *A. defectiva* strains were susceptible to ciprofloxacin, but only 17.4% of *Granulicatella* strains were susceptible to it.

Individual MIC values of *A. defectiva* and *Granulicatella* isolates to the antimicrobial agents were shown in Tables 1 and 2, respectively. Benzylpenicillin-nonsusceptible oral isolates of *A. defectiva* C1-2 and YK-3 were highly resistant to cefazolin and ceftazidime (both MICs = 16 μg/mL) and C1-2 showed additional resistance to cefaclor (MIC = 32 μg/mL), but were susceptible to ceftriaxone (MIC ≤ 1 μg/mL). Oral isolate of *G. adiacens* HHC3 was highly multi-drug resistant to ceftazidime, gentamycin, ciprofloxacin, and minocycline. The benzylpenicillin-nonsusceptible oral isolate of *G. adiacens* P7-4 was resistant to cephems, including ceftazidime, ceftriaxone, and cefaclor (all MICs = 4 μg/mL). Among the NVS isolates, only *G. elegans* DSM11693^T was resistant to vancomycin (MIC = 4 μg/mL).

4. Discussion

Abiotrophia and *Granulicatella* species are very common inhabitants in human normal oral microbiota, in spite of their fastidiousness in growth [9,11,18–20], and are significant causative pathogens of endocarditis, bacteremia, and other systemic infections [21–24]. They often cannot grow on commercial blood agar plates used for the usual clinical examination, and even if they could grow on supplemented culture plates, their colonies are sometimes small, 0.2 to 0.5 mm in diameter [1,25]. Therefore, these fastidious microorganisms have been overlooked in clinical specimens from foci of infective diseases, especially when they are concomitant with easily recovered bacteria

Medicines **2018**, *5*, 129

(such as *S. aureus*). Based on their phenotypic characteristics, *Abiotrophia* and *Granulicatella* spp. were initially classified as members of genus *Streptococcus*. Although genera *Abiotrophia* and *Granulicatella* were transferred and divided into two groups, based on the 16S rRNA sequence homology analysis, they have been treated as a same bacterial group of NVS in the field of clinical infectious diseases because they have common phenotypic characteristics, such as requiring vitamin B_6 analogs in growth and producing bacteriolytic enzymes. The human oral cavity is assumed to be a reservoir for the pathogens of many systemic infective diseases, so it is important to examine the antimicrobial susceptibilities of oral bacteria. In this study, we determined MICs of genetically identified seven *Abiotrophia* and 23 *Granulicatella* isolates (including oral isolates), according to the guideline from CLSI. Although NVS species have biochemical and phenotypic properties in common, and are difficult to distinguish without molecular genetical identification methods, the susceptibility profiles to antimicrobial agents were different among the species (Table 3).

Because of their fastidiousness, NVS species often were not recovered from the specimen in the usual clinical examination for infectious diseases caused by these bacteria. When no bacteria are recovered from the specimen of infective diseases, and that happens often, the empiric therapy with broad-spectrum antimicrobial agents (such as carbapenem, macrolide, quinolone, and tetracycline) is selected by the clinicians. As with the antimicrobials tested, all NVS isolates were susceptible to imipenem, and species-related differences were observed with respect to susceptibilities to ciprofloxacin and minocycline. The ciprofloxacin susceptibility rate for *A. defectiva* isolates was 100%, and that for *Granulicatella* isolates was 17.4%. In contrast, the susceptibility rate of minocycline for *Abiotrophia* isolates was 57.1%, and that for *Granulicatella* isolates was 95.7%. Species-related differences in susceptibility of antibiotics should be considered in the empiric therapy for NVS related infections.

In case of infective endocarditis (IE) caused by NVS, a combination of benzylpenicillin and gentamycin has been used for the antibiotic therapy [26–29]. However, 42.9% of *A. defectiva* isolates were not susceptible to benzylpenicillin and no strains of NVS isolates were susceptible to gentamycin in this study. Aminopenicillins, ampicillin, and amoxicillin showed better susceptible rates than benzylpenicillin and piperacillin. Ceftriaxone and ceftazidime are both third generation cephem, but the susceptible rates were contrary: Only three isolates of *G. elegans* (10.0% of the NVS isolates) were susceptible to ceftazidime. In contrast, 86.6% of the NVS isolates were susceptible to ceftriaxone (Table 3). According to the guidelines for endocarditis treatment by the British Society for Antimicrobial Chemotherapy, vancomycin can be used alone for the NVS IE patients with penicillin allergy [29]. The susceptibility rate of vancomycin for NVS isolates in our study was 96.7%. In the antimicrobial treatment of NVS IE, the recommended initial drugs (the combination of benzylpenicillin and gentamycin) may not be effective, and the regimen of initial drugs should be reconsidered.

Some isolates showed unique susceptibility profiles, for example, *A. defectiva* C1-2 showed multi-drug resistance to piperacillin, cefazolin, ceftazidime, cefaclor, gentamicin, erythromycin, and minocycline, but was susceptible to amoxicillin and ceftriaxone. Some *G. adiacens* isolates, such as HHC3, YTC1, and YTT3, were highly resistant to ceftazidime but susceptible to ceftriaxone, ampicillin, and amoxicillin. *G. adiacens* P7-4 was not susceptible to benzylpenicillin, piperacillin, and cefazolin, and was resistant to ceftriaxone, ceftazidime, and cefaclor, but was susceptible to ampicillin and amoxicillin. In the antimicrobial process, beta-lactams are bound to the penicillin binding protein (PBP) of the bacteria and inhibit their cell wall synthesis. The minor variations of PBP(s) may affect the antimicrobial susceptibilities of these isolates. Further molecular genetic research is needed to determine the mechanism of resistance in the NVS isolates with unique susceptibility profiles.

Author Contributions: T.K. and H.N. conceived the study. T.K. and S.T. performed the laboratory work. T.K. wrote the manuscript. All authors read and approved the final manuscript.

Funding: This study was supported by Department of Microbiology, St. Marianna University School of Medicine.

Acknowledgments: We thank Hiromu Takemura, for advice and stimulating discussions.

Conflicts of Interest: The authors declare no conflicts of interest.

References

1. Frenkel, A.; Hirsch, W. Spontaneous development of L forms of streptococci requiring secretions of other bacteria or sulphydryl compounds for normal growth. *Nature* **1961**, *191*, 728–730. [CrossRef] [PubMed]
2. Ruoff, K.L. Nutritionally variant streptococci. *Clin. Microbiol. Rev.* **1991**, *4*, 184–190. [CrossRef] [PubMed]
3. Kawamura, Y.; Hou, X.G.; Sultana, F.; Liu, S.; Yamamoto, H.; Ezaki, T. Transfer of *Streptococcus adjacens* and *Streptococcus defectivus* to *Abiotrophia* gen. nov. as *Abiotrophia adiacens* comb. nov. and *Abiotrophia defectiva* comb. nov., respectively. *Int. J. Syst. Bacteriol.* **1995**, *45*, 798–803. [CrossRef] [PubMed]
4. Collins, M.D.; Lawson, P.A. The genus *Abiotrophia* (Kawamura et al.) is not monophyletic: Proposal of *Granulicatella* gen. nov., *Granulicatella adiacens* comb. nov., *Granulicatella elegans* comb. nov. and *Granulicatella balaenopterae* comb. nov. *Int. J. Syst. Evol. Microbiol.* **2000**, *50 Pt 1*, 365–369. [CrossRef] [PubMed]
5. Casalta, J.P.; Habib, G.; La Scola, B.; Drancourt, M.; Caus, T.; Raoult, D. Molecular diagnosis of *Granulicatella elegans* on the cardiac valve of a patient with culture-negative endocarditis. *J. Clin. Microbiol.* **2002**, *40*, 1845–1847. [CrossRef] [PubMed]
6. Tattevin, P.; Watt, G.; Revest, M.; Arvieux, C.; Fournier, P.E. Update on blood culture-negative endocarditis. *Med. Mal. Infect.* **2015**, *45*, 1–8. [CrossRef] [PubMed]
7. Tellez, A.; Ambrosioni, J.; Llopis, J.; Pericas, J.M.; Falces, C.; Almela, M.; Garcia de la Maria, C.; Hernandez-Meneses, M.; Vidal, B.; Sandoval, E.; et al. Epidemiology, Clinical Features, and Outcome of Infective Endocarditis due to *Abiotrophia* Species and *Granulicatella* Species: Report of 76 Cases, 2000–2015. *Clin. Infect. Dis.* **2018**, *66*, 104–111. [CrossRef]
8. Coto, H.; Berk, S.L. Endocarditis caused by *Streptococcus morbillorum*. *Am. J. Med. Sci.* **1984**, *287*, 54–58. [CrossRef]
9. Kanamoto, T.; Eifuku-Koreeda, H.; Inoue, M. Isolation and properties of bacteriolytic enzyme-producing cocci from the human mouth. *FEMS Microbiol. Lett.* **1996**, *144*, 135–140. [CrossRef]
10. Kanamoto, T.; Sato, S.; Inoue, M. Genetic heterogeneities and phenotypic characteristics of strains of the genus *Abiotrophia* and proposal of *Abiotrophia para-adiacens* sp. nov. *J. Clin. Microbiol.* **2000**, *38*, 492–498.
11. Sato, S.; Kanamoto, T.; Inoue, M. *Abiotrophia elegans* strains comprise 8% of the nutritionally variant streptococci isolated from the human mouth. *J. Clin. Microbiol.* **1999**, *37*, 2553–2556. [PubMed]
12. Jorgensen, J.H.; Hindler, J.F. New consensus guidelines from the Clinical and Laboratory Standards Institute for antimicrobial susceptibility testing of infrequently isolated or fastidious bacteria. *Clin. Infect. Dis.* **2007**, *44*, 280–286. [CrossRef] [PubMed]
13. Bouvet, A.; Grimont, F.; Grimont, P.A.D. *Streptococcus defectivus* sp. nov. and *Streptococcus adjacens* sp. nov., nutritionally variant streptococci from human clinical specimens. *Int. J. Syst. Bacteriol.* **1989**, *39*, 290–294. [CrossRef]
14. van de Rijn, I.; George, M. Immunochemical study of nutritionally variant streptococci. *J. Immunol.* **1984**, *133*, 2220–2225. [PubMed]
15. Roggenkamp, A.; Abele-Horn, M.; Trebesius, K.H.; Tretter, U.; Autenrieth, I.B.; Heesemann, J. *Abiotrophia elegans* sp. nov., a possible pathogen in patients with culture-negative endocarditis. *J. Clin. Microbiol.* **1998**, *36*, 100–104. [PubMed]
16. CLSI. *Methods for Antimicrobial Dilution and Disk Susceptibility Testing of Infrequently Isolated or Fastidious Bacteria*; Approved Guideline M45-A; Clinical and Laboratory Standards Institute: Wayne, PA, USA, 2006; Volume 26, pp. 10–11.
17. CLSI. Methods for Dilution Antimicirobial Susceptibility Tests for Bacteria That Grow Aerobically; Approved Standard-Seventh Edition M7-A7. In *Performance Standards for Antimicrobial Susceptibility Testing*; Eighteenth Informational Supplement M100-S18; Wikler, M.A., Ed.; Clinical and Laboratory Standards Institute: Wayne, PA, USA, 2008; Volume 27, pp. 86–161.
18. Aas, J.A.; Paster, B.J.; Stokes, L.N.; Olsen, I.; Dewhirst, F.E. Defining the normal bacterial flora of the oral cavity. *J. Clin. Microbiol.* **2005**, *43*, 5721–5732. [CrossRef]
19. Diaz, P.I.; Chalmers, N.I.; Rickard, A.H.; Kong, C.; Milburn, C.L.; Palmer, R.J., Jr.; Kolenbrander, P.E. Molecular characterization of subject-specific oral microflora during initial colonization of enamel. *Appl. Environ. Microbiol.* **2006**, *72*, 2837–2848. [CrossRef]
20. Zaura, E.; Keijser, B.J.; Huse, S.M.; Crielaard, W. Defining the healthy "core microbiome" of oral microbial communities. *BMC Microbiol.* **2009**, *9*, 259. [CrossRef]

21. Brouqui, P.; Raoult, D. Endocarditis due to rare and fastidious bacteria. *Clin. Microbiol. Rev.* **2001**, *14*, 177–207. [CrossRef]
22. Woo, P.C.; To, A.P.; Lau, S.K.; Fung, A.M.; Yuen, K.Y. Phenotypic and molecular characterization of erythromycin resistance in four isolates of *Streptococcus*-like gram-positive cocci causing bacteremia. *J. Clin. Microbiol.* **2004**, *42*, 3303–3305. [CrossRef]
23. Senn, L.; Entenza, J.M.; Greub, G.; Jaton, K.; Wenger, A.; Bille, J.; Calandra, T.; Prod'hom, G. Bloodstream and endovascular infections due to *Abiotrophia defectiva* and *Granulicatella* species. *BMC Infect. Dis.* **2006**, *6*, 9. [CrossRef] [PubMed]
24. De Luca, M.; Amodio, D.; Chiurchiu, S.; Castelluzzo, M.A.; Rinelli, G.; Bernaschi, P.; Calo Carducci, F.I.; D'Argenio, P. *Granulicatella* bacteraemia in children: Two cases and review of the literature. *BMC Pediatr.* **2013**, *13*, 61. [CrossRef] [PubMed]
25. Reimer, L.G.; Reller, L.B. Growth of nutritionally variant streptococci on laboratory media supplemented with blood of eight animal species. *Med. Lab. Sci.* **1982**, *39*, 79–81. [PubMed]
26. Cargill, J.S.; Scott, K.S.; Gascoyne-Binzi, D.; Sandoe, J.A. *Granulicatella* infection: Diagnosis and management. *J. Med. Microbiol.* **2012**, *61*, 755–761. [CrossRef] [PubMed]
27. Ohara-Nemoto, Y.; Kishi, K.; Satho, M.; Tajika, S.; Sasaki, M.; Namioka, A.; Kimura, S. Infective endocarditis caused by *Granulicatella elegans* originating in the oral cavity. *J. Clin. Microbiol.* **2005**, *43*, 1405–1407. [CrossRef] [PubMed]
28. Lin, C.H.; Hsu, R.B. Infective endocarditis caused by nutritionally variant streptococci. *Am. J. Med. Sci.* **2007**, *334*, 235–239. [CrossRef] [PubMed]
29. Gould, F.K.; Denning, D.W.; Elliott, T.S.; Foweraker, J.; Perry, J.D.; Prendergast, B.D.; Sandoe, J.A.; Spry, M.J.; Watkin, R.W.; Working Party of the British Society for Antimicrobial Chemotherapy. Guidelines for the diagnosis and antibiotic treatment of endocarditis in adults: A report of the Working Party of the British Society for Antimicrobial Chemotherapy. *J. Antimicrob. Chemother.* **2012**, *67*, 269–289. [CrossRef] [PubMed]

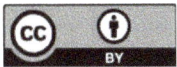

medicines

MDPI

Review

Kampo Therapies and the Use of Herbal Medicines in the Dentistry in Japan

Shuji Watanabe [1,2], Toshizo Toyama [1], Takenori Sato [1], Mitsuo Suzuki [1,3], Akira Morozumi [4], Hiroshi Sakagami [5] and Nobushiro Hamada [1,*]

[1]   Division of Microbiology, Department of Oral Science, Kanagawa Dental University, 82 Inaoka-cho,
      Yokosuka 238-8580, Japan; swatanabe2010@nifty.com (S.W.); toyama@kdu.ac.jp (T.T.); t.sato@kdu.ac.jp (T.S.);
      suzuki@d2clinic.jp (M.S.)
[2]   Odoriba Medical Center, Totsuka Green Dental Clinic, 1-10-46 Gumizawa, Totsuka-ku,
      Yokohama 245-0061, Japan
[3]   Dental Design Clinic, 3-7-10 Kita-aoyama, Minato-ku, Tokyo 107-0061, Japan
[4]   Morozumi Dental Clinic, 1-3-1 Miyamaedaira, Miyamae-ku, Kawasaki 216-0006, Japan;
      morozumident@gmail.com
[5]   Meikai University Research Institute of Odontology (M-RIO), 1-1 Keyakidai, Sakado,
      Saitama 350-0283, Japan; sakagami@dent.meikai.ac.jp
*   Correspondence: hamada@kdu.ac.jp; Tel./Fax: +81-46-822-8867

Received: 13 February 2019; Accepted: 25 February 2019; Published: 28 February 2019

Abstract: Dental caries and periodontal disease are two major diseases in the dentistry. As the society is aging, their pathological meaning has been changing. An increasing number of patients are displaying symptoms of systemic disease and so we need to pay more attention to immunologic aggression in our medical treatment. For this reason, we focused on natural products. Kampo consists of natural herbs—roots and barks—and has more than 3000 years of history. It was originated in China as traditional medicine and introduced to Japan. Over the years, Kampo medicine in Japan has been formulated in a way to suit Japan's natural features and ethnic characteristics. Based on this traditional Japanese Kampo medicine, we have manufactured a Kampo gargle and Mastic Gel dentifrice. In order to practically utilize the effectiveness of mastic, we have developed a dentifrice (product name: IMPLA CARE) and treated implant periodontitis and severe periodontitis.

Keywords: periodontitis; Kampo; traditional medicine; *Jixueteng*; *Juzentaihoto*; technical terms; gargle; tongue diagnosis; mastic; pathogenic factors

---

1. Introduction

Kampo medicine in Japan is the Oriental medicine which was originally brought from China through east Asia and the Korean peninsula as the ancient Chinese medicine. During the Nara period of Japan (AD 710-784), Japanese envoys were sent to Tang Dynasty (AD616-907) under the name of Kentoshi and it became a channel that Chinese medicine was directly brought to Japan. In the Kamakura period (AD1185-1333), it made a progress to become more practical medicine by being adopted more to Japan's natural environment, rather than a simple copy of Chinese medicine. In the Muromachi period (AD 1336-1573), a Japanese whose name was Sanki Tashiro studied in China during its Ming dynasty (AD1368-1644) and created the academic foundation of the Japanese Kampo medicine. Kampo was first used in higher social classes but since the 15th century it has provided general people natural material-based medicine. In the Edo period (AD 1603-1867), Western medicine was introduced to Japan from Netherland and was called Rangaku, innovating special characteristics such as abdominal diagnosis and contributed to the developments of medical diagnosis and treatment [1–3]. On the other hand, the traditional medicine which was primarily using herbal medicines was called Kampo medicine. In 1883, the Japanese government promulgated the regulation of the medical license that only those doctors who have mastered the Western medicine could prescribe the Kampo medicines and the Kampo medicine declined since then except for the practice by some facilities or individuals. In 1927, the book of Kokan Igaku (traditional Japanese and Chinese medicine) by Kyushin Yumoto was published and it triggered the subsequent revival of Kampo medicine. Following that in 1950, the academic society of "Japan Society of Oriental Medicine" of Kokan Igaku was established, which became the association of Oriental medicine including acupuncture and moxibustion treatments. Under the guidance of the Japan Medical Association, Kitasato University Oriental Medicine Research Centre was founded in 1972 and it has played a central role in the education of Oriental Medicine. Further in 2001, the model curriculum of medical education newly incorporated a course of study for "being capable of explaining Japanese and Chinese medicines." At present, all medical schools in Japan have the courses of study for Kampo medicine or Oriental medicine as part of their education program.

Kampo medicine has a unique character, which is different from Western medicine. Kampo uses as a combination drug of various herbal plants that have complementary physiological activities. In fact, 148 Kampo formulations are used for medicinal treatments and are covered by the Japanese National Health Insurance Program [4]. Since 2012, seven kinds of Kampo formulations were approved by Japan Dental Association within the National Health Insurance Drug Price Standard related with dental treatment [5]. In 2015, Kampo Education Plan of Dentistry was sent from the Japan Dental Association to all dental universities [6]. At the same time, the first author of this article (S.W.) established the Yokohama Kampo Dentistry Study Group for the continuing education of Kampo. This group has held 18 research sessions and symposiums by calling a special lecturer of Kampo and is planning to publish a side reader of 11 Kampo preparations for dental students from the Nanzando publishing company. There are two academic societies on Kampo in Japan: The Japan Society for Oriental Medicine and Japan Dental Society of Oriental Medicine. The latter showed previously different direction about *qigong* and massage but now changing to the same direction with the former.

Kampo prescriptions in dentistry has special characteristics due to the diverse symptoms such as the pain caused by the bad bite alignment or malocclusion (exogenous cause) and unidentified complaints. For Kampo prescriptions, it is important to understand the symptoms, by considering these special characteristics. It has also become known that the negative feedback functionality would not work when malocclusion and occlusal destruction become chronic with the sympathetic-nerve predominant state. We expect that Western medicine and the Oriental medicine will be used selectively and in parallel in many of the clinical cases in dentistry to ensure the best results for primary cares and that it would contribute to the dentistry medicine going forward.

In this review article, we firstly focus on the basic theory of Kampo medicine and then its biological activities and clinical effects in the dental treatments.

2. Basic Theory of Kampo Medicine

2.1. Concept of Oriental Medicine

Western medicine is a proof medicine that is based on the medical evidence, while Oriental medicine is a traditional medicine that has accumulated the evidence based on the experiences [7]. The modern medicine has made great advances by accumulating scientific evidences but it was at the same time a challenge to the limit of the medicine and it has added a new dimension of problems such as the side effects of medicines to cope up with the aggravation of diseases. In recent years, medical evidences of Kampo prescription (traditional medicine in Japan based on the traditional Chinese medicine), which is one of the pharmacotherapies of Oriental medicine, has become widely known. It is making it possible to include Kampo in the pharmacotherapy of the modern medicine, in consideration of its role as biological response modifiers (BRMs) of the vital balance. Oriental medicine was generated from the concept that the natural world consists of the opposing axis of *Yin* (Table A1) or "non-resistant" and *Yang* or "resistant," where the relativity of these axes maintains the qualitative balance of the workings of mother nature [3]. This principle is therefore called the "*Yin-Yang* theory." In the Kampo therapy, the body state and each internal organ are divided into *Yin* or *Yang* and it treats the patient so the *yin-yang* is balanced and can maintain the homeostasis (Figure 1).

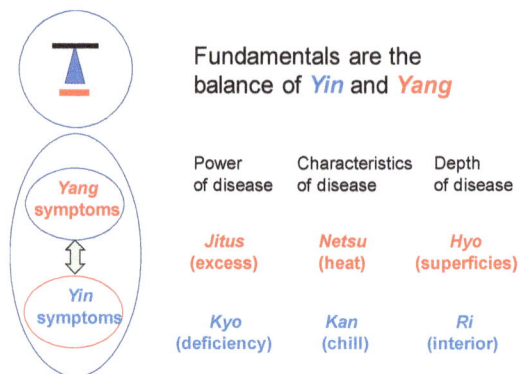

Fundamentals are the
balance of **Yin** and **Yang**

Power of disease	Characteristics of disease	Depth of disease
Jitus (excess)	*Netsu* (heat)	*Hyo* (superficies)
Kyo (deficiency)	*Kan* (chill)	*Ri* (interior)

Figure 1. Concepts of Kampo therapy. Kampo therapy begins with the knowledge of constitutional characteristics of patient's body. *In-Yo* or *Yin-Yang*: When the switch-over between two representative autonomic nerves, the sympathetic nerves (*yang*) and the parasympathetic nerves (*yin*), is good, the *yin-yang* balance is kept well. *Kyo-Jits* or asthenia and sthenia show physical strength, constitutional characteristics of body and the strength of resistance against disease. The reaction differs, depending on their *Kyo-Sho* or *Jitsu-Sho*. It is categorized into *Jitsu-Sho* (excess symptom), *Kyo-Sho* (deficiency symptom) and *Chukan-Sho* (symptom in-between the two). *Kan-Netsu* or chills and fever: *Kan* is *Yin* while *Netsu* is *Yang*. They are always in a relative relation. When *Yin* deteriorates, *Yang* predominates, called *Netsu-sho* (heat syndrome).

2.2. Differences from the Western Medicine

Oriental medicine and Western medicine are both medical sciences, fundamentally and equally. Oriental medicine identifies the disease mainly based on the pathological condition at the time of diagnosis. It understands that a part of the body appeals the problem and it spreads to the entire body and shows the symptom in that part. Therefore, the treatment aims at alleviating the symptom while improving the pathological condition itself. This pathological condition is called *Sho* or Kampo Diagnosis.

The Western medicine diagnoses based on the demonstrated symptom and it emphasizes the importance of the examinations in order to find out the condition of the appearing symptoms, then gives it a name and treats it accordingly. On the other hand, Kampo medicine improves the symptom by improving the pathological condition presented in the form of *Sho* [2,8]. *Sho* is the measure to know the characteristics, size and depth of the disease, which would indicate the cause of the disease and the treatment, is given by finding out the cause of the pathological condition by *Sho*. From this, Oriental medicine makes it possible to treat the patient as expressed in the phrase "Different treatments for one disease; identical treatment for different diseases." It means that different treatments will be given for the same disease name of patients if the *Sho* (Kampo diagnosis) is different. Likewise, the same treatment will be given to the different disease names of patients, if the *Sho* is the same. Here in this article, the disease name means the name of the disease under the modern medical science (Figure 2).

2.3. The Categories of Sho

Shoko (Kampo medical conditions, symptoms in Western medical terms) consists of *Yin*-Yang with *Kyo-Jitsu*, *Kan-Netsu* and *Hyo-Ri*. They reflect the current pathogenic condition. Table 1 shows the definitions and classifications of *Yin-Yang*, *Kyo-Jitsu* (asthenia and sthenia) and *Kan Netsu* (chills and fever). Table 2 shows the definitions of *Yin-Kyo*, *Yo-Kyo*, *Yin-Jitsu* and *Yo-Jitsu*. Figure 3 shows the condition categories of *Yin-Yang*, *Kyo-sho* and *Netsu-Kan* in the body.

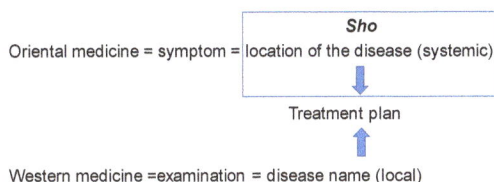

Figure 2. Characteristics of Oriental medicine and Western medicine therapy. *Sho* (Kampo Diagnosis): Capturing the *Shoko* (*yin-yang*, *Kyo-Jitsu* or deficiency and excess, *Kan-Netsu* or chills and fever, *Hyo-Ri* or superficies and interior) as the holistic symptom caused by the pathological condition and it shows the condition of the patient at the time of diagnosis. *Sho* changes depending on the bodily sensation.

Table 1. Definitions and classifications of *Yin-Yong*, *Kyo-Jitsu* and *Kan-Netsu*.

Categories	Yin-Yang	Kyo-Jitsu (Asthenia and Sthenia)	Kan-Netsu (Chills and Fever)
Definitions	Ability to resist the disease. The treatment differs, depending on whether the *sho* is *yang* and *yin*. *Yin* disease: The resistant power against the disease is weak. Treatment is given to recover the exhaustion of the body. It is called *honchi* or the systemic meridian treatment	The state of deficiency is *kyo-sho* or asthenia and excess is *jitsu-sho* or sthenia. *Kyo* (Asthenia): Deficiency of what is required for the body and shows the *sho* of *Yin-kyo* syndrome or *yang-kyo* syndrome	Actual feeling of chill and heat *Kyo-netsu* (asthenic heat): Heat coming from poor metabolism and retained inside the body, slight fever, internal fever, showing *yin*-syndrome.
Classification (According to the Orthodox Theory)	*Yang* disease: The resistant power against the disease is strong. Treatment which positivity attacks the disease is effective. It is called *hyochi* or local and symptomatic treatment.	*Jitsu* (Sthenia): Low metabolic rate due to the accumulation of toxic substance in the body and shows the *sho* of *yin-jitsu* or *yang-jitsu*.	*Jitsu-netsu* (sthenic heat): Chills that occurs by increasing the heat in the body. Observes pyrexia and showing *Yang*-syndrome.

Table 2. Definitions of *Yin-Kyo*, *Yo-Kyo*, *Yin-Jitsu* and *Yo-Jitsu*.

Categories	Yin-Kyo (yin deficiency)	Yo-Kyo (yang deficiency)	Yin-Jitsu (Yin excess)	Yo-Jitsu (Yang excess)
Definitions	*Yin* is insufficient and *yan* becomes relatively overactive; shows fever called asthenic fever; feverish symptom.	*Yang* is insufficient and *yin* relatively becomes overactive; asthenia cold; feeling chills.	Coldness comes from outside to constantly maintain the homeostasis of *yin* and *yang* and shows the state of chills, called *Jitsu-Kan* or sthenic cold; body is chilled and feeling cold.	Heat comes from outside to constantly maintain the homeostasis of *yin* and *yang*; and shows the state of heat, called *Jitsu-Netsu* or sthenic heat; feeling hot and excessive sw eating.

On the other hand, *Hyo-Ri* (superficies and interior) indicates where the disease exists in the body and shows the depth of *Sho*, depending on the part of the body. *Hyo-ri* is a unique concept of Kampo medicine, which indicates the seriousness of the disease, based on the location and depth of the disease. According to the classic literature "Shokan-ron," *Yin* and *Yang* are further divided into 3 layers by the degree of development and it calls them the "Three *Yin*" and the "Three *Yang*" of diseases [8]. The Three *Yang* stage indicates *Hyo* or the surface of the body such as skin but also includes the parts of the body that show the *Hyo* symptoms such as chill, fever, headache, joint pain and sweat. The three *Yin* stage indicates *Ri*. Mostly *Sho's* of the internal organs, including heart, lungs and digestive apparatus, are shown, where the symptoms are, for example, abdominal pain, constipation, diarrhoea, fullness of the abdomen, stomach tension. The middle part between the *Hyo-Ri* is called *Han-Hyo-Ri* or mesodermal.

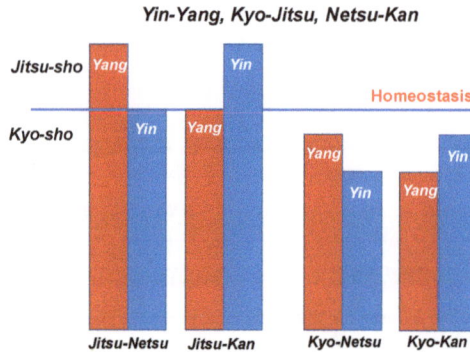

Figure 3. Condition categories of *Yin-Yang*, *Kyo-sho* and *Netsu-Kan* in the body.

2.4. Cause of Illness

Disease in Kampo medicine is the disorder of harmony of spirit and body. The living body has physiological functions to maintain the homeostasis of the organism against the changes of internal and external environment. This function is called *Shoki* or healthy *Ki*. *Shoki* is a function which would defend the body against disease and would induce natural healing ability, where the natural healing ability would seek for the harmony of *Ki*, *Ketsu* and *Sui* (vital energy, blood circulation and aqua). In contrast, the factor that attempts to destroy the homeostasis is called *Ja* or *Byoja* or stress or pathogen. It induces the climate, emotion or virus to cause various physical abnormalities which would lead to diseases. Causes of disease are categorized into endogenous, exogenous and other factors.

Endogenous factor means that the cause of disease comes from the inside of body. It may be common emotions of human beings. It is a physiological phenomenon and may be quintessential in life. However, it can cause abnormality in the functions of internal organs, when mental stress persists or when a sudden strong shock hits us, because it would collapse the balance of *Yin*, *Yang*, *Ki* and *Ketsu* on such occasions. It is called the *Seven Emotions* –joy, anger, anxiety, worry, grief, apprehension and fear.

Exogenous factor means that *ja* invades the body from outside. Diseases occur influenced by the mental or physical changes when the body cannot accept the natural environment such as pathogens, severe natural environment and sudden climate changes. It is called the *Six Pathogenic Agents* - wind, cold, heat, humidity, dryness and fire (fever).

These are other factors, which would cause diseases due to other causes such as inadequate eating-drinking, fatigue, overwork, injury, poisoning, parasite and heredity.

2.5. Explanation of Ki, Ketsu, Oketsu and Sui

The concept of *Ki* (vital energy), *Ketsu* (blood/blood circulatory function) and *Sui* (aqua) is the fundamental concept to understand the Kampo medicine [2,8] (Figure 4).

Ki indicates *yang* and *Ketsu* and *Sui* indicate *yin*. Patients reversibly show *Jitsu-Sho* (excessive) and *Kyo-Sho* (deficiency) (Table 3).

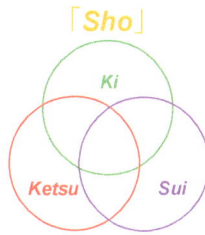

Figure 4. Diagrams of biological factors in *Sho*.

Table 3. Classifications of *Ki*, *Ketsu* and *Sui*.

Yin	Yang
Ketsu Sui	Ki

2.5.1. *Ki*, Vital Energy

Ki is the source of energy of the entire biological activities and it circulates blood and bodily fluid in the whole body [8]. Therefore, the inhibition of the workings of *Ki* would inhibit the workings of *Ketsu* (blood circulation) and *Sui* (bodily liquid) and thus a disease would occur. *Ki* belongs to *yang*. When these elements are excessively active, it is called *Jitsu* or excess and is called *Kyo* or deficiency when these are deficient. Excessive *Ki* is called *Ki-Gyaku* (*ki-Jitsu*) or hyperactive *ki*. It is called *Ki-Tai* when stagnated due to over excess, while *Ki-Kyo* when under hypersecretion.

2.5.2. *Ketsu*, Blood Circulation

Blood circulates through the body and supplies nutrition to the five parenchymatous viscera (heart, liver, spleen, lung and kidney) and the six hollow viscera [gallbladder, stomach, small intestine, large intestine, urinary bladder and triple heater (*sansho*, a passage that controls the flow of air, blood and water)]. *Ki* and *ketsu* are interdependent each other –*Ki* warms up the body in *Yang* and *ketsu* nourishes the body in *Yin*. There are three states of *Ketsu*, namely, *Ketsu-Netsu* (*Ketsu-Jitsu*) (blood-heat), *Oketsu* (*Ketsu-Tai*) (blood stagnation) and *Ketsu-Kyo* (blood deficiency). Symptoms of blood-heat shows hematemesis, bloody stools, nose bleeds, for example and shows bleeding from tissue, constipation and yellowish urine [8]. When heated blood (*ketsu-netsu*) goes up to the upper body, it causes not only *oketsu* (blood stagnation) but also affects emotions such as irritation. Blood deficiency is the decay of the recuperation ability of blood. It causes so-called anaemia but also shows other dysfunction such as anorexia and weakening of digestion and absorption and these are governed by *Ki*. Blood will not circulate the body if *Ki* is insufficient to operate the blood vessels. This *Ki* in each part of the body is called *Ei-ki* or *Yin*-energy. *Ki* initiates functions of each organ of the body. *Ketsu* belongs to *Yin*. The concept of *Oketsu* or blood stagnation is the most important concept. *Oketsu* is a pathological change that would cause diseases when the blood is stagnated in the entire body or in a local tissue (Figure 5).

Sansho (triple heater), one of the 12 main acupuncture channels in the body, responsible for moving energy between the upper body and the lower body.

2.5.3. Oketsu

Pathological condition of *Oketsu* (blood stagnation) is expressed in a unique way to Kampo medicine and it is the most important concept [8]. In the modern medicine, it is perhaps more commonly understood as one of the syndromes of disability of microcirculation mechanism (Figure 6). However, Kampo medicine does not simply diagnose the symptoms but it considers important to identify the pathological condition which caused the symptom and the following are considered the pathogenic *Sho* of *Oketsu* such as the changes in the blood vessels due to inflammation, accentuation of blood coagulation factors, blood congestion, polycythaemia, menstruation, pregnancy or child-delivery.

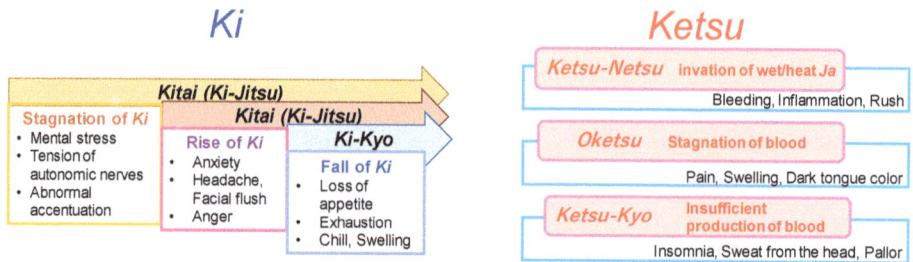

Figure 5. The concepts of *Ki* and *Ketsu*.

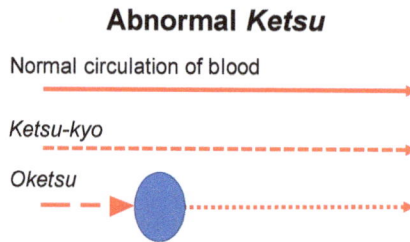

Figure 6. The Symptoms of *Oketsu*, in blood stagnation.

When the following symptoms are observed, we diagnose them *Oketsu*; the patient feels mouth dryness and would moisten the mouth with water but does not want to drink water; the patient feels stomach fullness though the abdominal distension is not observed; burning fever is felt locally or universally; purple spots appear on the skin or membrane; purple spots are appearing on the skin or membrane; dark purple spots appear on the edge of the tongue and lips are pale; stool is black; easy bleeding. The endogenous factor is in imbalance of autonomic nerve and the exogenous factor is coldness and bruise.

2.5.4. *Sui, Aua*

Sui is also called *Shin-Eki*. *Shin* is the relatively thin and pure fluids such as fluid component of blood, tissue fluids, sweat and urine, while *Eki* is relatively thick and sticky fluids among the intracellular and secretory fluids [8]. Each shows *Sho* of *Sui-Tai* (*Sui-Jitsu*) and *Sui-Kyo*. *Sui-tai* means stagnation of the body fluid (Figure 7).

Unevenly distributed *Sui* or aqua causes a local oedema. When it is linked with blood-heat, it becomes *Tan-In*-diseases and the fluid becomes sticky phlegm. As the blood-heat is understood as the inflammatory blood, it can appear when physical infection control is conducted. *Ko-Katsu* or mouth dryness is a symptom appearing when water is temporarily exhausted due to insufficient intake of water. Fever, thirst and tongue dryness are also systemically observed. It is called *Sui-Kyo* or aqua deficiency, which occurs from the temporal water exhaustion and shows dehydration. Xerostomia is a symptom of chronical insufficiency of water. Patients would feel mouth dryness and appeal lip dryness and cracks but would not want to drink water. It is mainly caused by the endogenous factors and systemically showing *Yin-Kyo* or *Yin*-deficiency and is diagnosed as *Oketsu-Sho*. It also shows the deterioration of kidney functions that is the symptom of deterioration of *Ki*.

Sui (*Shin-Eki*)

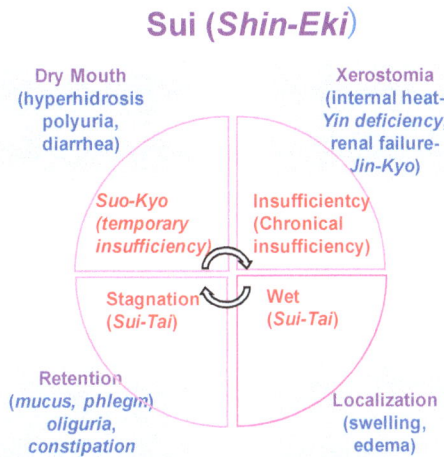

Dry Mouth
(hyperhidrosis
polyuria,
diarrhea)

Xerostomia
(internal heat-
Yin deficiency,
renal failure-
Jin-Kyo)

Suo-Kyo
(temporary
insufficiency)

Insufficientcy
(Chronical
insufficiency)

Stagnation
(*Sui-Tai*)

Wet
(*Sui-Tai*)

Retention
(*mucus, phlegm*)
oliguria,
constipation

Localization
(swelling,
edema)

Figure 7. The concepts of *Sui* (*Shin-Eki*).

2.5.5. Views on Periodontal Disease and Toothache

In the progress of periodontitis, the gingival blood circulation induces the loss of capillary vessels and become anaemia. This status is so-called *Ketsu-Kyo* (blood deficiency) in Kampo. *Ketsu-Kyo* affects the nutritional disorder of gingiva and reduces oral immune system. Consequently, microcirculatory dysfunction induces the loss of oral biological activity, increasing the numbers of compromised hosts. This status is called *Oketsu* (blood stasis) in Kampo. *Oketsu* was observed in 70% to 80% of the randomly chosen periodontal patients above age 40 (Figure 8).

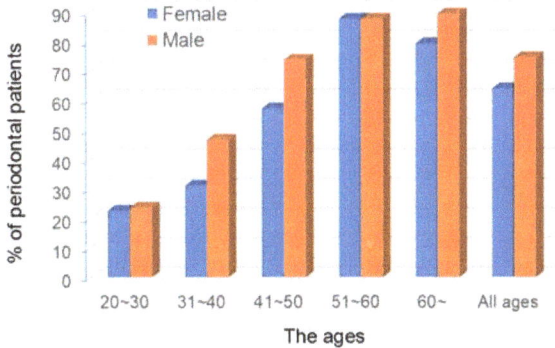

Figure 8. The proportions of poor blood circulation (*Oketu*) in the ages of the periodontal patients. Cited from [9] with permission.

Although there are Kampo medicines which contain analgesic effect but they are not comparable to the western medicines. In oriental medicine, pain is understood as the change of symptom to maintain the homeostasis of organism. The flows of *ki, ketsu, sui* (vital energy, blood circulation function and aqua) deteriorate and it causes the unwell condition from stagnation. Therefore, Kampo medicine emphasizes to recuperate the body condition to normal. The background of pain would include not only infections and injuries but also the environmental and mental stress, where psychological factor would cause anxiety and anger and can go back to the emotions in the past. Chinese proverb says that good circulation brings no pain (= stagnation), meaning that if it flows, no pain.

Occlusal trauma, occlusal destruction and traumatic occlusion are intraoral fragility and could cause systemic symptoms (Figure 9).

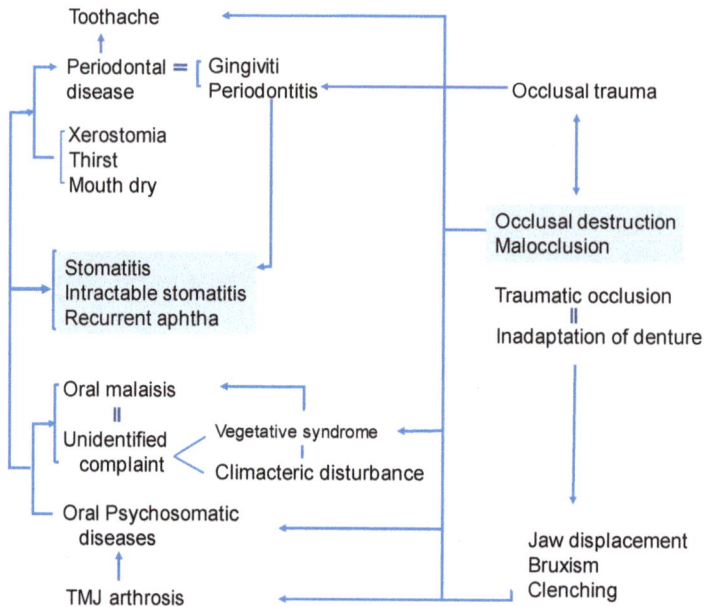

Figure 9. The correlations between occlusal-related troubles and oral diseases. (Watanabe S, unpublished data)

3. Tongue Diagnosis

Clinical tongue conditions reflect the diseases of internal organs. The important points of clinical observations are colours, coatings and volume of the tongue [8]. The tension of the tongue (shape and lustre) change to the depending on the fall and rise of *Ki-Ketsu and* the location and the depth of the pathogen in body. Coating of the tongue mostly indicates the stomach condition, especially, dampness-dryness, coldness-heat of the body. Normal and abnormal conditions are shown in Tables 4 and 5.

Table 4. The correlations between the colours and shapes in tongue.

Colour Tone	
	• *Pale tongue:* Paler colour than normal tongue; showing deficiency of *Ki* and *Ketsu*.
	• *Reddish tongue:* *Netsu-Sho* (heat) symptom; redder than normal tongue colour and often shows dryness of mouth and lips.
	• *Purplish tongue:* Systemic *Oketsu* due to stagnation of *Ki and Ketsu*; especially it is very likely when the dorsal lingual veins are over swelling.
	• If the tongue is wet, it is *Kan-Sho* (cold) symptom and the body is chilled. If dry, it shows *Netsu-Sho*.
Shape	
	• *Swelled tongue:* Tongue is swollen and shows tooth marks on peripheral; showing *Ki-Kyo* and *Sui-Tai* (deficiency of *Ki* and fluid stagnation).
	• *Thin tongue:* Tongue is dry and in deep purple colour; shows *Sui-Kyo*, *Yin-Yo-Kyo* (deficiency of *Sui*, *Kyo* of both *Yin and Yang*.
	• *Trembling tongue:* When moving the tongue, it trembles; it vibrates; showing *Netsu-Sho* and *Ki-Kyo* (*Ki* deficiency).

Table 5. The correlations between the colours and volumes in tongue.

Colour Tone	
	• *White tongue coating*: Pale white colour is considered normal but shows the changes in body condition, depending on the wetness
	• *Yellow tongue coating:* Shows stomach/intestine function deficiency; fever; lack of water due to fever
	• *Greyish black tongue coating*: Yellow tongue coating symptom progressed and disease worsened; related to infectious disease, high fever, dehydration
Volume	
	• *Thin tongue coating*: Normal
	• *No tongue coating*: Abnormal; chronical disease; protracted illness
	• *Thick tongue coating*: Abnormal; exacerbation of disease, growth of bacteria due to defective metabolism of tongue coating

Kampo promotes the metabolism involved in the physical growth, development and physiological activity. Kampo moderate *Ketsu* and *Sui*, so that the blood runs in blood vessels and prevents blood from leaking outside. Kampo produces *Ki* that works to produce *Ketsu* and *Sui*, thus converting fluids into sweat and urine.

Changes in the internal organs (liver, heart, lienogastric, lung and kidney) are reflected on the tongue (Figure 10). It tells the *Sho* of disease, namely, *Kyo, Jitsu, Hyo* and *Ri*. Tongue diagnosis is very important among the empirical diagnostic techniques. Systematic diagnosis theory has been formed based on the empirical evidences over several thousands of years. The rise and fall of *Ki, Ketsu* and *Sui* reflect the advance or retreat of illness. Severity of the disease can be seen on the tongue. Therefore, pathological changes of a disease are shown in the change of the tongue at its early stage. It is called *Mibyo* or pre-symptomatic in Kampo medicine. It is important diagnostic criteria and is recognized as a clue to find the cause of the illness at an early stage in the primary care.

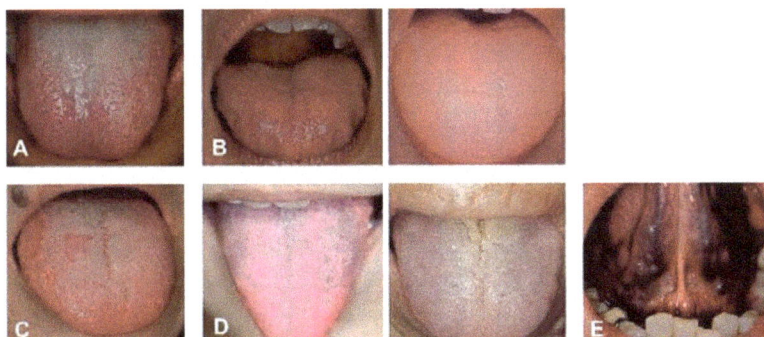

Figure 10. Tongue diagnosis of patients. (**A**) *Clinical observation of Healthy tongue*. Properly moistened: tongue coating white colour, thinly spread across the tongue. Light pink colour, Shape: fitting within the mouth. Back of tongue: sublingual vein is not over swelling. (**B**) *Abnormal tongue (Sui)*. Tongue peripheral impression, swelling tongue (oedema). Left: *Sui-Tai* or water stagnationis oedema, tongue peripheral impression. Pressure impression by the teeth on the edge of the tongue where water is sustained. Right: *Sui-Kyo* (insufficient water): oedema, water is not flowing well; big and swollen. (**C**) *Abnormal Ki (vital energy)*. Map-like tongue, insufficient Ki, slow circulation of *Ki*. Warming: Workings of warm-up and circulation; central of *Ki*. Defence: Workings to promote natural healing; protects skin and membrane and defends the body from the cause of disease. (**D**) *Abnormal tongue (Ketsu-Kyo and Kyo-Netsu)*. *Ketsu* (blood circulation) indicate the body of the tongue and sublingual vein that are in reddish purple, colour change of the tongue coating (*Ketsu-Kyo, Kyo-Netsu*). Left: *Ketsu-Kyo*: Tongue is thin and lean; Nutrition, water and blood circulation were insufficient. Right: *Kyo-Netsu*: Sticky blood; stagnated; Nutrition. water and blood body fluids were insufficient. Body is dry, since

the heat remains to circulate internally. (**E**) *Abnormal tongue (Okesu)*. Blood heat condition in tongue. Ischemia (tongue: cyanosis) and over-swelling of sublingual veins. Systemically impaired flow of blood. These photos were taken, after obtaining the informed consent from the patients, under the condition that the patients are not identified. (Watanabe S, unpublished data)

4. Therapeutic Effect of *Juzentaihoto*

Periodontitis is the most common chronic inflammatory disease in humans and is characterized by alveolar bone loss and connective tissue destruction. Periodontitis is exacerbated by risk factors including age, gender, smoking, systematic diseases and psychological stress [10]. The stress response mediates the interaction between unfavourable psychological conditions and inflammatory periodontal disease. There is a higher prevalence of chronic destructive periodontal disease in individuals with psychological stress, which may be associated with acute necrotizing periodontal disease [11]. Psychological stress downregulates the cellular immune response, which may link the stress to periodontal disease [12]. Herbal medicines, such as *Juzentaihoto* (JTT), have good therapeutic effects for stress-related systematic diseases and minimal side effects. JTT consists of 10 herbs: *Ginseng radix*, *Astragali radix*, *Angelicae radix*, *Rehmanniae radix*, *Atractylodis lanceae rhizoma*, *Cinnamomi cortex*, *Poria*, *Paeoniae radix*, *Ligustici rhizome* and *Glycyrrhizae radix*. JTT is traditionally used for anaemia, rheumatoid arthritis, chronic fatigue syndrome and inflammatory bowel disease. It is widely used to prevent cancer metastasis and infection in immunocompromised patients [13]. We had examined the efficacy of JTT to prevent periodontitis.

4.1. Biological Activity (in Vitro)

4.1.1. Bactericidal Effect of JTT on *P. gingivalis*

We evaluated the bactericidal effect of JTT on *P. gingivalis*. Treatment of *P. gingivalis* with 0.1 to 10 mg/mL JTT reduced the number of viable cells in a dose-dependent manner. In particular, bacterial reduction by 10 mg/mL JTT was greater than that of 0 (control), 0.1 and 1 mg/mL JTX treatment at 60 minutes [14] (Figure 11), suggesting that JTT may suppress virulence factors from periodontal bacteria and prevent the progression of periodontitis. Some herbs from JTT and their ingredients have antimicrobial effects [15]. Compounds from *Glycyrrhizae radix* inhibit the growth of *P. gingivalis* [16]. *Glycyrrhizae radix* may have an important role in the bactericidal effect of JTT on *P. gingivalis*.

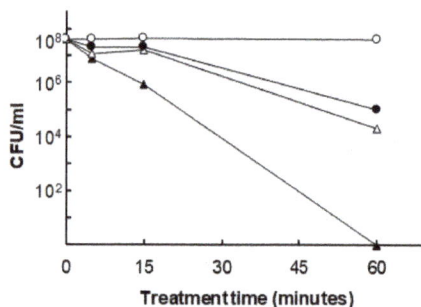

Figure 11. Antibacterial effect of JTT on *P. gingivalis*. Bacterial cells were treated with 10 mg/mL (▲), 1 mg/mL (△) or 0.1 mg/mL of JTT (●) or 0 mg/mL of JTT (○) for the indicated period. At the end of the incubation period, a 10-fold serial dilution was performed in phosphate-buffered saline (PBS; pH 7.4) and spread onto a BHI blood agar plate broth supplemented with hemin (5 µg/mL), vitamin K_1 (0.2 µg/mL) and yeast extract (5 mg/mL). The number of CFU (colony forming unit) was determined after 7 days of incubation under anaerobic conditions (CO_2: 10%, H_2: 10%, N_2: 80%) at 37°C. Cited from [14] with permission.

4.1.2. Anti-osteoclastogenesis Effect of JTT

We investigated whether JTT inhibits the osteoclast differentiation using a mouse co-culture system, according to the guideline of the intramural Committee of Ethics on Animal Experiments. Bone marrow cells (1.5×10^5 cells/well) obtained from the tibiae of 5–8-week-old BALB/c mice and pre-adipose cell line MC3T3-G2/PA6 cells (1.5×10^4 cells/well) were co-cultured for 7 days in the presence of 10 nM 1a,25-$(OH)_2D_3$ (calcitriol) and 10 nM dexamethasone in α modification of Minimum Essential Medium (α-MEM) supplemented with 20% FBS (foetal bovine serum) in 48-well plates under a 5% CO_2 atmosphere. Osteoclast was defined as tartrate-resistant acid phosphatase (TRAP)-positive multinucleated cells containing three or more nuclei. Treatment with JTT at concentrations of 10, 1 and 0.1 μg/mL significantly inhibited osteoclast formation (Figure 12A) [14]. A low concentration (0.1 μg/mL) of JTX significantly inhibited the osteoclast formation compared to control (Figure 12B). *Angelicae gigantis radix*, one of the components in JTT, significantly decreased osteoclast formation [17]. Therefore, JTT can be a therapeutic drug that prevents periodontitis.

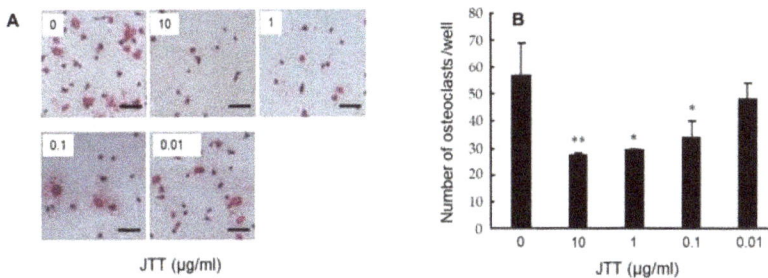

Figure 12. JTT inhibits osteoclast differentiation of BALB/c mouse bone marrow cells co-cultured with MC3T3-G2/PA6 cells. After incubation for 7 days, co-cultured cells were stained for TRAP (**A**) and determination of TRAP-positive multinucleated cells containing three or more nuclei (**B**). Results are expressed as the mean ±SD of triplicate cultures. **$p < 0.01$, *$p < 0.05$. Cited from [14] with permission.

4.2. Clinical of JTT

Kampo medicine and adjustment of denture were effective for a patient (80 years old, female, cervical cancer operated 25 years ago with good prognosis), with symptom of spinal canal stenosis, cervical vertebra stenosis, dizziness, unsteadiness and oppression on the chest. She was diagnosed as inadaptation of the denture, oral malaise (tongue), dysfunction of masticatory and xerostomia. Her *oketsu* (blood stagnation) was improved by taking JTT mornings and evenings – 2 doses before meals. Swelling and oedema of the tongue was improved by taking *Goreisan* (GRS) before going to bed. Medical consultation resulted in the improvement of mental condition. Two Kampo medicines, GRS (that improves *Sui-Tai* or fluid retention symptom caused by poor metabolism of water) and JTT [that enhances *ki* (vital energy) and *ketsu* (blood circulation function) and improve fatigue, anaemia, low appetite, night sweat, cold hands and feet which accompany the decondition] were administered in this case. In the initial diagnosis, prescription of GRS showed no progress in 2 weeks, then additionally JTT *was* administered. After 1 month later (Figure 13A), the filling pain when chewing with denture stopped jaws gliding and oppression on throat while sleeping. Two months later, she could bite off and eat food. She had no sensation of tongue torsion, stopped waking up at night due to the neck pain. Administration of GRS stopped due to frequent urination. Four months later (Figure 13B), upon the mounting of dentures, she felt neck strain and torsion of denture and tongue. The administration of GRS was restarted. Eight months later (Figure 13C), she became able to chew any food, with no sensation of tongue swells. She did not wake up at night. Twelve months later (Figure 13D), the administration of GRS was stopped but that of JTT was continued (Figure 13).

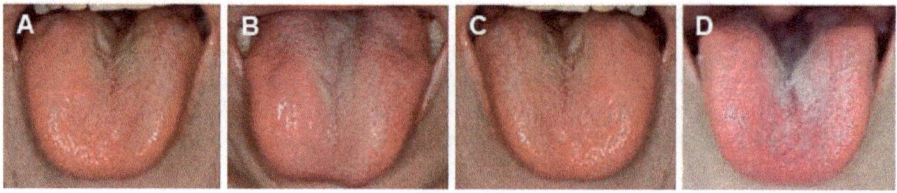

Figure 13. Changes of the tongue surfaces at 1 (**A**), 4 (**B**), 8 (**C**) or 12 (**D**) months after GRS + JTT treatment. (Presented in Kanagawa Dental College Society 53rd General Assembly: A case in which Kampo and denture adjustment was successful for patients complaining of denture). Photos were taken, after obtaining the informed consent from the patient. (Watanabe S, unpublished data)

When making dental prosthesis, it is necessary to pay attention to the intraoral environment. In the case above, we observed the lower jaw denture floated due to tongue oedema and swelling and that the denture instability caused the occlusal pain and dysfunction of masticatory. We therefore prescribed Kampo medicines that would improve these symptoms. In this clinical case, we considered that the improvement of *sui-tai* (fluid stagnation) should be the target of *Hyo-Chi*, a local and symptomatic treatment, to improve the tongue oedema, so GRS was administered. However, we could not get the expected results, so JTT was also administered in the morning and before going to bed and it presented the trend of improvements from the next day. JTT is a Kampo medicine for *hon-chi*, that is, the systemic treatment of the fundamental cause of the disease. It is often observed in the dentistry and intraoral medicine that patient's conditions change until the symptom finally surfaces due to the chronical deficiencies. Especially, the entire body is psychologically and mentally affected when malocclusion exists. Under the situation that malocclusion lasts long, it is known that glucocorticoid appears in blood chronically due to the chronical stress from the malocclusion which would induce the malfunction of negative feedback. The Oriental medicine explains that the symptoms of *Ki* and *Ketsu* occur and they worsen as the time elapses. In our case above, GRS manifested its effect at early timing by the simultaneous administration of JTT. It not only cured the oedema of the tongue but also mentally stabilized the patient.

JTT is known to improve the pathological condition of the blood circulation and mental stability. When the condition of the disease is found difficult to improve, Kampo medicine of *hon-chi* (treatment of fundamental cause), in combination would relieve the symptoms.

5. Therapeutic Effects of *Jixueteng*

5.1. Bactericidal Effect of Jixueteng

Jixueteng is prepared from the dried stems of *Spatholobus suberectus* (*S. suberectus*) Dunn of the family Leguminosae. *Jixueteng* has beneficial pharmacological properties such as increasing circulation, analgesia and the number of red and white blood cells [18]. *Jixueteng* contains various types of flavonoids such as flavone, isoflavones, flavanones, flavanonols and chalcone [19]. Flavonoids are natural products that show antibacterial [20] and antioxidant activities [21]. Production of reactive oxygen species (ROS) is decreased by *Jixueteng* in a dose-dependent manner [22]. Therefore, we focused on the bactericidal effect of *Jixueteng* on oral bacteria. The gram-positive species, *Streptococcus mutans* Ingbritt (*S. mutans*) and the gram-negative species, *Aggregatibacter actinomycetemcomitans* ATCC 29523 (*A. actinomycetemcomitans*), *Fusobacterium nucleatum* ATCC 25586 (*F. nucleatum*), *Porphyromonas gingivalis* ATCC 33277 (*P. gingivalis*) and *Veillonella parvula* GAI-0580 (*V. parvula*), were grown in BHI broth and suspended in PBS to an optical density of 1.0 at 600 nm. Fifty µL of bacterial suspension was exposed for 1, 15 and 60 min in the presence of 0, 0.2, 2.0 or 8% *Jixueteng* extract. The same volume of PBS was used as a control. At the end of the incubation period, a 10-fold serial dilution was inoculated onto BHI sheep blood agar plates and incubated anaerobically at 37°C for 7 days. The bactericidal effect of *Jixueteng* was determined by counting the number of bacterial cells. *Jixueteng* extract reduced the number of viable bacterial cells, such as *S. mutans* (Figure 14A), *P. gingivalis* (Figure 14B), *V. parvula* (Figure 14C) and *F. nucleatum* (Figure 14D) (Figure 14). In particular, the bactericidal effects of *Jixueteng* against *F. nucleatum* (Figure 14D) was higher than those of other oral bacteria. After treatment with 8% *Jixueteng* extract for 60 min, the number of *P. gingivalis* was decreased from 4.61×10^9 to 2.90×10^6 per millilitre (Figure 14B) [23]. Gram-negative periodontal pathogens are late colonizers of dental plaque and promote inflammatory tissue destruction in the oral cavity [24]. Thus, *Jixueteng* extract may act selectively on periodontal bacteria and break down dental plaque accumulation.

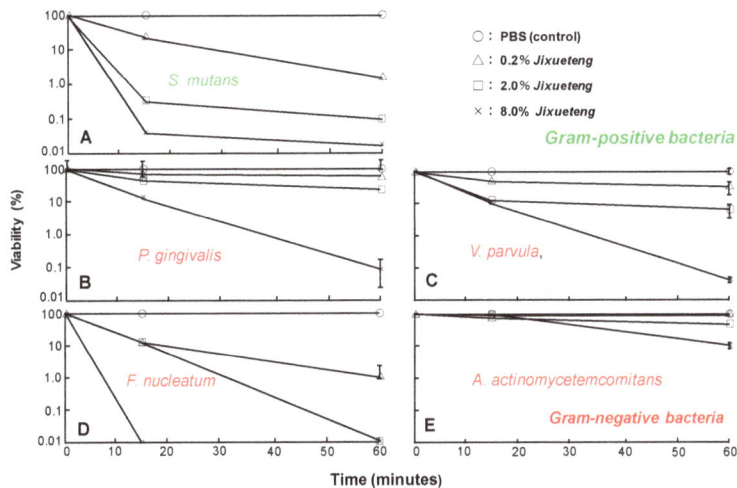

Figure 14. Bactericidal effect of *Jixueteng* against Gram-positive and -negative bacteria. Gram-positive bacteria (*S. mutans*) (**A**) and gram-negative bacteria (**B**: *P. gingivalis*, **C**: *V. parvula*, **D**: *F. nucleatum*, **E**: *A. actinomycetemcomitans*.) were treated by 0.2, 2 and 8% of the *Jixueteng* extract for 1, 15 or 60 min. The suspensions were treated by PBS as a control. Cell viability was expressed as a percentage relative to control. Cited from [23] with permission.

5.2. Inhibitory Effect of Jixueteng on Osteoblast Differentiation

In periodontitis, several cytokines, such as interleukin (IL)-1, prostaglandin (PG) E_2 and RANKL (receptor activator of NF-κB ligand), promote osteoclast differentiation. RANKL, a tumour necrosis factor (TNF)-family member, binds to its receptor RANK, which is on the surface of osteoclasts and preosteoclasts. The interaction between RANK and RANKL signalling is important for osteoclastogenesis [25]. To examine the influence of *Jixueteng* on osteoclastogenesis, we used mouse co-cultured cells in the presence of $1\alpha,25$-$(OH)_2D_3$ and dexamethasone. *Jixueteng* extracts were added to co-cultured cells at a final concentration of 0.1%, 0.01%, 0.001% and 0.0001% and cultivated for 7 days under 5% CO_2 atmosphere. After 7 days, cells were fixed and stained for TRAP. TRAP-positive multinucleated cells containing three of more nuclei were counted as osteoclasts. The treatment of *Jixueteng* extract (at concentrations of 0.1% and 0.01%) significantly inhibited osteoclast formation ($P < 0.01$). Addition of 0.1% extract completely inhibited TRAP-positive cells and multinucleated osteoclasts. In addition, the inhibitory effect of *Jixueteng* on osteoclast survival was determined by mouse co-cultured cells in the presence of RANKL and PGE_2. The number of osteoclasts was decreased with 0.001 to 0.1 mg/mL *Jixueteng* in a dose-dependent manner [26]. These results suggest that *Jixueteng* inhibits osteoclastogenesis and reduces osteoclast activity in periodontitis.

5.3. Inhibitiory Effect of Alveolar Bone Resorption by Jixueteng on Mice Experimental Periodontitis

Flavonoids are effective ingredients for the inhibition of inflammatory bone resorption [27]. We evaluated the inhibitory effect of alveolar bone resorption by *Jixueteng* using an experimental periodontitis model, under the guideline of the intramural Committee of Ethics on Animal Experiments. Fifty-four male C57BL/6N 4-week-old mice were used. Mice were given sulfamethoxazole (1 mg/mL) and trimethoprim (200 mg/mL) in their drinking water for 4 days to reduce original oral flora followed by 3 days of an antibiotic-free period before bacterial infection. The bacteria used was *P. gingivalis* A, which was inoculated in BHI broth under anaerobic conditions. Animals were randomly divided into the following three groups: Group A received only 5% carboxymethylcellulose (CMC) (sham-infected group), group B was infected orally with *P. gingivalis* and group C was administered *Jixueteng* extract in drinking water and was infected orally with *P. gingivalis*. Each mouse in group B and group C was infected orally with *P. gingivalis*, which was suspended in 5% CMC and received 0.1 ml (1.0×10^{10} cells/mL) of bacterial suspension. The bacterial infection was given by oral gavage (three times) at 48 h intervals. The mice were sacrificed 2, 4 and 6 weeks after the final bacterial infection to examine the change in alveolar bone resorption every 2 weeks. The left sides of the horizontal alveolar bone resorption around the maxillary molars were evaluated morphometrically as dry specimens to measure horizontal alveolar bone loss. The distance between the cemento-enamel junction (CEJ) and the alveolar bone crest (ABC) was measured at seven palatal sites per mouse. Measurements were made under a dissecting microscope (40× magnification) fitted with a digital high-definition system, standardized to provide measurements in millimetres. The right sides of the upper jaws were analysed for histology. The samples were fixed, decalcified and embedded in paraffin. The paraffin section was cut serially into 5-mm sections in a mesial–distal direction. The sections were stained for haematoxylin–eosin (H–E) and TRAP. In particular, TRAP-positive multinucleated cells were defined as osteoclasts and examined under an optical microscope (40× magnification). The number of osteoclasts was counted in the area of the periodontal tissue between the mesial root of the first molar and the distal root of the third molars. We found apparent horizontal bone loss in C57BL/6N mice challenged with *P. gingivalis* (group B) but not in the control (group A) or the *Jixueteng*-administered group (group C) (Figure 15A). Figure 15B shows the mean values ± standard error (SEM) of the CEJ to ABC derived from seven measurement sites in weeks 2, 4 and 6 after infection. Induction of alveolar bone loss was more reproducible with an infection by *P. gingivalis* by oral gavage (group B) ($p < 0.01$) than in the sham-infected control (group A) 4 weeks after infection, whereas no difference was observed 2 weeks after infection. In all experimental groups, the maximum resorption of alveolar bone was observed at the end of the experiment and the mean bone levels of the sham-infected control (group A) and *P. gingivalis* infection group (group B) were 0.194 ± 0.001 mm and 0.228 ± 0.010 mm, respectively. Alveolar bone loss was significantly lower in the *Jixueteng* group (group C) ($p < 0.01$) than that of group B in weeks 4 and 6. The mean bone level of group C in week 6 was 0.188 ± 0.003 mm, which was comparable to that of the control group A (Figure 15) [28].

By histopathological examination, osteoclasts were observed along the alveolar septum in mice periodontal tissues (Figure 16). Table 6 shows the number of osteoclasts in the alveolar bone crest. No significant difference in the number of osteoclasts was observed among the experimental groups 2 weeks after infection.

Table 6. Effects of *Jixueteng* on osteoclast formation in periodontal tissues.

Groups	Number of Osteoclasts		
	2W	4W	6W
Control	14.25 ± 1.71	16.00 ± 1.00	10.33 ± 0.58
P. gingivalis	18.50 ± 5.45	29.00 ± 8.25 **	23.33 ±1.53 **
Jixueteng + *P. gingivalis*	15.75 ± 7.41	17.00 ± 2.94	12.33 ± 3.21

** Significantly different ($p < 0.01$) from Group A and C. The number of osteoclasts was examined in the section from right maxillary specimen stained of tartrate-resistant acid phosphatase. The results were expressed as mean ± standard deviation. Group A, control (non- infected with *P. gingivalis*); group B, orally infected with *P. gingivalis*; group C, administered *Jixueteng* and orally infected *with P. gingivalis*. Cited from [28] with permission.

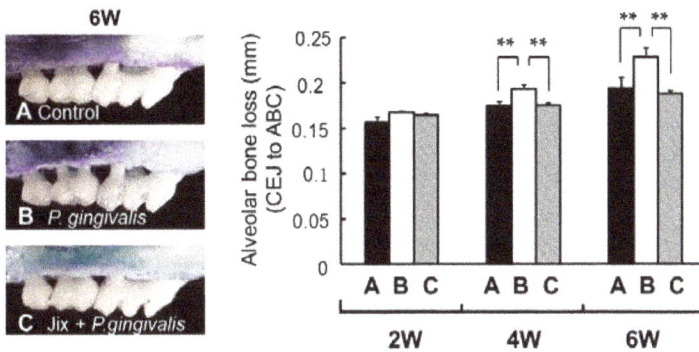

Figure 15. Morphometric bone levels of 6 week after *P. gingivalis* infection (left) and alveolar bone levels at 2, 4 and 6 weeks after *P. gingivalis* infection (right). **A**, non-infected control; **B**, infected with *P. gingivalis*; **C**, Jixueteng administered group along with *P. gingivalis* infection. Bone levels were evaluated by measuring the distance from the cemento-enamel junction (CEJ) to the alveolar bone crest (ABC) at seven palatal sites per mouse. Values indicate the mean bone loss levels ± standard error of the mean (n = 6/group). **: significantly different ($p < 0.01$). Cited from [28] with permission.

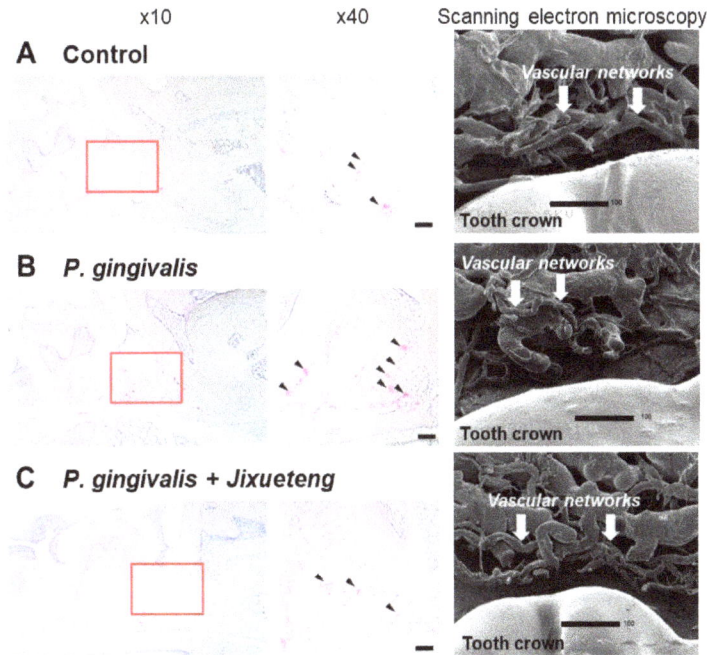

Figure 16. Histopathological examination of mice periodontal tissues. Specimens obtained from the maxillary bone of mice were evaluated with TRAP staining. Osteoclasts (arrows) were observed along the alveolar septum of the maxillary molars. **A**, con-infected control; **B**, infected with *P. gingivalis*; **C**, administered *Jixueteng* and infected with *P. gingivalis*. Original magnification: × 10 and × 40. Bars: 100 μm. Scanning electron microscopy shows that compared to the normal group (**A**), morphological degeneration of vessels in vascular networks and abnormality of the vascular lumen caused by *P. gingivalis* infection were observed (**B**). However, improvement in degeneration of these vascular networks and prolongation of the vascular plexus were observed by administration of *Jixueteng* (**C**). Cited from [28] with permission.

After 4 weeks, the number of osteoclasts in the *P. gingivalis*-infected group B was significantly higher than that of sham-infected group (group A) and the *Jixueteng*-administered group (group C) (*p* < 0.01) [28]. *P. gingivalis* has virulent factors that induce inflammatory responses and alveolar bone resorption [29]. This bacterium also invades and survives in host cells, inducing a network of inflammatory responses [30]. *P. gingivalis* also increases the likelihood of systemic diseases such as diabetes and cardiovascular disease [31]. We previously reported that *Jixueteng* improves gingival vascular networks in a *P. gingivalis*-induced periodontitis [28] (Figure 15). *Jixueteng* may inhibit the adherence and colonization of *P. gingivalis* in mice oral cavities. Therefore, our findings suggest that *Jixueteng* reduces the inflammatory destruction in periodontitis. *Jixueteng* has bactericidal effects against oral bacteria, inhibits the osteoclastogenesis and reduces the alveolar bone resorption induced by *P. gingivalis*. *Jixueteng* reduces the inflammatory tissue destruction in periodontitis and *Jixueteng* may be a useful ingredient to prevent periodontitis.

6. Therapeutic Effects of *Mastic*

6.1. History of Mastic (Kampo Name: Yo-Nyuko olibanum)

Mastic is the resin collected from the naturally growing trees in only Chios Island in southeast Aegean Sea of Greece. It was initially called frankincense. Mastic has a long history, it is written in the Old Testament (Genesis 37:25) and many ancient Greek literatures mentioned the medical effect of mastic. Christopher Columbus, before he stayed in Portugal, visited Chios Island during his voyage to the Orient as recorded in his diary in 1474–1475 and he described about mastic; it is sticky sap extracted from tree and becomes resin when solidified. There has been a habit of chewing this in Greece since more than 5000 years ago and it was known that those people who had this habit rarely had digestive diseases. In China's classical Kampo medicine masterpiece of "Zu-Kei Honzo" (masterpiece of plant diagrams) also described it as *Kun-roku-ko*, kuduruka. The substance called frankincense today is the resin from the trees of *Boswellia* genus of the *Burseraceae* family that grow in north-eastern Africa or Arabian coast and it is different from the mastic from Greece. Traditional frankincense to present is the same kuduruka in the book of Honzo and they grow in the Mediterranean coast areas. Resin from the tree that belongs to the *Anacardiaceae* family is considered *MASTICHE RESINA*. This is called "mastic" or *Yo-Nyuko* in Kampo and is known as *Pistacia lentiscus* locally (Figure 17).

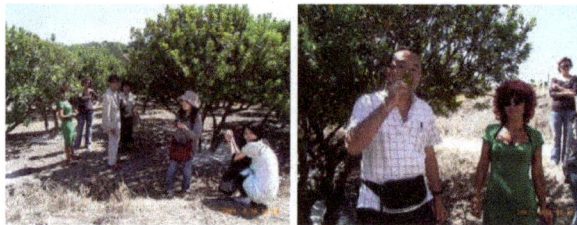

Figure 17. Mastic tree (*Pistacia lentiscus*). (photos taken at Chios island, Greece, 2007)

It is empirically proven that herbs that are used in folk therapies, including the herbal medicines constituting Kampo, have multifunctional medicinal effects. Mastic resin has a unique shape and various efficacy and has been used to promote health from old time. In addition, mastic resin has been used in chewing gums as a material for oral health and hygiene and indicated antiplaque activities. Recently in Japan, mastic has been receiving attention as material for oral cares and many companies are developing and selling mastic-formulated oral gels for toothbrushing paste.

Mastic has been forming a market of high-end products of oral cares. Also, dentists have been paying attentions to its effect and mastic is securing its position in the clinical medicine as the primary care product for oral cavity cares. To cope with the improvements of adult diseases and systemic diseases associated with the oral hygiene in the aging society of Japan and further to improve the oral health in Asia, a group of dentists launched an NPO called "Mastic Clinical Study Group." It has been running the public awareness building programs of the oral hygiene including preventive dentistry. Presently, many dentists are making use of mastic in the clinical studies and are promoting its use in the treatment of patients and to spread the awareness of the primary cares.

6.2. Component of Mastic

Essential oils, obtained by hydrodistillation of aerial parts of *Pistacia lentiscus* var *chia*, were determined for their oil composition using gas chromatography-mass spectrometry (GC/MS). Most abundant component was α-pinene (72.93% of the total oil composition), followed by β-myrcene (13.57%) > β-pinene (2.58%) > limonene (0.89%) > linalool (0.73%) > camphene (0.58%), methylanisol (0.58%) > α-pinene oxide (0.56%) > sabinene (0.30%), β-caryophyllene (0.30%) > verbenone (0.26%) > pinocarveol (0.21%) > myrtenol (0.18%) > pinocarvone (0.10%) [32].

6.3. Biological Activity of Mastic Gum (Resin)

6.3.1. Antimicrobial Activity

Compared with the group, which used the PBS mouthwash, the group that used the mastic-formulated gums showed the significant inhibition of the increase of oral bacteria (Figure 18). Compared with the group that used the gums without mastic formulation, it inhibited the increase of the pathogenic bacteria and the effect was equivalent of benzalkonium chloride.

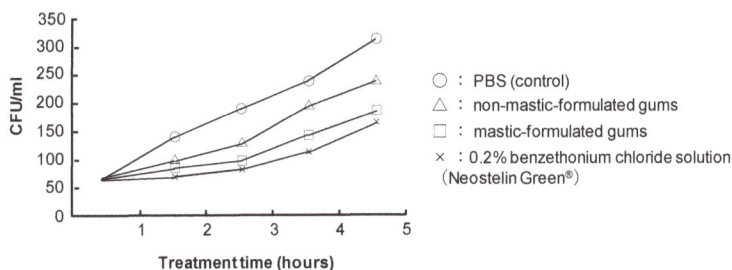

Figure 18. Bactericidal effect of mastic gum against oral bacteria. (Hamada N, unpublished data)

Stick examined the antibacterial effect against gram-negative bacteria. The result of the examination of the minimum inhibitory concentration (MIC) of mastic resin oil against the oral bacterial groups showed it had antibacterial effect (< 0.05%) for adult periodontal bacteria, *P. gingivalis*. Mastic rein oil also showed great selective effect at < 0.05% against *Fusobacterium nucleatum* (Tables 7 and 8). *F. nucleatum* is an important periodontal bacterium that derives the bacterial agglutination on the dental plaque formation. Mastic rein oil can reduce the dental plaque and promote the prevention of periodontitis.

Mastic showed selective antimicrobial activity against *Porphyromonas gingivalis* and *Prevotella melaninogenica*, as compared with that against the growth of *Actinomyces viscosus*, *Streptococcus gordonii*, *Streptococcus mutans*, *Capnocytophaga ochracea*, *Fusobacterium nucleatum*, *Prevotella intermedia*, *Staphylococcus aureus*, *Escherichia coli* and *Candida albicans* [33]. When mastic gum was fractionated with successive extractions with organic solvents with increasing water-solubility into hexane, ethyl acetate, n-butanol extracts and remaining water layer, the ethyl acetate extractable fraction showed eight or nine times higher anti-bacterial activity against *Streptococcus mutans* (IC_{50} = 104 μg/mL), as compared with other fractions (831–936 μg/mL). The most sensitive bacterium was *P. gingivalis* (IC_{50} = 32.7 μg/mL), followed by *S. mutans* (IC_{50} = 104 μg/mL), *S. aureus* (IC_{50} = 609.4 μg/mL), *F. nucleatum* (IC_{50} = 759.6 μg/mL) and *E. coli* (IC_{50} = 907.4 μg/mL) [34]. Ethyl acetate extract of mastic, which has higher antibacterial activity than unfractionated mastic, may be appropriate for the treatment of periodontal diseases.

Table 7. Minimum inhibitory concentration (MIC) of mastic resin oil. (Hamada N, unpublished data).

Oral Bacteria	MIC (%)
Streptococcus mutans	0.4
Streptococcus sanguinis	0.4
Streptococcus mitis	0.4
Lactobacillus species	0.2
Staphylococcus aureus	0.8
Bacillus species	0.2
Actinomyces species	0.2
Porphyromonas gingivalis	< 0.05
Porphyromonas endodontalis	1.6
Prevotella intermedia	1.6
Fusobacterium nucleatum	< 0.05
Aggregatibacter actinomycetemcomitans	0.2

Table 8. Plaque formation on the tooth surface and effect of inhibition of gingivitis of mastic gums. (Hamada N, unpublished data).

Group	Plaque Index		Gingivitis Index	
	Baseline	1 week	Baseline	1 week
Mastic gum (n = 10)	1.06 ± 0.29	2.69 ± 0.29 **	0	0.44 ± 0.15*
Placebo gum (n = 10)	1.19 ± 0.19	3.15 ± 0.24 **	0	0.66 ± 0.23*

These data are represented as mean ± standard deviation. No statistical difference was observed between the groups at baseline. $p < 0.05$* $p < 0.001$** comparison with the baseline using Student' test. The data are determined as the lowest concentrations of mastic resin oil.

The MIC of polymers from mastic gum of *Pistacia lentiscose* (MW: 50-130 kD), isolated by gel permeation chromatography against gram-negative bacteria (*Escherichia coli* type 1, *Salmonella typhimurium*, *Serratia marscens*. *Pseudomonas aeruginosa*, *Alcaligenes faecalis*, *Enterobacter aerogenes*, *Pseudomonas fluorescens*, *Proteus vulgaris*, *Porphyromonas*. *gingivalis*) and gram-positive bacteria (*Bacillus cereus*, *Staphylococcus aureus*, *Streptococcus faecalis*, *Staphylococcus epidermidis*, *Bacillus subtilis*, *Corynebacterium sp*) was 200–250 and 1000 µg/mL, respectively. The MIC of polymer of β-myrcene (MW 50–500 kD), synthesized by incubation with cyclohexane and *sec*-butyl lithium, against gram-negative and -positive bacteria was 100 and 1000 µg/mL, respectively [35]. Chewing mastic gum decreased the total viable bacteria, *S. mutans* and *lactobacilli* in saliva in orthodontically treated patients with fixed appliances, suggesting the usefulness of chewing mastic gum in preventing caries lesions [36].

6.3.2. Antiviral Activity

Anti-HIV activity was determined by the selectivity index (SI), based on the ratio of 50% cytotoxic concentration (CC_{50}) against mock-infected CD4-positive human T-cell line MT-4 cells to 50% protective concentration (EC_{50}) against HIV-infected MT-4 cells. All mastic extracts did not prevent HIV-induced cytopathic effects on MT-4 cells (SI <1), whereas three anti-HIV agents (azidothymidine, dideoxycytidine, curdlan sulphate) showed excellent anti-HIV activity (SI = 5624, 3868, 7142). All mastic extracts partially but significantly reduced the HSV-induced cytopathic effects on Vero cells, recovering the cell viability up to 43.2 ± 5.3% of mock-infected cells [34].

6.3.3. Anti-tumour Activity

Mastic showed very low antitumor activity against four human oral squamous cell carcinoma cell lines (Ca9-22, HSC-2, HSC-3, HSC-4) (CC_{50} = 13.5–24.4 µg/mL) as compared with three human normal oral cells (gingival fibroblast HGF, periodontal ligament fibroblast HPLF, pulp cells HPC) (CC_{50} = 28.1–84.8 μg/mL), with the tumour-specificity value (TS, determined by the ratio of CC_{50} against normal cells to CC_{50} against tumour cells) of only 1.4 to 2.4. Among 5 extracts, ethyl acetate extract showed the highest TS values (TS = 2.6), although its values were two-order lower than that of doxorubicin (TS = 244.7) [34]. However, mastic showed approximately 5-fold higher cytotoxicity against human leukemic cell lines: promyelocytic HL-60 (19 μg/mL), myeloblastic ML-1 (25 μg/mL), myeloblastic KG-1 (27 μg/mL), erythroleukemia K-562 (30 μg/mL), as compared with normal cells (HGF, HPLF, HPC) (93–155 μg/mL). Mastic induced apoptotic cell death (internucleosomal DNA fragmentation, caspase-3 activation, decline in the intracellular concentration of putrescine) in HL-60 promyelocytic leukaemia, while it inhibited the spontaneous apoptosis of oral polymorphonuclear leukocytes. Mastic showed hydroxyl radical scavenging activity, suggesting the beneficial effects of mastic on oral health [33]. Mastic gum (200 mg/kg) inhibited the growth of colorectal tumour xenografts by approximately 35%, when the optimal experimental conditions were chosen [37].

Recently, apoptosis induction by mastic in COLO205 human colonic adenocarcinoma [38], MCF-7 human breast cancer cells [39], LT97 human colon adenoma cells [40], FTC-133 (human follicular thyroid carcinoma) [41], H-SY5Y, SK-N-BE(2)C human neuroblastoma [42] and YD-10B human oral squamous carcinoma [43] has been reported, however, most of these studies have not mentioned the tumour-specificity of mastic.

6.3.4. Anti-inflammatory Activity

Essential oil of mastic showed a strong iron chelating activity (IC_{50} = 20 μg/mL) and actively scavenged hydroxyl radical (IC_{50} = 3 μg/mL) and protected *tert*-butyl hydroperoxide-treated lymphocyte [44]. Mastic inhibited the production of nitric oxide (NO) and prostaglandin (PG)E$_2$, as well as expression of inducible NO synthase (iNOS) and cyclooxygenase (COX)-2 protein and mRNA, induced by lipopolysaccharide (LPS)-activated mouse macrophage-like RAW264.7 cells. Mastic scavenged hydroxyl radical more potently than NO and superoxide radicals. The narrow range of effective concentration of mastic due to its cytotoxicity may limit its potential application as an anti-inflammatory agent [45].

6.3.5. Inhibition of CYPs

Five days oral treatment with *Pistacia lentiscus* oil 100 μL per mice did not show any undesirable effect on the function of kidney and liver but significantly inhibited the enzyme activity and expression of CYP1A1, CYP1A2, CYP2E1 and CYP3A4, especially in the liver tissue [46]. The result suggests the possibility that when mastic is used in combination with other pharmacological agents, the biological action of the latter may be more enhanced.

Among five masic fractions, *n*-hexane extract exhibited the highest CYP3A4-inhibitory activity (IC_{50} = 3.1 μg/mL), followed by methanol extract (macerated) (IC_{50} = 4.1 μg/mL), *n*-butanol extract (IC_{50} = 12.1 μg/mL), unfractionated sample (IC_{50} = 14.3 μg/mL), ethyl acetate extract (IC_{50}=14.8 μg/ml) (C) and, finally, methanol extract (refluxed) (IC_{50} = 24.4 μg/ml). Washing out these CYP3A4 inhibitory substance with *n*-hexane may reduce these pharmacological action or side-effects of combined drugs [34].

6.3.6. Oral Application of Mastic Gel

Salivary bacteria create healthy microbiomes when the intraoral condition becomes good. In order to maintain the good intraoral environment, we developed a gel toothpaste with mastic (*Boswellia carterii*, Kampo name: Yo-Nyuko), a mouthwash with Kampo herbs formulated (Figure 19).

Since the patient had lost the freedom of his hands thus the prevention infection control after treatment would be difficult, it was decided to try treatments using dental laser and Kampo mouth wash and mastic gel to improve the gingival tissue [47–49]. Then, we show a clinical case using the mastic gel in oral cavity. The following is the clinical report of patients treated with mastic in our dental clinic, after obtaining the informed consent from the patient, under the condition that the patient is not identified (Figure 20).

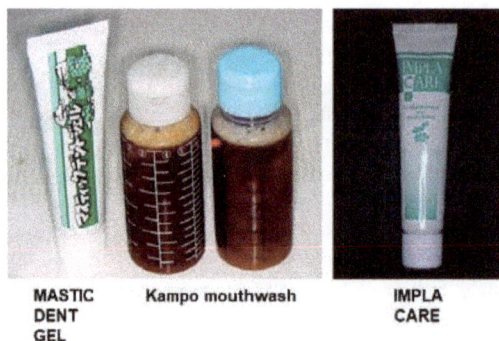

MASTIC DENT GEL   Kampo mouthwash   IMPLA CARE

Figure 19. Toothpaste and mouth-rinse including mastic and IMPLA CARE. (unpublished data)

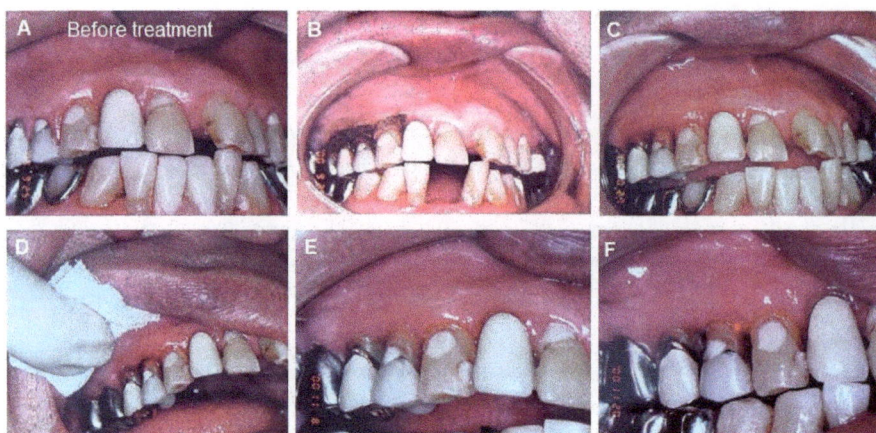

Figure 20. The clinical observation of periodontal tissue around the upper 4th and 5th teeth before and after treatment with laser and mastic gel. (**A**) Before treatment (at the first visited time); (**B**) First time after the laser treatment. Mastic gel was applied after carbonized laser treatment. (**C**) Second times after the laser treatment. After the laser treatment, chlorhexidine was used to prevent bacterial infection and mastic gel was applied at the gingiva. (**D**) Third times after the laser treatment. Mastic gel was applied after light coagulation layer was added by laser. (**E**) Fourth times after the laser treatment. Mastic gel was applied around the inflammatory gingival area. (**F**) Inflammatory gingival area between upper 4th and 5th are improved by using the mastic gel. Photos were taken, after obtaining the informed consent from the patient. (Watanabe S, unpublished data)

The patient was a 66 years old male. Showing bleeding due to the mobility of upper right 4th and 5th teeth. He visited us due to his chief complaint of mastication disorder. He had a stroke 3 years ago and is currently seeing the physician once a month. The condition is stable. As his hands tremble, the mouth cleaning was poor and the breath was bad. Poor oral hygiene, bleeding from the gums (+++), red swelling on the gums and inflammation were observed. As it was necessary to create the environment that treatment can be done, Kampo mouthwash and application of mastic gel toothpaste was conducted for three times a day before and after the treatment. Next, we showed the improvement of the chief complaint by the initial treatment. When the patient came to the clinic, his 4th and 5th teeth in upper right were showing medium level of mobility but it was judged from the observation using X-ray that the bone absorption was not bad.

We used the dentifrice that mastic was formulated and expected the effect of preventing the fixation of pathogen bacteria before and after the treatment. Considering that the oral hygiene significantly influences the management of the entire body, the biological study of the natural products is critically important from now on [50–52].

7. Development of A Dentifrice Gel Containing A Mastic Resin and *Jixueteng*

Periodontitis is the second most common dental disease worldwide after dental decay. Periodontitis is caused by microorganisms that adhere and grow on tooth surfaces and by an aggressive immune response against these microorganisms. The mouth contains a wide variety of oral bacteria, which is an ideal environment for their growth. Nutrition is supplied from food residues and saliva, nitrogen and amino acids mix in gingival crevicular fluids. Periodontitis is triggered by a complex microbial biofilm in the subgingival area that houses over 700 bacterial species and phylotypes [47]. Bacteria from the red complex group, such as *P. gingivalis*, predominate in gingivitis and periodontal disease patients by PCR analysis. Three microorganisms are mainly associated with periodontal disease, *Treponema denticola*, *Tannerella forsythia* and *P. gingivalis* and they usually form a complex called red complex bacteria (RCB). These bacteria are Gram negative, non-spore-forming anaerobic organisms and they may be found as pure or mixed infections [48]. RCB possess several virulence factors including fimbriae, proteinases, exopolysaccharides and hemin-binding proteins [49]. RCB have been detected in both subgingival plaque and in the apical root canal and cause periodontal and endodontic diseases [48,53,54]. *P. gingivalis* is a pathogen that causes periodontal disease, which is a common chronic inflammatory disease [55–57].

Jixueteng is a herbal medicine with pharmacological properties, such as increasing circulation, analgesia and the number of red and white blood cells and is composed of the dried stems of *Spatholobus suberectus* Dunn and *Millettia dielsiana* Harms, both family Leguminosae [58,59]. *Jixueteng* has potent local anti-infection effects on oral indigenous bacteria and inhibits alveolar bone loss [23,39]. These findings suggest that *Jixueteng* is a safe and effective therapeutic agent for periodontal disease because of its antibacterial and immune activities and its ability to improve circulation. However, *Jixueteng* has not been clinically used in the oral field and its effects on reactive oxygen species (ROS) in inflamed regions and the detailed mechanisms underlying these pharmacological actions remain unclear. ROS is involved in various physiological and pathological events. Overproduction of ROS causes oxidative damage to biomolecules, such as lipids, proteins and DNA, which ultimately results in many chronic diseases in humans such as atherosclerosis, cancer, diabetes, rheumatoid arthritis, post-ischemic perfusion injury, myocardial infarction, cardiovascular diseases, chronic inflammation, stroke, septic shock, aging and other degenerative diseases [60,61].

Because, *Jixueteng* extract inhibits osteoclast differentiation and survival in a dose-dependent manner, neutralizes oxygen species and improves blood flow, we developed a dentifrice containing *Jixueteng* in this study. However, *Jixueteng* alone did not have a satisfactory bactericidal effect on periodontopathic bacteria and fungi. Therefore, the antimicrobial effect was supplemented with a mastic, which effectively suppresses pathogenic bacteria. Furthermore, as a result of searching for plant-derived components that suppress periodontopathic bacteria, we found that antibacterial lotuses had comprehensive and effective antibacterial effects on pathogenic bacteria and fungi. We are commercializing a dentifrice containing these ingredients and named it "IMPLA CARE" (Figure 19).

At our hospital, dental hygienists do not invasively remove dental calculus in primary care. Patients were supplied with an IMPLA CARE at night-time and the dental calculus was removed after the gums were healthy and tight. Improving gingiva before treatment with IMPLA CARE reduced the risk of bacteraemia. IMPLA CARE was important for subsequent treatment, postoperative management and may help prevent systemic diseases such as diabetes, cerebral infarction and myocardial infarction. We investigated natural products with antimicrobial activity. First, the minimum inhibitory concentrations (MIC) of *Jixueteng*, *Sasa veitchii* and lotus on oral bacteria were measured. The natural products were dissolved in sterilized phosphate-buffered saline (PBS; pH 7.4) and two-fold serial dilutions were aliquoted in small volumes in microwell plates. Bacterial cells were grown in brain heart infusion (BHI) broth supplemented with hemin (5 µg/mL), vitamin K_1 (0.2 µg/mL) and yeast extract (5 mg/mL) under anaerobic conditions (CO_2: 10%, H_2: 10%, N_2: 80%) at 37°C for 18 h. Bacterial cells were washed and suspended in PBS to an optical density of 1.0 at 600 nm. The bacterial suspension was exposed for 40 h to two-fold serial dilutions of the natural products. The same volume of PBS was used as a control. *Jixueteng* had bactericidal effects on *S. mutans, L. casei, S. gordonii, F. nucleatum* and *S. aureus*. *Sasa veitchii* had a strong bactericidal effect on the fungus *C. albicans* (Table 9). Therefore, the IMPLA CARE contained a mixture of *Jixueteng, Sasa veitchii*, grapefruit and lotus in the mastic resin.

Table 9. Minimum inhibitory concentration (MIC) of five natural products. (Hamada N, unpublished data).

Tested bacteria	*Jixueteng*	Sasa Veitchii	Grapefruit	Propolis	Lotus
Streptococcus mutans	4	> 8192	512	256	8192
Streptococcus gordonii	8	4	2048	8192	> 8192
Lactobacillus casei	4	> 8192	512	256	8192
Staphylococcus aureus	32	> 8192	4096	> 8192	> 8192
Actinomyces viscosus	32	4	4096	256	8192
Porphyromonas gingivalis	> 8192	512	4096	> 8192	> 8192
Prevotella nigresecens	> 8192	128	> 8192	> 8192	> 8192
Fusobacterium nucleatum	16	8	4096	2048	> 8192
Escherichia coli	> 8192	> 8192	1024	16	8192
Candida albicans	64	8	8192	2048	> 8192

Six patients with periodontal disease, peri-implant inflammation or both were examined. Results were measured after using IMPLA CARE and 1–3 times daily tooth brushing and 1–3 months of light massage of the affected part with fingers (Tables 9 and 10). Periodontal disease improved in all patients (Table 11, Figure 21).

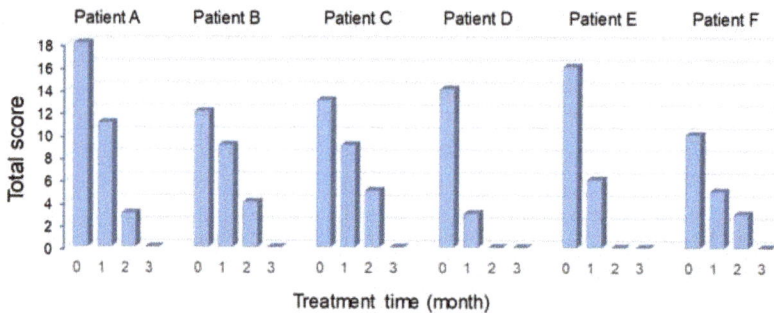

Figure 21. Effects of the IMPLA CARE. (Watanabe S, unpublished data)

Table 10. Scores showing the progress of periodontal disease.

Score	Swollen Pus	Redness	Bleeding	Pus Discharge	Gingival Colour	Mobility	Patient's Opinion
			Examination Criteria				
5	Papilla and adhering to gingiva	Extending to the papilla and gingival gums	Naturally bleeding	Naturally draining	Dark red purple	Upper and lower lip and tongue immobile	No change
3	Papilla and extending to the gingival margin	Papilla and tooth inflammation	Bleeding by acupressure	Acupressure-induced draining	Dark red	Strongly immobile	Improved a little
1	Part of the papilla	Part of the papilla	Slight bleeding with acupressure	Slight draining with acupressure	Brilliant	Slightly immobile	Tightened
0	None at all	No redness	None at all	No discharge at all	Light pink	Within a physiological range	Improved a lot

Table 11. Improvement of periodontal disease after administration of the IMPLA CARE. (Watanabe S, unpublished data).

Examination Items	Patient A				Patient B				Patient C				Patient D				Patient E				Patient F			
								Scores at 0, 1, 2 or 3 Months Later																
	0	1	2	3	0	1	2	3	0	1	2	3	0	1	2	3	0	1	2	3	0	1	2	3
Swollen pus	1	0	0	0	1	0	0	0	3	2	1	0	3	0	0	0	5	3	0	0	1	1	0	0
Redness	5	3	1	0	3	3	1	0	3	2	1	0	3	0	0	0	3	1	0	0	3	1	1	0
Bleeding	5	3	1	0	3	2	1	0	2	1	1	0	2	0	0	0	3	0	0	0	1	0	0	0
Pus discharge	1	0	0	0	1	0	0	0	3	2	1	0	3	0	0	0	1	0	0	0	1	0	0	0
Gingival colour	3	1	0	0	3	2	1	0	2	1	0	0	2	3	0	0	3	1	0	0	3	1	1	0
Mobility	3	0	1	0	1	0	0	0	0	0	0	0	0	0	0	0	1	0	0	0	1	1	1	0
Patient's opinion	3	1	0	0	1	3	0	0	1	1	0	0	0	0	0	0	1	1	0	0	1	0	0	0
Total score	18	11	3	0	12	9	4	0	13	9	5	0	14	3	0	0	16	6	0	0	10	5	3	0

We evaluated patients who were not examined by dentists and found a self-reported improvement (Figure 22). Patient satisfaction also increased, which suggests that IMPLA CARE can be used as a primary care tool after treatment.

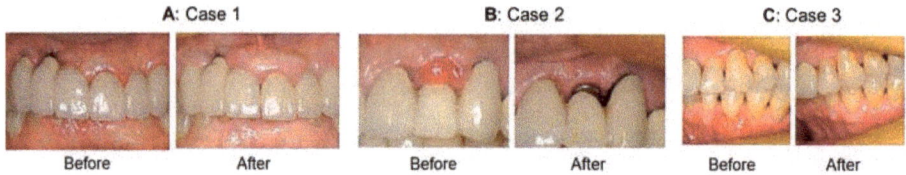

Figure 22. Case 1: A patient who was developing diabetes and hypertension (**A**), Case 2: A patient with peri-implantitis (**B**), Case3: A patient with an ulcer from sleep deprivation and work stress (**C**). (Suzuki M, unpublished data)

Case 1: A patient who was developing diabetes and hypertension. The patient had an implant in the anterior teeth of the maxilla and had teeth cleaned regularly at a dental clinic but gingivitis persisted. The doctor instructed the patient to use the IMPLA CARE before going to bed every night. Gingivitis improved gradually (Figure 22A).

Case 2: A patient with peri-implantitis. After insertion of an implant at 65 years old, a secondary operation was performed but peri-implantitis developed after the second operation. The doctor instructed the patient to use the IMPLA CARE himself before going to bed every night. Conditions gradually improved and a superstructure was formed after one month (Figure 22B).

Case3: A patient with an ulcer from sleep deprivation and work stress. A patient developed an ulcer from work stress and sleep deprivation. An IMPLA CARE was used daily in the morning and evening and improvements were observed with a week, which suggests that the IMPLA CARE containing traditional Chinese medicines did not cause gingival recession (Figure 22C).

8. Conclusions and Future Studies

Kampo is a historic traditional medicine that has been adjusted to Japanese culture. The concept of Kampo emphasizes the relationship between the human body and its social and natural environments [2]. Our experiments concluded that Kampo (JTX and *Jixueteng*) reduce a great effect on oral bacteria and inhibited the bacteria-induced alveolar bone loss. Kampo also suppressed the osteoclast differentiation. Furthermore, Kampo improved the inflammatory response in the periodontal tissues of patients. These findings suggest that Kampo is an effective agent for the prevention of dental caries and periodontitis. The administration of Kampo may ameliorate to infected oral tissue environment.

Oral health is related to life-style such as diet in many ways. The development of dental caries requires high sugar intakes [62]. On the other hand, the high consumptions of smoking and alcohol and the loss of vitamin D affects metabolic functions of periodontal tissue and induce periodontitis. Previous review has been reported that psychological stress reduces human immune system and promotes chronic inflammation in periodontal tissue [63]. Our result demonstrated that JTX affected the correlation between restraint stress and bacteria-induced periodontal destruction [6,14]. Recently, psychological stress is a risk factor of toothache, especially non-odontogenic pain [64]. Odontogenic pain is generally derived from pulpal or periodontal tissue. However, non-odontogenic pain is not often originated from the orofacial regions. The characteristics of non-odontogenic pain indicate various types of symptoms; very mild, intermittent and severe, sharp pain and continuous. The general dentists are difficult to be specified the pain regions, that confuse the exact pain control in any case. In the clinical suggestion of effective pain control, the use of Kampo is expected to reduce the non-odontogenic pain [65]. In the future, the mixed concept of Western medicine and Kampo medicine will contribute in the treatment and prevention of several oral diseases.

Supplementation of alkaline extract of *Sasa sp.* leaves (SE), which can alleviate the deoxorubicin-induced keratinocyte cytotoxicity [66] and paclitaxel-induced neurotoxicity [67] by promoting hermetic cell growth. and have anti-HIV activity [68], may enhance the potential of mastic gel tooth paste (Figure 23).

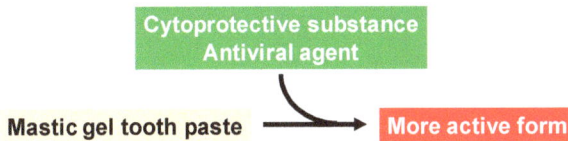

Figure 23. Manufacturing of advanced mastic gel tooth paste.

Author Contributions: S.W., N.H. and H.S. writing the paper; T.T., T.S., M.S. and A.M. collecting the data.

Funding: This work was partially supported by KAKENHI from the Japan Society for the Promotion of Science (JSPS): Sakagami H, 16K11519.

Acknowledgments: The authors acknowledge Tsumura Co. Ltd for the supply of Kampo and Katsushi Tamaki and Atsushi Shimada of the Division of Prosthodontic dentistry function of TMJ and Occlusion, Kanagawa Dental University and Atsushi Ishige and Jing Yu of Herbal medicine biology laboratory, Chinese herbal medicine department, Yokohama College of Pharmacy for the support for the research.

Conflicts of Interest: The authors declare no conflict of interest.

Abbreviations

ABC	alveolar bone crest
CC_{50}	50% cytotoxic concentrations
CEJ	cemento-enamel junction
CFU	colony forming unit
CMC	carboxymethylcellulose
COX	cyclooxygenase
CYP	cytochrome P450
EC_{50}	50% effective concentration
FBS	foetal bovine serum
GC/M	gas chromatography-mass spectrometry
GRS	goreisan
HGF	human gingival fibroblast
HIV	human immunodeficiency virus
HPC	human pulp cell
HPLF	human periodontal ligament fibroblast
HSV	herpes simplex virus
IC_{50}	50% inhibitory concentration
kD	kilo dalton
LPS	lipopolysaccharide
MIC	minimum inhibitory concentration
NO	nitric oxide
PGE_2	prostaglandin E_2
RANKL	receptor activator of NF-κB ligand
RCB	red complex bacteria
SI	selectivity index, determined by the ratio of CC_{50}/EC_{50}
TNF	tumour necrosis factor
TRAP	tartrate-resistant acid phosphatase
TS	tumour specificity, determined by ratio of CC_{50} for normal cells to CC_{50} for tumour cells

Appendix A

Table A1. Kampo terminology.

Byo-ja	Pathogen, disease inducing factor
Ei-ki	Ying energy, *Ki* which operates the blood flows in the blood vessels. Without *ki*, blood does not circulate
Honchi	Systemic meridian treatment for systemic route cause of the disease
Hyo	Superficies, Surface of the body
Hyochi	Local and symptomatic treatment for symptoms derived by the rout cause
Hyo-sho	Pathological condition which appears on the surface of the boy
In	*Yin*, the state opposite of *Yang*, including *ri, kan, kyo, shuren* (convergence) and *yukei* (tangible)
In-Yo	*Yin-Yang*, Bipolar nature of all phenomena or viewing the phenomena from bipolar aspect
Ja	Stress/pathogenic factor, disease-inducing factor that is harmful to the body; endogenous factor, exogenous factor, neither endogenous or exogenous factor
Jitsu	Excess of required substance of body being a disease inducing factor or its pathological condition
Jitsu-kan	Sthenic chill; *Kan-ja* inhibits *yang-ki* (heat energy) in body and deteriorates body functions
Jitsu-netsu	Sthenic heat/excess heat, affected by the exogenous cause of heat; or heat from dental stress and intemperance
Jitsu-sho	Robust/excess constitution, condition or characteristics of over-reaction caused by *byo-ja*
Kan	Chill, symptom showing coldness
Kan-netsu	Chills and fever, pathological condition of chill and heat
Kan-sho	*Kan-sho*, pathological condition showing chilly feeling
Kekkyo	*Ketsu-kyo*, pathological condition of *ketsu* insufficiency
Ketsu-netsu	Blood-heat, *ketsu* (blood) affected by heat-ja and shows *kyo-netsu*
Ki	Vital energy that operates body functions
Ki-gyaku	Pathological condition of *ki* regression
Ki-kyo	*Ki* deficiency, state of insufficient or deficient *ki*
Ki-kyo	*Ki* deficiency, state of insufficient or deficient *ki*
Ki-tai	*Ki* stagnation, pathological condition of *ki* stagnation
Ko-kan	Xerostomia, feeling mouth dryness but not wanting to drink water; tends to occur with mental strain
Ko-katsu	Mouth dryness, feeling thirst and wanting to drink water
Kyo	Deficiency/asthenia, insufficiency of functions or physiological substance that physical body requires
Kyo-kan	Asthenia-cold, *kyo-sho* symptom and belongs to Kan; insufficient *yang-ki* (heat) to warm up the body
Kyo-netsu	Asthenic heat-syndrome, where *yin-eki* is insufficient and relatively *yang* becomes overactive feeling feverish
Kyo-sho	asthenia constitution; Pathological condition of insufficiency of fundamental substances that operate body functions
Nai-netsu	Internal heat-syndrome, generated as a relative result of the imbalance of *yin-yang*; *jitsu-netsu, kyo-netsu*
Okets	Blood stagnation, symptom caused by the stagnation of the blood flow
Ri	Interior of the entire body
Sansho	a passage that controls the flow of air, blood and water, called "triple heater "

Table A1. *Cont.*

Shin-eki	Bodily transparent fluid which constitutes the human body
Shitsu	Dampness of morbidly sustained fluid in the body as a disease inducing factor
Sho	Kampo diagnosis, set of holistic pattern of a patient's pathological symptoms that cause disease
Shoko	Kampo medical conditions, symptoms in Western medical terms
Tan	phlegm, sticky fluid locally pooled due to poor water metabolism
Tan-in	Diseases due to pathological accumulation of fluids in the body
Tongue coating	Mossy substance covering the surface of the tongue
yang	Chinese term for *Yo*
Yin	Chinese term for *In*
Yin-eki	Fluid consisting of human body and composed of transparent *shin-eki* and red blood
Yang	Yin-deficiency Symptom of heat due to insufficient Yin-eki
Yo	Yang, the state opposite of *Yin*, including *hyo, netsu, jitsu, hassan* (divergence) and *mukei* (intangible)
Yo-kyo	Yang-deficiency, pathological condition that chill of *ki-kyo* is worsened
Yo-sho	Yang-sho, condition that has characteristics of excitement, activity and warm-heat
Shokan-ron	A treatise on Shang han, a form of an acute infectious disease

References

1. Motoo, Y.; Arai, I.; Tsutani, K. Use of Kampo diagnosis in randomized controlled trials of Kampo products in Japan: A systematic review. *PLoS ONE* **2014**, *9*, e104422. [CrossRef] [PubMed]
2. Yu, F.; Takahashi, T.; Moriya, J.; Kawaura, K.; Yamakawa, J.; Kusaka, K.; Itoh, T.; Morimoto, S.; Yamaguchi, N.; Kanda, T. Traditional Chinese medicine and Kampo: A review from the distant past for the future. *J. Int. Med. Res.* **2006**, *34*, 231–239. [CrossRef] [PubMed]
3. Yakubo, S.; Ito, M.; Ueda, Y.; Okamoto, H.; Kimura, Y.; Amano, Y.; Togo, T.; Adachi, H.; Mitsuma, T.; Watanabe, K. Pattern classification in kampo medicine. *Evid. Based Complement. Alternat. Med.* **2014**, *2014*, 535146. [CrossRef] [PubMed]
4. Katayama, K.; Yoshino, T.; Munakata, K.; Yamaguchi, R.; Imoto, S.; Miyano, S.; Watanabe, K. Prescription of kampo drugs in the Japanese health care insurance program. *Evid. Based Complement. Alternat. Med.* **2013**, *2013*, 576973. [CrossRef] [PubMed]
5. Wang, P.L.; Sunagawa, M.; Yamaguchi, K.; Kameyama, A.; Kaneko, A. EBM of Kampo medicine in oral surgery. *Oral Ther. Pharmacol.* **2015**, *34*, 23–30. (In Japanese)
6. Wang, P.L.; Kaneko, A. Introduction to Kampo medicine for dental treatment—Oral pharmacotherapy that utilizes the advantages of Western and Kampo medicines. *Jpn. Dent. Sci. Rev.* **2018**, *54*, 197–204. [CrossRef] [PubMed]
7. Dong, J. The Relationship between Traditional Chinese Medicine and Modern Medicine. *Evid. Based Complement. Alternat. Med.* **2013**, *2013*, 153148. [CrossRef] [PubMed]
8. Terasawa, K. Evidence-based Reconstruction of Kampo Medicine: Part II-The Concept of Sho. *Evid. Based Complement. Alternat. Med.* **2004**, *1*, 119–123. [CrossRef] [PubMed]
9. Miyata, T. Prescription of Chinese medicine in clinical dentistry. Introduction of tongue diagnostics for dental physician and dental hygienist. In *The Nippon Dental Review*; Hyoron Publishers, Inc.: Tokyo, Japan, 2001; pp. 145–151. (In Japanese)
10. Al Jehani, Y.A. Risk factors of periodontal disease: Review of the literature. *Int. J. Dent.* **2014**, *2014*, 182513.
11. Warren, K.R.; Postolache, T.T.; Groer, M.E.; Pinjari, O.; Kelly, DL.; Reynolds, M.A. Role of chronic stress and depression in periodontal diseases. *Periodontology 2000* **2014**, *64*, 127–138. [CrossRef] [PubMed]

12. Stoeken, J.E.; Paraskevas, S.; van der Weijden, G.A. The long-term effect of a mouthrinse containing essential oils on dental plaque and gingivitis: A systematic review. *J. Periodontol.* **2007**, *78*, 1218–1228. [CrossRef] [PubMed]

13. Watanabe, S.; Imanishi, J.; Satoh, M.; Ozasa, K. Unique place of Kampo (Japanese traditional medicine) in complementary and alternative medicine: A survey of doctors belonging to the regional medical association in Japan. *Tohoku J. Exp. Med.* **2001**, *194*, 55–63. [CrossRef] [PubMed]

14. Takeda, O.; Toyama, T.; Watanabe, K.; Sato, T.; Sasaguri, K.; Akimoto, S.; Sato, S.; Kawata, T.; Hamada, N. Ameliorating effects of *Juzentaihoto* on restraint stress and *P. gingivalis*-induced alveolar bone loss. *Arch. Oral Biol.* **2014**, *59*, 1130–1138. [CrossRef] [PubMed]

15. Tan, B.K.; Vanitha, J. Immunomodulatory and antimicrobial effects of some traditional Chinese medicinal herbs: A review. *Curr. Med. Chem.* **2004**, *11*, 1423–1430. [CrossRef] [PubMed]

16. Gafner, S.; Bergeron, C.; Villinski, J.R.; Godejohann, M.; Kessler, P.; Cardellina, J.H.; Ferreira, D.; Feghali, K.; Grenier, D. Isoflavonoids and coumarins from Glycyrrhiza uralensis: Antibacterial activity against oral pathogens and conversion of isoflavans into isoflavan-quinones during purification. *J. Nat. Prod.* **2011**, *74*, 2514–2519. [CrossRef] [PubMed]

17. Kil, J.S.; Kim, M.G.; Choi, H.M.; Lim, J.P.; Boo, Y.; Kim, E.H.; Kim, J.B.; Kim, H.K.; Leem, K.H. Inhibitory effects of Angelicae Gigantis Radix on osteoclast formation. *Phytother. Res.* **2008**, *22*, 472–476. [CrossRef] [PubMed]

18. Huang, K.C. *The Pharmacology of Chinese Herbs*; CRC Press: Boca Raton, FL, USA, 1993; p. 146.

19. Yoon, J.S.; Sung, S.H.; Park, J.H.; Kim, Y.C. Flavonoids from *Spatholobus suberectus*. *Arch. Pharm. Res.* **2004**, *27*, 589–592. [CrossRef] [PubMed]

20. Farhadi, F.; Khameneh, B.; Iranshahi, M.; Iranshahy, M. Antibacterial activity of flavonoids and their structure-activity relationship: An update review. *Phytother. Res.* **2019**, *33*, 13–40. [CrossRef] [PubMed]

21. Saxena, M.; Saxena, J.; Pradhan, A. Flavonoids and phenolic acids as antioxidants in plants and human health. *Int. J. Pharm. Sci. Rev. Res.* **2012**, *16*, 130–134.

22. Toyama, T.; Wada-Takahashi, S.; Takamichi, M.; Watanabe, K.; Yoshida, A.; Yoshino, F.; Miyamoto, C.; Maehata, Y.; Sugiyama, S.; Takahashi, S.S.; et al. Reactive oxygen species scavenging activity of *Jixueteng* evaluated by electron spin resonance (ESR) and photon emission. *Nat. Prod. Commun.* **2014**, *9*, 1755–1759. [PubMed]

23. Toyama, T.; Sawada, T.; Takahashi, Y.; Todoki, K.; Lee, M.C.; Hamada, N. Bactericidal activities of the *Jixueteng* against cariogenic and periodontal pathogens. *Oral Therap. Pharmacol.* **2011**, *30*, 51–56. (In Japanese)

24. Ximénez-Fyvie, L.A.; Haffajee, A.D.; Socransky, S.S. Comparison of the microbiota of supra- and subgingival plaque in health and periodontitis. *J. Clin. Periodontol.* **2000**, *27*, 648–657. [CrossRef] [PubMed]

25. Takayanagi, H.; Kim, S.; Taniguchi, T. Signaling crosstalk between RANKL and interferons in osteoclast differentiation. *Arthritis Res.* **2002**, *4* (Suppl. 3), S227–S232. [CrossRef] [PubMed]

26. Toyama, T.; Todoki, K.; Takahashi, Y.; Watanabe, K.; Takahashi, S.S.; Sugiyama, S.; Lee, M.C.; Hamada, N. Inhibitory effects of *Jixueteng* on *P. gingivalis*-induced bone loss and osteoclast differentiation. *Arch. Oral Biol.* **2012**, *57*, 1529–1536. [CrossRef] [PubMed]

27. Weaver, C.M.; Alekel, D.L.; Ward, W.E.; Ronis, M.J. Flavonoid intake and bone health. *J. Nutr. Gerontol. Geriatr.* **2012**, *31*, 239–253. [CrossRef] [PubMed]

28. Suzuki, M.; Toyama, T.; Watanabe, K.; Sasaki, H.; Sugiyama, S.; Yoshino, F.; Yoshida, A.; Takahashi, S.S.; Wada-Takahashi, S.; Matsuo, M.; et al. Ameliorating effects of *Jixueteng* in a mouse model of *Porphyromonas gingivalis*-induced periodontitis: Analysis based on gingival microcirculatory system. *Nat. Prod. Commun.* **2018**, in press.

29. Bostanci, N.; Belibasakis, G.N. *Porphyromonas gingivalis*: An invasive and evasive opportunistic oral pathogen. *FEMS Microbiol. Lett.* **2012**, *333*, 1–9. [CrossRef] [PubMed]

30. Hajishengallis, G. *Porphyromonas gingivalis*-host interactions: Open war or intelligent guerilla tactics? *Microb. Infect.* **2009**, *11*, 637–645. [CrossRef] [PubMed]

31. Kim, J.; Amar, S. Periodontal disease and systemic conditions: A bidirectional relationship. *Odontology* **2006**, *94*, 10–21. [CrossRef] [PubMed]

32. Buriani, A.; Fortinguerra, S.; Sorrenti, V.; Dall'Acqua, S.; Innocenti, G.; Montopoli, M.; Gabbia, D.; Carrara, M. Human adenocarcinoma cell line sensitivity to essential oil phytocomplexes from pistacia species: A multivariate approach. *Molecules* **2017**, *22*, 1336. [CrossRef]

33. Sakagami, H.; Kishino, K.; Kobayashi, M.; Hashimoto, K.; Iida, S.; Shimetani, A.; Nakamura, Y.; Takahashi, K.; Ikarashi, T.; Fukamachi, H.; et al. Selective antibacterial and apoptosis-modulating activities of mastic. *In Vivo* **2009**, *23*, 215–223.

34. Suzuki, R.; Sakagami, H.; Amano, S.; Fukuchi, K.; Sunaga, K.; Kanamoto, T.; Terakubo, S.; Nakashima, H.; Shirataki, Y.; Tomomura, M.; et al. Evaluation of Biological Activity of Mastic Extracts Based on Chemotherapeutic Indices. *In Vivo* **2017**, *31*, 591–598. [PubMed]

35. Sharifi, M.S.; Ebrahimi, D.; Hibbert, D.B.; Hook, J.; Hazell, S.L. Bio-activity of natural polymers from the genus Pistacia: A validated model for their antimicrobial action. *Glob. J. Health Sci.* **2011**, *4*, 149–161. [CrossRef] [PubMed]

36. Aksoy, A.; Duran, N.; Toroglu, S.; Koksal, F. Short-term effect of mastic gum on salivary concentrations of cariogenic bacteria in orthodontic patients. *Angle Orthod.* **2007**, *77*, 124–128. [CrossRef] [PubMed]

37. Dimas, K.; Hatziantoniou, S.; Wyche, J.H.; Pantazis, P. A mastic gum extract induces suppression of growth of human colorectal tumor xenografts in immunodeficient mice. *In Vivo* **2009**, *23*, 63–68. [PubMed]

38. Rahman, H.S. Phytochemical analysis and antioxidant and anticancer activities of mastic gum resin from Pistacia atlantica subspecies kurdica. *Onco Targets Ther.* **2018**, *11*, 4559–4572. [CrossRef] [PubMed]

39. Seifaddinipour, M.; Farghadani, R.; Namvar, F.; Mohamad, J.; Abdul Kadir, H. Cytotoxic effects and anti-angiogenesis potential of pistachio (*Pistacia vera* L.) hulls against MCF-7 human breast cancer cells. *Molecules* **2018**, *23*, 110. [CrossRef] [PubMed]

40. Glei, M.; Ludwig, D.; Lamberty, J.; Fischer, S.; Lorkowski, S.; Schlörmann, W. Chemopreventive potential of raw and roasted pistachios regarding colon carcinogenesis. *Nutrients* **2017**, *9*, 1368. [CrossRef]

41. Catalani, S.; Palma, F.; Battistelli, S.; Benedetti, S. Oxidative stress and apoptosis induction in human thyroid carcinoma cells exposed to the essential oil from *Pistacia lentiscus* aerial parts. *PLoS ONE* **2017**, *12*, e0172138. [CrossRef] [PubMed]

42. Piccolella, S.; Nocera, P.; Carillo, P.; Woodrow, P.; Greco, V.; Manti, L.; Fiorentino, A.; Pacifico, S. An apolar *Pistacia lentiscus* L. leaf extract: GC-MS metabolic profiling and evaluation of cytotoxicity and apoptosis inducing effects on SH-SY5Y and SK-N-BE(2)C cell lines. *Food Chem. Toxicol.* **2016**, *95*, 64–74. [CrossRef] [PubMed]

43. Li, S.; Cha, I.H.; Nam, W. Chios mastic gum extracts as a potent antitumor agent that inhibits growth and induces apoptosis of oral cancer cells. *Asian Pac. J. Cancer Prev.* **2011**, *12*, 1877–1880. [PubMed]

44. Smeriglio, A.; Denaro, M.; Barreca, D.; Calderaro, A.; Bisignano, C.; Ginestra, G.; Bellocco, E.; Trombetta, D. In vitro evaluation of the antioxidant, cytoprotective, and antimicrobial properties of essential oil from *Pistacia vera* L. Variety Bronte Hull. *Int. J. Mol. Sci.* **2017**, *18*, 1212. [CrossRef] [PubMed]

45. Zhou, L.; Satoh, K.; Takahashi, K.; Watanabe, S.; Nakamura, W.; Maki, J.; Hatano, H.; Takekawa, F.; Shimada, C.; Sakagami, H. Re-evaluation of anti-inflammatory activity of mastic using activated macrophages. *In Vivo* **2009**, *23*, 583–589. [PubMed]

46. Attoub, S.; Karam, S.M.; Nemmar, A.; Arafat, K.; John, A.; Al-Dhaheri, W.; Al Sultan, M.A.; Raza, H. Short-term effects of oral administration of *Pistacia lentiscus* oil on tissue-specific toxicity and drug metabolizing enzymes in mice. *Cell Physiol. Biochem.* **2014**, *33*, 1400–1410. [CrossRef] [PubMed]

47. Paster, B.J.; Olsen, I.; Aas, J.A.; Dewhirst, F.E. The breadth of bacterial diversity in the human periodontal pocket and other oral sites. *Periodontology 2000* **2006**, *42*, 80–87. [CrossRef] [PubMed]

48. Socransky, S.S.; Haffajee, A.D.; Cugini, M.A.; Smith, C.; Kent, R.L., Jr. Microbial complexesin subgingival plaque. *J. Clin. Periodontol.* **1998**, *25*, 134–144. [CrossRef] [PubMed]

49. Holt, S.C.; Ebersole, J.L. *Porphyromonas gingivalis*, *Treponema denticola*, and *Tannerella forsythia*: The "red complex", a prototype polybacterial pathogenic consortium in periodontitis. *Periodontology 2000* **2005**, *38*, 72–122. [CrossRef] [PubMed]

50. Watanabe, S. Study and development of the prevention of the periodontal diseases using Kampo mouth wash. In *Shika Iryo*; Dai-ichi Shika Shuppan Publications: Tokyo, Japan, 2003; Volume Spring, pp. 87–97. (In Japanese)

51. Watanabe, S. Study and development of the prevention of the periodontal diseases using Kampo mouth wash. In *Shika Iryo*; Dai-ichi Shika Shuppan Publications: Tokyo, Japan, 2003; Volume Summer, pp. 61–67. (In Japanese)

52. Watanabe, S. Study and development of the prevention of the periodontal diseases using Kampo mouth wash. In *Shika Iryo*; Dai-ichi Shika Shuppan Publications: Tokyo, Japan, 2004; Volume Winter. (In Japanese)

53. Baumgartner, J.C.; Khemaleelakul, S.U.; Xia, T. Identi fication of spirochetes (treponemes) in endodontic infections. *J. Endod.* **2003**, *29*, 794–797. [CrossRef] [PubMed]

54. Foschi, F.; Cavrini, F.; Montebugnoli, L.; Stashenko, P.; Sambri, V.; Prati, C. Detection of bacteria in endodontic samples by polymerase chain reaction assays and association with defined clinical signs in Italian patients. *Oral Microbiol. Immunol.* **2005**, *20*, 289–295. [CrossRef] [PubMed]

55. Zambon, J.J. Periodontal diseases: Microbial factors. *Ann. Periodontol.* **1996**, *1*, 879–925. [CrossRef] [PubMed]

56. Lamont, R.J.; Jenkinson, H.F. Life below the gum line: Pathogenic mechanisms of *Porphyromonas gingivalis*. *Microbiol. Mol. Biol. Rev.* **1998**, *62*, 1244–1263. [PubMed]

57. Landi, L.; Amar, S.; Polins, A.S.; Van, D.T. Host mechanisms in the pathogenesis of periodontal disease. *Curr. Opin. Periodontol.* **1997**, *4*, 3–10. [PubMed]

58. Li, R.W.; David Lin, G.; Myers, S.P.; Leach, D.N. Anti-inflammatory activity of Chinese medicinal vine plants. *J. Ethnopharmacol.* **2003**, *85*, 61–67. [CrossRef]

59. Wang, D.X.; Liu, P.; Chen, Y.H.; Chen, R.Y.; Guo, D.H.; Ren, H.Y.; Chen, M.L. Stimulating effect of catechin, an active component of *Spatholobus suberectus* Dunn, on bioactivity of hematopoietic growth factor. *Chi-Med. J.* **2008**, *121*, 752–755. [CrossRef]

60. Freidovich, I. Fundamental aspects of reactive oxygen species, or what's the matter with oxygen? *Ann. N. Y. Acad. Sci.* **1999**, *893*, 13–18. [CrossRef]

61. Fang, Y.Z.; Yang, S.; Wu, G. Free radicals, antioxidants, and nutrition. *Nutrition* **2002**, *18*, 872–879. [CrossRef]

62. Moynihan, P.; Petersen, P.E. Diet, nutrition and the prevention of dental diseases. *Public Health Nutr.* **2004**, *7*, 201–226. [CrossRef] [PubMed]

63. Genco, R.J.; Borgnakke, W.S. Risk factors for periodontal disease. *Periodontology 2000* **2013**, *62*, 59–94. [CrossRef] [PubMed]

64. Sajjanhar, I.; Goel, A.; Tikku, A.P.; Chandra, A. Odontogenic pain of non-odontogenic origin: A review. *Int. J. Appl. Dent. Sci.* **2017**, *3*, 1–4.

65. Japanese Society of Orofacial Pain. *Clinical Practice Guideline for Nonodontogenic Toothache*; Japan Dental Association: Tokyo, Japan, 2011.

66. Sakagami, H.; Okudaira, N.; Masuda, Y.; Amano, O.; Yokose, S.; Kanda, Y.; Suguro, M.; Natori, T.; Oizumi, H.; Oizumi, T. Induction of apoptosis in human oral keratinocyte by doxorubicin. *Anticancer Res.* **2017**, *37*, 1023–1029. [PubMed]

67. Sakagami, H.; Shi, H.; Bandow, K.; Tomomura, M.; Tomomura, A.; Horiuchi, M.; Fujisawa, T.; Oizumi, T. Search of neuroprotective polyphenols using the "overlay" isolation method. *Molecules* **2018**, *23*, 1840. [CrossRef] [PubMed]

68. Sakagami, H.; Watanabe, T.; Hoshino, T.; Suda, N.; Mori, K.; Yasui, T.; Yamauchi, N.; Kashiwagi, H.; Gomi, T.; Oizumi, T.; et al. Recent progress of basic studies of natural products and their dental application. *Medicines* **2018**, *6*, 4. [CrossRef] [PubMed]

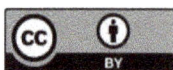

medicines

MDPI

Review

Kampo (Traditional Japanese Herbal) Formulae for Treatment of Stomatitis and Oral Mucositis

Masataka Sunagawa [ID], Kojiro Yamaguchi [ID], Mana Tsukada, Nachi Ebihara, Hideshi Ikemoto and Tadashi Hisamitsu *[ID]

Department of physiology, School of medicine, Showa University, Tokyo 142-8555, Japan;
suna@med.showa-u.ac.jp (M.S.); kampo5260@icloud.com (K.Y.); m-tsukada@med.showa-u.ac.jp (M.T.);
BYS00426@nifty.com (N.E.); h_ikemoto@med.showa-u.ac.jp (H.I.)
* Correspondence: tadashi@med.showa-u.ac.jp; Tel.: +81-3-3784-8110

Received: 10 November 2018; Accepted: 29 November 2018; Published: 10 December 2018

Abstract: Stomatitis is occasionally multiple, recurrent, and refractory. Currently, mucositis induced by chemotherapy and radiation therapy in patients with cancer has become a significant clinical problem. Effective treatments have not been established and the treatment of numerous cases remains a challenge for physicians. Traditional Japanese herbal medicines termed Kampo formulae (i.e., Hangeshashinto, Orengedoku, Inchinkoto, Orento, Byakkokaninjinto, Juzentaihoto, Hochuekkito, and Shosaikoto) are used for treating various types of stomatitis and mucositis. Its use has been based on the Kampo medical theories—empirical rules established over thousands of years. However, recently, clinical and basic research studies investigating these formulae have been conducted to obtain scientific evidence. Clinical studies investigating efficacies of Shosaikoto and Orento for the treatment of cryptogenic stomatitis and acute aphthous stomatitis and those investigating the effects of Hangeshashinto, Orengedoku, and Juzentaihoto on chemotherapy- or radiotherapy-induced mucositis have been conducted. The Kampo formulae comprise several crude drugs, whose mechanisms of action are gradually being clarified. Most of these drugs that are used for the treatment of stomatitis possess anti-inflammatory, analgesic, and antioxidative properties. In this review, we introduce the clinical applications and summarize the available evidence on the Kampo formulae for the treatment of stomatitis and oral mucositis.

Keywords: kampo formula; traditional Japanese herbal medicine; stomatitis; mucositis; Hangeshashinto

1. Introduction

Stomatitis is a sore and often recurrent inflammatory condition of the oral mucosa, characterized by various symptoms such as the presence of vesicles, erosions, aphthae, and ulcerations. Stomatitis is caused by various factors such as viral, fungal, and bacterial infections, allergic reactions, loose-fitting dental prosthetics, and systemic diseases. Occasionally, stomatitis is multiple, recurrent, and refractory. Currently, mucositis induced by chemotherapy and radiation therapy in patients with cancer has become a significant clinical problem [1]. The pain associated with mucositis often affects a patient's functional status and quality of life.

Kampo formula, a traditional Japanese herbal medicine, has its root in ancient Chinese medicine, and the antecedent form of medicine was introduced to Japan between the 5th and 6th century. It was developed into an individual form of medicine adapting the constitutions of the Japanese people. Kampo formulae have been reported to be effective for the treatment of stomatitis and mucositis [2,3]. The objective of this review was to introduce the clinical applications and summarize the available evidence on the Kampo formulae for the treatment of these two conditions.

2. Clinical Applications

We conducted a questionnaire survey regarding the treatment of stomatitis using the Kampo formulae. According to the results, formulae such as Hangeshashinto (HST), Orengedokuto (OGT), Inchinkoto (ICT), Orento (ORT), Byakkokaninjinto (BKN), Juzentaihoto (JTT), Hochuekkito (HET), and Shosaikoto (SST) were used (Figure 1) [4]. The Kampo formulae are generally composed of at least two kinds of crude drugs and these combinations may suppress the development of infections, inflammation, concomitant oxidative stress, and the underlying causes of stomatitis. The chief ingredient and principal effects of each crude drug included in the formulae frequently used for the treatment of stomatitis are shown in Table 1. Many of these agents possess anti-inflammatory and/or analgesic properties. Of note, *Astragali* Radix, *Scutellariae* Radix, *Phellodendri* Cortex, *Coptidis* Rhizoma, *Glycyrrhizae* Radix, *Bupleuri* Radix, *Paeoniae* Radix, *Artemisiae Lanceae* Rhizoma, *Cimicifugae* Rhizoma, *Cnidii* Rhizoma, *Angelicae* Radix, and *Poria* exert anti-inflammatory effects. Moreover, *Cinnamomi* Cortex, *Cimicifugae* Rhizoma, *Paeoniae* Radix, *Glycyrrhizae* Radix, *Cnidii* Rhizoma, *Angelicae* Radix, *Zingiberis* Rhizoma Processum, and *Magnoliae* Cortex exert analgesic effects [5]. The occurrence of stomatitis is related to the generation of reactive oxygen species (ROS) [6]. Therefore, anti-oxidants contained in these medicinal herbs may effectively mitigate this damaging effect. Dragland et al. [7] assessed the contribution of culinary and medicinal herbs to the total dietary intake of anti-oxidants (Table 1). Notably, *Cinnamomi* Cortex, *Scutellariae* Radix, *Cimicifugae* Rhizoma, *Paeoniae* Radix, *Aurantii Nobilis* Pericarpium, and *Glycyrrhizae* Radix contain high concentrations of anti-oxidants.

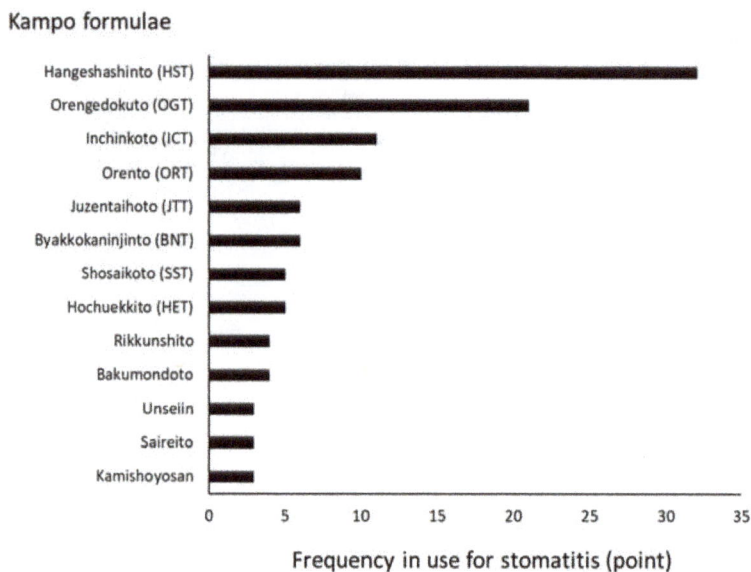

Figure 1. Kampo formulae frequently used for the treatment of stomatitis [4]. The trends in the use of the Kampo formulae at hospitals and faculties of oral surgery of dental/medical universities in Japan were surveyed. A total of 55 hospitals participated in the survey and rated the frequency of Kampo formulae use via a scale from 0 to 3. This graphic summarizes the results of rating.

Table 1. The Kampo formulae frequently used for the treatment of stomatitis and their corresponding crude drugs.

Crude Drug/ Japanese Name		Kampo Formulae										Antioxidant [7] (mmol/100 g)	Chief Ingredient	Principal Effects
		Hangeshashinto (HST)	Orento (ORT)	Orengedokuto (OGT)	Byakkokaninjinto (BKN)	Shosaikoto (SST)	Inchinkoto (ICT)	Heiisan (HIS)	Juzentaihoto (JTT)	Hochuekkito (HET)				
Cinnamomi Cortex	Keihi		○						○		120.2	cinnamaldehyde	antipyresis, perspiration, analgesia
Scutellariae Radix	Ogon	○		○		○					111.5	baicalin	anti-inflammation, antipyresis, laxative
Cimicifugae Rhizoma	Shoma									○	64.3	cimigenol	anti-inflammation, antipyresis, analgesia, antiedema
Paeoniae Radix	Shakuyaku								○		55.1	paeoniflorin	analgesia, spasmolysis, anti-inflammation
Aurantii Nobilis Pericarpium	Chinpi							○		○	17.5	hesperidin	stomachic, antitussive
Glycyrrhizae Radix	Kanzo	○	○		○	○		○	○	○	11.6	glycyrrhizin	anti-inflammation, analgesia, detoxification
Zingiberis Rhizoma	Shokyo	○				○		○		○	7.5	gingerol	stomachic, antinausea
Atractylodis Lanceae Rhizoma	Sojutsu							○	○	○	7.4	atractylodin	anti-inflammation, stomachic, diuresis
Cnidii Rhizoma	Senkyu								○		6.7	cnidilide	analeptic, nourishing, anti-inflammation, analgesia
Zizyphi Fructus	Taiso	○	○			○		○		○	5.9	zizyphus saponin	analeptic, nourishing, stomachic
Bupleuri Radix	Saiko					○				○	5.7	saikosaponin	anti-inflammation, antipyresis
Astragali Radix	Ogi								○	○	4.9	formononetin	anti-inflammation, analeptic, diuresis, hypotensive
Rhemanniae Radix	Jio								○		3.9	catalpol	nourishing, diuresis
Angelicae Radix	Toki								○	○	3.0	ligustilide	analeptic, nourishing, anti-inflammation, analgesia
Hoelen	Bukuryo								○		2.8	eburicoic acid	antiedema, stomachic
Ginseng Radix	Ninjin	○	○		○	○			○	○	1.5	ginsenoside	stomachic, nourishing, antinausea

Table 1. Cont.

Crude Drug/ Japanese Name		Kampo Formulae									Antioxidant [7] (mmol/100 g)	Chief Ingredient	Principal Effects
		Hangeshashinto (HST)	Orento (ORT)	Orengedokuto (OGT)	Byakkokaninjinto (BKN)	Shosaikoto (SST)	Inchinkoto (ICT)	Heiisan (HIS)	Juzentaihoto (JTT)	Hochuekkito (HET)			
Pinelliae Tuber	Hange	O	O			O					0.3	homogentisic acid	sedation, antinausea, antitussive
Zingiberis Rhizoma Processum	Kankyo	O	O									shogaol	warming, analgesia
Coptidis Rhizoma	Oren	O	O	O								berberine	anti-inflammation, stomachic, antibacterial, spasmolysis
Phellodendri Cortex	Obaku			O								berberine	anti-inflammation, stomachic
Gardeniae Fructus	Sanshishi			O			O					geniposide	anti-inflammation, antipyresis, choleresis
Artemisiae Capillaris Flos	Inchinko						O					capillarisin	anti-inflammation, antipyresis, choleresis
Rhei Rhizoma	Daio						O					sennoside	laxative, blood fluidity improving
Magnoliae Cortex	Koboku							O				magnolol	stomachic, analgesia, spasmolysis
Gypsum	Sekko				O							calcium sulfate	anti-inflammation, antipyresis, sedation
Oryzae Fructus	Kobei				O							starch	stomachic, nourishing
Anemarrhenae Rhizoma	Chimo				O							timosaponin AIII	antipyresis, hypoglycemia

Regarding the antioxidative effects of these formulae, only herbs that Dragland, et al. [7] assessed are described.

In addition, *Cinnamomi* Cortex, *Scutellariae* Radix, *Glycyrrhizae* Radix, *Astragali* Radix, *Coptidis* Rhizoma, and *Phellodendri* Cortex inhibit several bacterial infections. Moreover, *Cinnamomi* Cortex, *Scutellariae* Radix, and *Anemarrhenae* Rhizome exert antifungal effects. Furthermore, *Scutellariae* Radix and *Glycyrrhizae* Radix have been shown to inhibit viral infections [8].

In Kampo medicine, the approach to the treatment of stomatitis differs depending on the nature of the symptoms (i.e., acute or chronic). Furthermore, the most appropriate treatment is determined according to the presence of oral and general symptoms. The effectiveness of each Kampo formula according to the pathognomonic symptoms of patients is shown in Table 2. In the acute type, formulae exerting cooling effects (i.e., HST, ORT, OGT, BNT, SST, and ICT) are used. In the chronic type, formulae such as HIS, JTT, and HET are used [3]. The JTT and HET supply energy in patients with symptoms of tiredness, fatigue, or lowered/suppressed immunity [9,10]. The oral cavity is a part of the digestive system; thus, digestive symptoms are important selection criteria for the Kampo formulae. The HST, ORT, OGT, SST, ICT, HIS, JTT, and HET are applied for the treatment of gastrointestinal diseases and symptoms by the national health insurance in Japan.

Table 2. The effectiveness of each Kampo formula according to the pathognomonic symptoms of patients.

Kampo Formulae	Pathognomonic Symptoms
Hangeshashinto (HST)	multiple stomatitis irritation, anxiety, insomnia, rush of blood to the head, anorexia, diarrhea, epigastric discomfort and resistance
Orento (ORT)	multiple stomatitis rush of blood to the head, anorexia, decrease in digestive function, abdominal chill symptom, abdominalgia due to chill, epigastric discomfort and resistance
Orengedokuto (OGT)	multiple stomatitis irritation, insomnia, rush of blood to the head
Byakkokaninjinto (BKN)	thirstiness, dry mouth hyperidrosis, polyuria
Shosaikoto (SST)	bitter in the mouth irritation, depression, anorexia, hypochondriac discomfort and distension, nausea
Inchinkoto (ICT)	multiple stomatitis, dry mouth irritation, insomnia, constipation, oliguria
Heiisan (HIS)	multiple stomatitis anorexia, decrease in digestive function, abdominal distension
Juzentaihoto (JTT)	chronic and repetitive stomatitis, dry mouth depressed, fatigue, dullness, macies, hot sensation, night sweat, anemia, anorexia, decrease in digestive function
Hochuekkito (HET)	chronic and repetitive stomatitis depressed, fatigue, dullness, anorexia, decrease in digestive function

3. Clinical Studies

Use of the Kampo formulae has been based on the Kampo medical theories—empirical rules established over thousands of years. In recent years, clinical and basic research studies investigating the Kampo formulae have been performed to obtain scientific evidence.

For our literature review, PubMed (National Center for Biotechnology Information, Bethesda, MD, USA) and ICHUSHI (Japan Medical Abstracts Society, Tokyo, Japan) were used to identify relevant evidence. Reports of clinical studies (randomized controlled trials, case-control studies, and case series studies) identified through this search are summarized in Table 3.

Ogino, et al. [11] showed that the efficacy of SSK administered to patients with cryptogenic stomatitis accompanied by pain (n = 10) was 80%. SSK was particularly effective against symptoms such as erosion and redness. Oka [12] investigated the effect of ORT in patients with acute aphthous stomatitis (n = 39). The numbers of days until the resolution of pain (2.6 days) and complete cure

(6.3 days) were reduced in patients treated with ORT compared with those observed in patients treated with a steroid ointment (pain: 7.5 days; cure: 12.3 days).

Currently, there are effective treatment options for chemotherapy- or radiotherapy-induced stomatitis. HST exerts a preventive effect against these types of stomatitis. Yuki, et al. [13] administered OGT for the treatment of chemotherapy-induced stomatitis and diarrhea in patients with acute myeloblastic or lymphoblastic leukemia (n = 40). The incidence of stomatitis in ORG-treated patients (n = 14) was significantly lower compared with that reported in those who received a gargle consisting of allopurinol, sodium gualenate, and povidone-iodine (n = 25) (27.9% vs. 71.6%, respectively; $p < 0.0001$). Moreover, the incidence of diarrhea was significantly lower (9.3% vs. 31.7%, respectively; $p < 0.005$). HST has been administered for the treatment of chemotherapy-induced mucositis in patients with various types of cancers, such as colorectal [14–17], gastric [16–18], and renal cancers [19]. In all studies, HST extract granules (TJ-14; Tsumura, Tokyo, Japan) were dissolved in drinking water and subjects rinsed their oral cavity with the solution thrice daily. Kono, et al. [14] reported that 92.8% of patients (13/14 patients) with chemotherapy-induced oral mucositis (COM) during treatment with mFOLFOX6 or FOLFIRI for metastasis of advanced colorectal cancer showed significant improvement following a 1-week topical application of HST. Moreover, a significantly decreased mean Common Terminology Criteria for Adverse Events grade was reported in patients treated with HST ($p = 0.0012$). Aoyama, et al. [18] conducted a double-blinded, placebo-controlled, randomized study of HST for the treatment of COM in patients with gastric cancer (n = 91). Although treatment with HST did not reduce the incidence of grade ≥ 2 COM, a trend toward the reduction of the risk of grade 1 COM by HST was observed during the screening cycle. Matsuda, et al. [15] also conducted a double-blinded, randomized study investigating the effect of HST against mucositis induced by infusional fluorinated-pyrimidine-based colorectal cancer chemotherapy (n = 93). Although the incidence of grade ≥ 2 mucositis was lower in patients treated with HST than in those treated with placebo, the difference was not statistically significant (48.8% vs. 57.4%, respectively; $p = 0.41$). The median duration of grade ≥ 2 mucositis was 5.5 days versus 10.5 days, respectively ($p = 0.018$). Nishikawa, et al. [17] demonstrated similar results in patients with gastric and colorectal cancer (n = 181), with a median time to improvement from grade ≥ 2 to grade < 1 COM of 8 days versus 15 days in the HST and placebo groups, respectively ($p = 0.072$). Yoshida, et al. [16] and Ohoka, et al. [19] also administered HST to patients with various types of cancer, demonstrating significant decreases in the Common Terminology Criteria for Adverse Events (v4.0) grades. The findings of these studies suggested that HST may be effective for the treatment of chemotherapy- or radiotherapy-induced stomatitis.

A previous study investigated the administration of JTT for the treatment of radiation-induced stomatitis in patients with oral cancer, in whom oral ingestion was not possible (n = 15) [20]. The mean period during which oral ingestion was not possible in these patients showed a reducing trend (i.e., 17.9 ± 7.1 days vs. 26.0 ± 11.6 days in the JTT-treated (n = 8) and non-treated (n = 7) groups, respectively ($p < 0.121$)). The clinical use of HST for the treatment of radiation-induced stomatitis has also been reported [21,22].

Table 3. Clinical studies reporting the use of the Kampo formulae for the treatment of stomatitis.

No.	First Author, Year [Reference No.]	Kampo Formula	Study Design	Target Patient	Principal Result
1	Ogino, 1992 [11]	Shosaikoto (SSK)	case series study	cryptogenic stomatitis (n = 10)	Efficacy rate was 80%. (very effective = 2, effective = 4, slightly effective = 2, no change = 2)
2	Oka, 2007 [12]	Orento (ORT)	RCT	acute aphthous stomatitis (n = 39) > non-treated (n = 6), steroid ointment-treated (n = 6) and ORT-treated (n = 27) groups	The administration of Orento reduced the number of days until the disappearance of pain and the complete cure compared to other groups.
3	Yuki, 2003 [13]	Orengedokuto (OGT)	case-control (retrospective) study	chemotherapy-induced stomatitis in patients with acute leukemia (n = 40) > ORG-treated (n = 15) and gargling (n = 25) groups	Incidence of stomatitis was 27.9% in the ORG-treated group, which was significantly lower compared with 71.6% in those who received a gargle consisting of allopurinol, sodium gualenate, and povidone-iodine (*p* < 0.0001).
4	Kono, 2010 [14]		case series study	chemotherapy-induced oral mucositis during mFOLFOX6 or FOLFIRI treatment for metastasis of advanced colorectal cancer (n = 14)	Thirteen patients (92.8%) showed improvements in oral mucositis, with significantly decreased mean CTCAE grades (*p* = 0.0012).
5	Aoyama, 2014 [18]		RCT	gastric cancer chemotherapy-induced oral mucositis (COM) (n = 91) > HST-treated (n = 45) and placebo (n = 46) groups	Although HST treatment did not reduce the incidence of ≥grade 2 COM, a trend was observed in which HST reduced the risk of COM in the patients who developed grade 1 COM.
6	Matsuda, 2015 [15]	Hangeshashinto (HST)	RCT	infusional fluorinated-pyrimidine-based colorectal cancer chemotherapy-induced oral mucositis (n = 93) > HST-treated (n = 46) and placebo (n = 47) groups	Although the incidence of grade ≥2 mucositis was lower for patients treated with HST compared to those treated with placebo, there was no significant difference (48.8 vs. 57.4%; *p* = 0.41). The median duration of grade ≥2 mucositis was 5.5 versus 10.5 days (*p* = 0.018).
7	Yoshida, 2017 [16]		case series study	cancer chemotherapy-induced oral mucositis (grade ≥ 2) (n = 50)	Thirty-seven patients (74%) showed improvements in oral mucositis, with significantly decreased mean NRS and CTC-grade (*p* < 0.001).
8	Nishikawa, 2018 [17]		RCT	chemotherapy-induced oral mucositis (COM) in patients with gastric cancer and colorectal cancer (n = 181) > HST-treated (n = 88) and placebo (n = 93) groups	The incidence of grade ≥2 COM in the HST group was 55.7%, while that in the placebo group was 53.8% (*p* = 0.796). The median time to remission of grade ≥ 2 COM to grade < 1 was 8 days in the HST group and 15 days in the placebo group (*p* = 0.072).
9	Ohoka, 2018 [19]		RCT	sunitinib-induced oral mucositis (OM) in patients with metastatic renal cancer (n = 22) > HST-gargling (n = 12) and non-gargling (n = 10) groups	The gargling with HST significantly improved OM grade and eating status (Global self assessment) (*p* = 0.002).
10	Wada, 2004 [20]	Juzentaihoto (JTT)	RCT	radiation (40 Gy >)-induced stomatitis in patients with oral cancer (n = 15) > JTT-treated (n = 8) and non-treated (n = 7) groups	The mean period that patients could not ingest orally was 17.9 ± 7.1 days in the JTT-treated group, while that in the non-treated group was 26.0 ± 11.6 day (*p* = 0.121).

RCT: randomized controlled trial.

4. Basic Studies of HST

Stomatitis and oral mucositis are induced by various factors, such as infection, inflammation, concomitant oxidative stress, suppressed immunity, depressed function of the digestive tract, malnutrition, psychological stress, and physical stress. Regarding chemotherapy- and radiotherapy-induced mucositis, these treatments induce DNA and non-DNA damage that results in injury of basal epithelial, submucosal, and endothelial cells. In response to this damage, oxidative stress results in the formation of ROS. The presence of ROS damages cell membranes, induces proinflammatory cytokines such as tumor necrosis factor-α, prostaglandin (PG) E_2, interleukin-6, and interleukin-1β, and upregulates cyclooxygenase (COX)-2 in submucosal fibroblasts and endothelial cells leading to mucosal ulceration [23,24]. Furthermore, chemotherapy and radiotherapy reduce immunity, facilitating the development of infectious diseases [25].

Hitomi, et al. [26] conducted in-vivo studies evaluating the analgesic effects of HST using an oral ulcer rat model treated with acetic acid. The topical application of HST in ulcerative oral mucosa suppressed mechanical pain hypersensitivity without exerting effects on healthy mucosa. Moreover, Kamide, et al. [27] assessed the effectiveness of HST for the prevention of radiation-induced mucositis using a hamster model. Administration of HST significantly reduced the severity of mucositis. The percentage of severe mucositis (score $\geq$ 3) was 100% and 16.7% in the untreated and HST groups, respectively. Moreover, HST inhibited the infiltration of neutrophils and expression of COX-2 in irradiated mucosa.

As mentioned earlier in this review, the main characteristic of the Kampo formulae is the combination of several crude drugs (Table 1). These combinations may suppress multiple causes of stomatitis and mucositis. Of note, HST is composed of seven herbs, namely *Scutellariae* Radix, *Glycyrrhizae* Radix, *Zizyphi* Fructus, *Ginseng* Radix, *Pinelliae* Tuber, *Zingiberis* Rhizoma Processum, and *Coptidis* Rhizoma. These constituents, except *Pinelliae* Tuber, exert antioxidative effects [7,28]. Matsumoto, et al. [28] reported that *Glycyrrhizae* Radix, *Ginseng* Radix, and *Zizyphi* Fructus demonstrated scavenging activity for hydroxyl radical, while *Scutellariae* Radix, *Glycyrrhizae* Radix, *Zingiberis* Rhizoma Processum, and *Coptidis* Rhizoma eliminated superoxide. Moreover, *Scutellariae* Radix and *Coptidis* Rhizoma have been shown to eliminate nitroxyl radical.

Regarding its antibacterial action, in vitro studies demonstrated that HST extract inhibited the growth of Gram-negative bacteria including Fusobacterium nucleatum, Porphyromonas gingivalis, Porphyromonas endodontalis, Prevotella intermedia, Prevotella melaninogenica, Tannerella forsythia, Treponema denticola, and Porphyromonas asaccharolytica. However, these inhibitory effects were less pronounced in Gram-positive bacteria and Candida albicans. These effects are thought to be induced by *Scutellariae* Radix (baicalein), *Pinelliae* Tuber (homogentisic acid), *Zingiberis* Rhizoma Processum ([6]-shogaol) and *Coptidis* Rhizoma (berberine, coptisine) [29]. Furthermore, *Glycyrrhizae* Radix [30,31], *Pinelliae* Tuber [31], *Coptidis* Rhizoma [32], and *Ginseng* Radix may enhance immunity. In particular, *Ginseng* Radix was reported to increase the activity of natural killer cells in mice treated orally with it [33,34].

Regarding its anti-inflammatory effect, HST inhibited the production of PGE_2 and suppressed the expression of COX-2 protein. In vitro studies show that *Scutellariae* Radix, *Glycyrrhizae* Radix, *Zingiberis* Rhizoma Processum, and *Coptidis* Rhizoma are involved in these effects [35–38]. As stated earlier in this review, Hitomi, et al. reported the analgesic action of HST [26] and subsequently found through in vitro and in vivo studies that blockage of Na^+ channels by components of *Zingiberis* Rhizoma Processum ([6]-gingerol and ([6]-shogaol) play an essential role in HST-associated analgesia. Moreover, the *Ginseng* Radix extract demonstrated an acceleration of substance permeability into the tissue of the oral ulcer and enhanced the analgesic action of *Zingiberis* Rhizoma Processum [39]. Baicalein—an active constituent of *Scutellariae* Radix—alleviated mechanical allodynia in rats with cancer-induced bone pain [40]. Glycyrrhizin—an active constituent of *Glycyrrhizae* Radix—ameliorated inflammatory pain by inhibiting the microglial activation-mediated inflammatory response in mice with inflammatory pain [41]. HST induces its analgesic effect through the synergistic actions of certain crude drugs.

Therefore, HST exerts a combination of antioxidative, anti-inflammatory, immunostimulatory, and analgesic effects. Moreover, HST is able to control the symptoms and simultaneously eliminate the underlying causes of the condition (Figure 2).

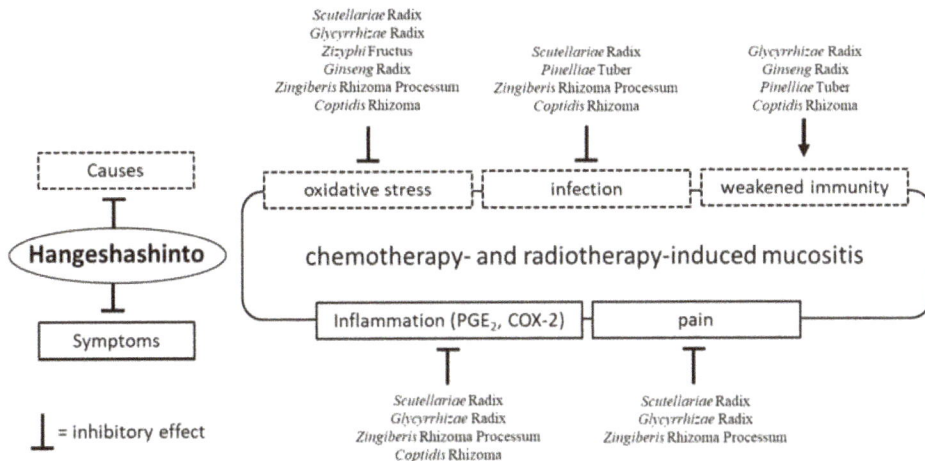

Figure 2. The effects of Hangeshashinto (HST) and the crude drugs on chemotherapy- and radiotherapy-induced mucositis. HST exerts antioxidative, anti-inflammatory, immunostimulatory, and analgesic effects. Moreover, HST is able to control the symptoms and simultaneously eliminate the underlying causes of the condition. PGE_2; prostaglandin E_2. COX-2; cyclooxygenase-2.

5. Conclusions

In general, western medicines such as steroid ointments, nonsteroidal anti-inflammatory drugs, and antiviral and antifungal drugs are applied for stomatitis and oral mucositis according to the causes and symptoms. In contrast to western medicines which generally include a single component, the Kampo formulae contain multiple components and their effects are exerted through complex mechanisms of action. Use of the Kampo formulae may be an alternative treatment option for patients who failed to respond to conventional therapies. In addition, the concomitant use of Kampo formulae with western medicines may be useful. Kobayashi [42] reported effective cases in which the concomitant use of HST with steroid ointment was applied. In this review, we introduced the clinical applications and summarized the available evidence of the Kampo formulae for the treatment of stomatitis and oral mucositis. Despite the availability of clinical reports, the evidence (except for that related to treatment with HST) is limited. Future clinical and basic research studies are warranted to further investigate the effectiveness on the Kampo formulae against these conditions.

Author Contributions: T.H. designed and supervised the work. M.S. wrote the initial draft with support from M.T., N.E. and H.I., and K.Y. edited the manuscript. All authors approved the final version of the manuscript.

Funding: This research received no external funding.

Acknowledgments: The authors would like to thank Shigemasa Kubo for his valuable assistance during the preparation of this manuscript and Enago (www.enago.jp) for English language review.

Conflicts of Interest: The authors declare no conflict of interest.

Abbreviations

BKN	Byakkokaninjinto
COM	chemotherapy-induced oral mucositis
COX	cyclooxygenase
HET	Hochuekkito

HST	Hangeshashinto
ICT	Inchinkoto
IL	interleukin
JTT	Juzentaihoto
OGT	Orengedokuto
ORT	Orento
PG	prostaglandin
RCT	randomized controlled trial
ROS	reactive oxygen species
SST	Shosaikoto

References

1. Curra, M.; Junior, S.; Valente, L.A.; Martins, M.D.; Santos, P.S.D.S. Chemotherapy protocols and incidence of oral mucositis. An integrative review. *Einstein* **2018**, *16*, eRW4007. [CrossRef] [PubMed]
2. Zheng, L.W.; Hua, H.; Cheung, L.K. Traditional Chinese medicine and oral diseases: Today and tomorrow. *Oral Dis.* **2011**, *17*, 7–12. [CrossRef] [PubMed]
3. Yamaguchi, K. Traditional Japanese herbal medicines for treatment of odontopathy. *Front. Pharmacol.* **2015**, *6*, 176. [CrossRef] [PubMed]
4. Sunagawa, M.; Wang, P.L.; Yohkoh, N.; Kameyama, A.; Mukunashi, K.; Mori, S.; Makiishi, T.; Takahashi, S. Survey on trends in the use of Kampo medicines in dentistry and oral surgery among the hospitals of universities. *J. Jpn. Dent. Soc. Orient. Med.* **2011**, *30*, 8–17. (In Japanese)
5. Kenkyukai, K.C. *Clinical Research of Chinese Traditional Medicine—Pharmacognosy*, 1st ed.; Ishiyaku Publishers, Inc.: Tokyo, Japan, 1992; pp. 36–553. ISBN 4-263-73065-8. (In Japanese)
6. Tugrul, S.; Koçyiğit, A.; Doğan, R.; Eren, S.B.; Senturk, E.; Ozturan, O.; Ozar, O.F. Total antioxidant status and oxidative stress in recurrent aphthous stomatitis. *Int. J. Dermatol.* **2016**, *55*, e130–e135. [CrossRef] [PubMed]
7. Dragland, S.; Senoo, H.; Wake, K.; Holte, K.; Blomhoff, R. Several culinary and medicinal herbs are important sources of dietary antioxidants. *J. Nutr.* **2003**, *133*, 1286–1290. [CrossRef] [PubMed]
8. Toriizuka, K. *Monographs of Pharmacological Research on Traditional Herbal Medicine*; Ishiyaku Publishers, Inc.: Tokyo, Japan, 2003; pp. 9–379. ISBN 978-4-263-20188-6. (In Japanese)
9. Ikemoto, T.; Shimada, M.; Iwahashi, S.; Saito, Y.; Kanamoto, M.; Mori, H.; Morine, Y.; Imura, S.; Utsunomiya, T. Changes of immunological parameters with administration of Japanese Kampo medicine (Juzen-Taihoto/TJ-48) in patients with advanced pancreatic cancer. *Int. J. Clin. Oncol.* **2014**, *19*, 81–86. [CrossRef]
10. Kuroiwa, A.; Liou, S.; Yan, H.; Eshita, A.; Naitoh, S.; Nagayama, A. Effect of a traditional Japanese herbal medicine, hochu-ekki-to (Bu-Zhong-Yi-Qi Tang), on immunity in elderly persons. *Int. Immunopharmacol.* **2004**, *4*, 317–324. [CrossRef]
11. Ogino, S.; Harada, T. The effects of Tsumura Shosaikoto on stomatitis. *J. New Rem. Clin.* **1992**, *41*, 592–595. (In Japanese)
12. Oka, S. The effects of Oren-to on Stomatitis. *Pharm. Med.* **2007**, *25*, 35–38. (In Japanese)
13. Yuki, F.; Kawaguchi, T.; Hazemoto, K.; Asou, N. Preventive effects of oren-gedoku-to on mucositis caused by anticancer agents in patients with acute leukemia. *Jpn. Cancer Chemother.* **2003**, *30*, 1303–1307. (In Japanese)
14. Kono, T.; Satomi, M.; Chisato, N.; Ebisawa, Y.; Suno, M.; Asama, T.; Karasaki, H.; Matsubara, K.; Furukawa, H. Topical Application of Hangeshashinto (TJ-14) in the Treatment of Chemotherapy-Induced Oral Mucositis. *World J. Oncol.* **2010**, *1*, 232–235. [PubMed]
15. Matsuda, C.; Munemoto, Y.; Mishima, H.; Nagata, N.; Oshiro, M.; Kataoka, M.; Sakamoto, J.; Aoyama, T.; Morita, S.; Kono, T. Double-blind, placebo-controlled, randomized phase II study of TJ-14 (Hangeshashinto) for infusional fluorinated-pyrimidine-based colorectal cancer chemotherapy-induced oral mucositis. *Cancer Chemother. Pharmacol.* **2015**, *76*, 97–103. [CrossRef] [PubMed]
16. Yoshida, N.; Taguchi, T.; Okayama, T.; Ishikawa, T.; Naito, Y.; Kanazawa, M.; Kanbayashi, Y.; Hosokawa, T.; Kohno, R.; Ito, Y. The effects of Hangeshashinto infiltration method for cancer chemotherapy-induced oral mucositis. *Prog. Med.* **2017**, *37*, 1339–1343. (In Japanese)

17. Nishikawa, K.; Aoyama, T.; Oba, M.S.; Yoshikawa, T.; Matsuda, C.; Munemoto, Y.; Takiguchi, N.; Tanabe, K.; Nagata, N.; Imano, M.; et al. The clinical impact of Hangeshashinto (TJ-14) in the treatment of chemotherapy-induced oral mucositis in gastric cancer and colorectal cancer: Analyses of pooled data from two phase II randomized clinical trials (HANGESHA-G and HANGESHA-C). *J. Cancer* **2018**, *9*, 1725–1730. [CrossRef]

18. Aoyama, T.; Nishikawa, K.; Takiguchi, N.; Tanabe, K.; Imano, M.; Fukushima, R.; Sakamoto, J.; Oba, M.S.; Morita, S.; Kono, T.; et al. Double-blind, placebo-controlled, randomized phase II study of TJ-14 (hangeshashinto) for gastric cancer chemotherapy-induced oral mucositis. *Cancer Chemother. Pharmacol.* **2014**, *73*, 1047–1054. [CrossRef] [PubMed]

19. Ohoka, H. The Clinical Usefulness of Gargling with Hangeshashinto for Treatment of Oral Mucositis Caused by Sunitinib in Patients with Metastatic Renal Cancer. *Kampo Med.* **2018**, *69*, 1–6. (In Japanese) [CrossRef]

20. Wada, S.; Furuta, I. The preventive effects of Juzentaihoto on side effects of radiation therapy for oral cancer. *Sci. Kampo Med.* **2004**, *28*, 76–78. (In Japanese)

21. Nagai, A.; Ogawa, K.; Miura, J.; Kobayashi, K. Therapeutic effects of Hangeshashinto, a Japanese Kampo medicine, on radiation-induced enteritis and oral mucositis: Case series. *Kampo Med.* **2014**, *65*, 108–114. (In Japanese) [CrossRef]

22. Tanaka, Y.; Yamashita, T.; Matsunobu, T.; Shiotani, A. Two Cases of Radiotherapy-induced Oral Mucositis Alleviated with Hange-shashin-to. *Pract. Oto-Rhino-Laryngol.* **2012**, *105*, 1199–1203. (In Japanese) [CrossRef]

23. Logan, R.M.; Gibson, R.J.; Sonis, S.T.; Keefe, D.M. Nuclear factor-kappaB (NF-kappaB) and cyclooxygenase-2 (COX-2) expression in the oral mucosa following cancer chemotherapy. *Oral Oncol.* **2007**, *43*, 395–401. [CrossRef] [PubMed]

24. Al-Dasooqi, N.; Gibson, R.J.; Bowen, J.M.; Logan, R.M.; Stringer, A.M.; Keefe, D.M. Matrix metalloproteinases are possible mediators for the development of alimentary tract mucositis in the dark agouti rat. *Exp. Biol. Med.* **2010**, *235*, 1244–1256. [CrossRef] [PubMed]

25. Al-Ansari, S.; Zecha, J.A.; Barasch, A.; de Lange, J.; Rozema, F.R.; Raber-Durlacher, J.E. Oral Mucositis Induced by Anticancer Therapies. *Curr. Oral Health Rep.* **2015**, *2*, 202–211. [CrossRef] [PubMed]

26. Hitomi, S.; Ono, K.; Yamaguchi, K.; Terawaki, K.; Imai, R.; Kubota, K.; Omiya, Y.; Hattori, T.; Kase, Y.; Inenaga, K. The traditional Japanese medicine hangeshashinto alleviates oral ulcer-induced pain in a rat model. *Arch. Oral Biol.* **2016**, *66*, 30–37. [CrossRef] [PubMed]

27. Kamide, D.; Yamashita, T.; Araki, K.; Tomifuji, M.; Shiotani, A. Hangeshashinto (TJ-14) prevents radiation-induced mucositis by suppressing cyclooxygenase-2 expression and chemotaxis of inflammatory cells. *Clin. Transl. Oncol.* **2017**, *19*, 1329–1336. [CrossRef]

28. Matsumoto, C.; Sekine-Suzuki, E.; Nyui, M.; Ueno, M.; Nakanishi, I.; Omiya, Y.; Fukutake, M.; Kase, Y.; Matsumoto, K. Analysis of the antioxidative function of the radioprotective Japanese traditional (Kampo) medicine, hangeshashinto, in an aqueous phase. *J. Radiat. Res.* **2015**, *56*, 669–677. [CrossRef]

29. Fukamachi, H.; Matsumoto, C.; Omiya, Y.; Arimoto, T.; Morisaki, H.; Kataoka, H.; Kadena, M.; Funatsu, T.; Fukutake, M.; Kase, Y.; et al. Effects of Hangeshashinto on Growth of Oral Microorganisms. *Evid. Based Complement. Alternat. Med.* **2015**, *2015*, 512947. [CrossRef]

30. Chan, A.; Pang, H.; Yip, E.C.; Tam, Y.K.; Wong, Y.H. The aqueous extract of Radix Glycyrrhizae stimulates mitogen-activated protein kinases and nuclear factor-kappaB in Jurkat T-cells and THP-1 monocytic cells. *Am. J. Chin. Med.* **2006**, *34*, 263–278. [CrossRef]

31. Matsuura, K.; Kawakita, T.; Nakai, S.; Saito, Y.; Suzuki, A.; Nomoto, K. Role of B-lymphocytes in the immunopharmacological effects of a traditional Chinese medicine, xiao-chai-hu-tang (shosaiko-to). *Int. J. Immunopharmacol.* **1993**, *15*, 237–243. [CrossRef]

32. Zhou, X.; Peng, Y.; Li, L.; He, K.; Huang, T.; Mou, S.; Feng, M.; Han, B.; Ye, X.; Li, X. Effects of dietary supplementations with the fibrous root of *Rhizoma Coptidis* and its main alkaloids on non-specific immunity and disease resistance of common carp. *Vet. Immunol. Immunopathol.* **2016**, *173*, 34–38. [CrossRef]

33. Jang, A.Y.; Song, E.J.; Shin, S.H.; Hwang, P.H.; Kim, S.Y.; Jin, Y.W.; Lee, E.K.; Lim, M.J.; Oh, I.S.; Ahn, J.Y.; et al. Potentiation of natural killer (NK) cell activity by methanol extract of cultured cambial meristematic cells of wild ginseng and its mechanism. *Life Sci.* **2015**, *135*, 138–146. [CrossRef] [PubMed]

34. Liou, C.J.; Huang, W.C.; Tseng, J. Short-term oral administration of ginseng extract induces type-1 cytokine production. *Immunopharmacol. Immunotoxicol.* **2006**, *28*, 227–240. [CrossRef] [PubMed]

35. Kato, T.; Segami, N.; Sakagami, H. Anti-inflammatory Activity of Hangeshashinto in IL-1β-stimulated Gingival and Periodontal Ligament Fibroblasts. *In Vivo* **2016**, *30*, 257–263. [PubMed]
36. Kaneko, T.; Chiba, H.; Horie, N.; Kato, T.; Kobayashi, M.; Hashimoto, K.; Kusama, K.; Sakagami, H. Effect of Scutellariae radix ingredients on prostaglandin E(2) production and COX-2 expression by LPS-activated macrophage. *In Vivo* **2009**, *23*, 577–581. [PubMed]
37. Kase, Y.; Saitoh, K.; Ishige, A.; Komatsu, Y. Mechanisms by which Hange-shashin-to reduces prostaglandin E2 levels. *Biol. Pharm. Bull.* **1998**, *21*, 1277–1281. [CrossRef] [PubMed]
38. Kono, T.; Kaneko, A.; Matsumoto, C.; Miyagi, C.; Ohbuchi, K.; Mizuhara, Y.; Miyano, K.; Uezono, Y. Multitargeted effects of hangeshashinto for treatment of chemotherapy-induced oral mucositis on inducible prostaglandin E2 production in human oral keratinocytes. *Integr. Cancer Ther.* **2014**, *13*, 435–445. [CrossRef] [PubMed]
39. Hitomi, S.; Ono, K.; Terawaki, K.; Matsumoto, C.; Mizuno, K.; Yamaguchi, K.; Imai, R.; Omiya, Y.; Hattori, T.; Kase, Y.; et al. [6]-gingerol and [6]-shogaol, active ingredients of the traditional Japanese medicine hangeshashinto, relief oral ulcerative mucositis-induced pain via action on Na^+ channels. *Pharmacol. Res.* **2017**, *117*, 288–302. [CrossRef] [PubMed]
40. Hu, S.; Chen, Y.; Wang, Z.F.; Mao-Ying, Q.L.; Mi, W.L.; Jiang, J.W.; Wu, G.C.; Wang, Y.Q. The Analgesic and Antineuroinflammatory Effect of Baicalein in Cancer-Induced Bone Pain. *Evid. Based Complement. Altern. Med.* **2015**, *2015*, 973524. [CrossRef]
41. Sun, X.; Zeng, H.; Wang, Q.; Yu, Q.; Wu, J.; Feng, Y.; Deng, P.; Zhang, H. Glycyrrhizin ameliorates inflammatory pain by inhibiting microglial activation-mediated inflammatory response via blockage of the HMGB1-TLR4-NF-kB pathway. *Exp. Cell Res.* **2018**, *369*, 112–119. [CrossRef]
42. Kobayashi, E. Clinical study on 184 cases of stomatitis. *J. Kampo Med.* **2007**, *54*, 108–115. (In Japanese)

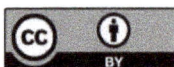

medicines

MDPI

Review

Search for Drugs Used in Hospitals to Treat Stomatitis

Yaeko Hara [1],*, Hiroshi Shiratuchi [2], Tadayoshi Kaneko [2] and Hiroshi Sakagami [3]

[1]   Second Division of Oral and Maxillofacial Surgery, Department of Diagnostic and Therapeutic Sciences,
     Meikai University School of Dentistry, 1-1 Keyakidai, Sakado, Saitama 350-0283, Japan
[2]   Department of Oral Maxillofacial Surgery, Nihon University School of Dentistry; 1-8-13 Kanda Surugadai,
     Chiyoda-ku, Tokyo 101-8310, Japan; shiratsuchi.hiroshi@nihon-u.ac.jp (H.S.);
     kaneko.tadayoshi@nihon-u.ac.jp (T.K.)
[3]   Meikai University Research Institute of Odontology (M-RIO), 1-1 Keyakidai, Sakado,
     Saitama 350-0283, Japan; sakagami@dent.meikai.ac.jp
*   Correspondence: hara.yaeko@dent.meikai.ac.jp; Tel.: +81-49-279-2758

Received: 4 January 2019; Accepted: 26 January 2019; Published: 29 January 2019

Abstract: Stomatitis is an inflammatory disease of the oral mucosa, often accompanied by pain. Usually it is represented by aphthous stomatitis, for which treatment steroid ointment is commonly used. However, in the cases of refractory or recurrent stomatitis, traditional herbal medicines have been used with favorable therapeutic effects. Chemotherapy, especially in the head and neck region, induces stomatitis at higher frequency, which directly affects the patient's quality of life and treatment schedule. However, effective treatment for stomatitis has yet to be established. This article presents the clinical report of Kampo medicines on the stomatitis patients in the Nihon university, and then reviews the literature of traditional medicines for the treatment of stomatitis. Among eighteen Kampo medicines, Hangeshashinto has been the most popular for the treatment of stomatitis, due to its prominent anti-inflammatory activity. It was unexpected that clinical data of Hangeshashinto on stomatitis from Chinese hospital are not available. Kampo medicines have been most exclusively administered to elder person, as compared to pediatric population. Supplementation of alkaline plant extracts rich in lignin-carbohydrate complex may further extend the applicability of Kampo medicines to viral diseases.

Keywords: Chinese herbal remedies; stomatitis

---

1. Introduction

Stomatitis is an inflammation induced by various factors such as trauma, viruses and bacterial infections, genetic factors, stress and vitamin deficiency [1–3]. Chemotherapy and radiotherapy may produce active oxygen species and free radicals, that cause oxidative injury, inflammation of the oral mucosa and pain [4,5]. Like the digestive tract, oral mucosa membrane is susceptible to stress, and prone to be deteriorated by contact with teeth and unsanitary oral hygiene. Therefore, anti-stomatitis therapy with herbal medicines should be based on their anti-stress, anti-oxidative, mucous membrane protection and regeneration activities.

Western medicine usually consists of a single active ingredient and is prescribed to eradicate the causal diseases, based on the main complaint and examination data of the patients. In contrast, herbal medicines such as Japanese traditional medicine (Kampo) and Traditional Chinese Medicine (TCM) are mixtures of at least two kinds of constitutional plant extracts, are therefore applicable to various diseases [6]. "Oriental medicine" includes TCM, Korean medicine, Ayurveda (traditional Indian medicine) and Japanese Kampo medicine. TCM and medical texts were first brought to Japan from China during the 5–6th centuries. Until the 14–16th centuries, diagnosis and treatment were performed according to the theory of TCM, and thereafter developed, evolved and established independently in Japan, as a system of medicine that matches the environment and climate of Japan as well as the physical constitution and lifestyle of the Japanese population [6].

Currently, various clinical and fundamental studies have been conducted to elucidate the mechanism of the action of traditional medicines. This article presented the clinical report of Kampo medicines on the stomatitis patients in the Nihon university, and then reviewed the literature of traditional medicines for the treatment of stomatitis, based on the search by PubMed (National Center for Biotechnology Information, Bethesda, MD, USA) and Ichushi (Japan Medical Abstracts Society, Tokyo, Japan).

2. Kampo Medicines Prescribed in the Hospital of Nihon University School of Dentistry

We have surveyed approximately 400 patients with stomatitis in our hospital of the Nihon University School of Dentistry from January 2014 to October 2018. Number of patients with stomatitis progressively declined (Figure 1A), while the number of Kampo medicines prescribed to stomatitis patients was increased (Figure 1B). When the percent of Kampo medicines prescribed to stomatitis patient was calculated, it was found to be increased sharply in 2018 (Figure 1C). The most frequently prescribed Kampo medicine was Hangeshashinto (Figure 1D) (Figure 1).

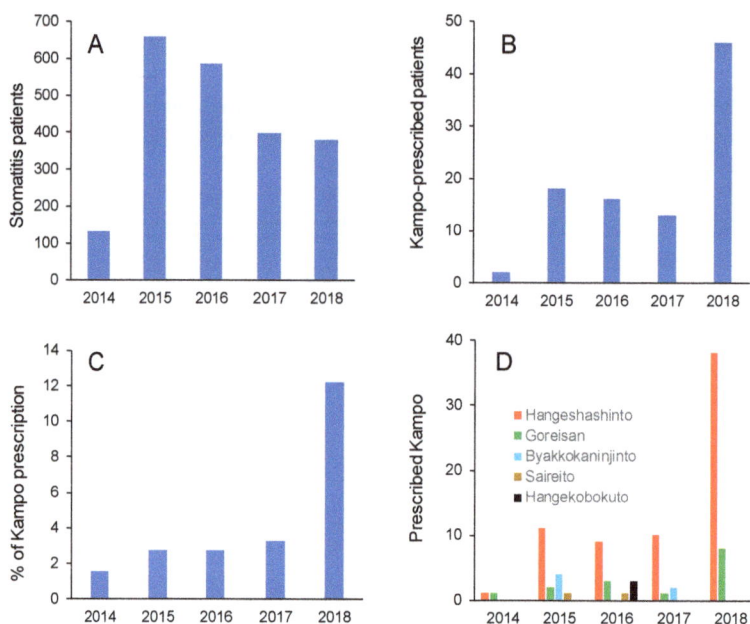

Figure 1. Changes in number of stomatitis patients (**A**), number of Kampo-prescribed stomatitis patients (**B**), percent of Kampo prescription (**C**) and number of prescribed Kampo medicines (**D**) during 2014 to 2018 (Data from hospital of Nihon University School of Dentistry).

During 12 months of years, the incidence of stomatitis was higher in winter season, peaked in March (Figure 2A), and the prescription of Kampo medicines peaked on April and May (Figure 2B), possibly to combat against the increasing numbers of stomatitis patients (Figure 2).

Byakkokaninjinto, Goreisan, Hangekobokuto, Hangeshashinto and Saireito extract granules used in our hospital contains 5, 5, 5, 7 and 11 constituent plant extracts, respectively (Table 1). It should be noted that each extract contains numerous numbers of compounds.

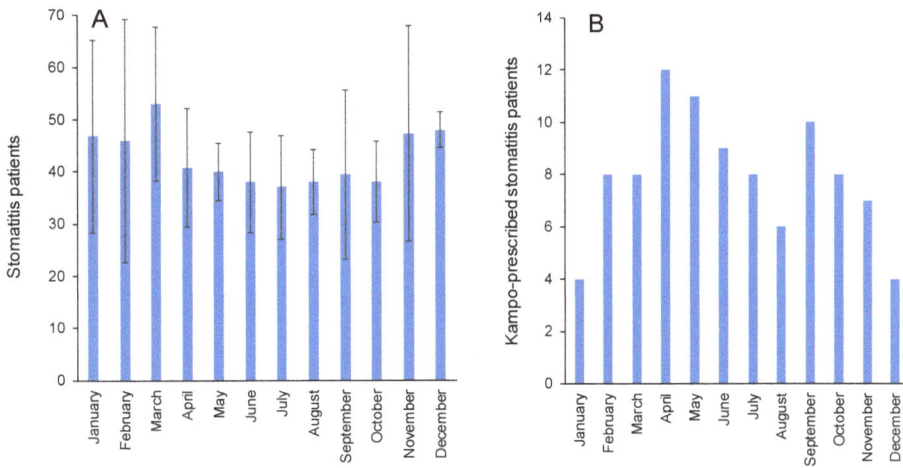

Figure 2. Number of stomatitis patients (**A**) and prescribed Kampo medicines in the hospital of Nihon University School of Dentistry (**B**).

Table 1. Kampo medicines and their constituent plant extracts used for treatment of stomatitis in the hospital of Nihon University School of Dentistry. BKTN, Byakkokaninjinto; GRS, Goreisan; HKT, Hangekobokuto; HST, Hangeshashinto; SRT, Saireito.

Constituent Plant Extracts	Kampo Medicines				
	BKNT	GRS	HKT	HST	SRT
Alisma Rhizome		○			○
Anemarrhena Rhizome	○				
Astractylodes Lancea Rhizome		○			○
Brown Rice	○				
Bupleurum Root					○
Cinnamon Bark		○			○
Coptis Rhizome				○	
Ginger			○	○	○
Ginseng	○			○	○
Glycyrrhiza	○			○	○
Gypsum	○				
Jujube				○	○
Magnolia Bark			○		
Perilla Herb			○		
Pinellia Tuber			○	○	○
Polyporus Sclerotium		○			
Poria Sclerotium		○	○		○
Scutellaria Root				○	○

During 5 years (2014–2018), 40 patients were treated with Hangeshashinto extract granules 2.5 g alone, while 27 patients were treated with hangeshashinto together with other Kampo medicines (Goreisan), gargle [sodium gualenate hydrate (azunol® gargle liquid 4%), 0.2% benzethonium chloride solution (Neostelin Green 0.2% mouthwash solution)], anti-inflammatory agent (dexamethasone, triamicinolone acetonide, loxoprofen), or antimicrobial agent (miconazole gel) (Table 2). We first dissolve Hangeshashinto in water, and patients swallow it after gargling. When bitterness is too strong for the patients, we prescribe steroid ointment or azunol gargle in addition to Hangeshashinto, since azunol gargle protects the mucous membrane [7]. If mouth rinse is difficult, we will use other medicines.

Table 2. Kampo medicines prescribed for stomatitis in the hospital of Nihon University School of Dentistry. All Kampo medicines are extract granules. BKTN, Byakkokaninjinto; BMZ, betamethasone; DX, dexamethasone, GRS, Goreisan; HKT, Hangekobokuto; HST, Hangeshashinto; SRT, Saireito; SC, Salcoat Capsule for oral spray; TAC, triamcinolone acetonide.

Kampo Medicine Prescribed	Number of Prescribed Kampo					
	2014	2015	2016	2017	2018	Total
HST 2.5 g/packet	0	8	5	9	18	40
HST 2.5 g/packet, SC 50 µg	0	1	0	0	0	1
GRS 2.5 g/packet	0	0	2	0	3	5
GRS 2.5 g + HST 2.5 g	0	0	1	0	0	1
BKTN 3 g + SC 50 µg	0	0	0	1	0	1
Azunol gargle 4% (10 mL) + HST 2.5 g	0	0	0	0	3	3
Azunol gargle 4% (10 mL) + HST 2.5 g + SC	0	0	0	0	2	2
Azunol gargle 4% (5 mL) + HST 2.5 g	0	1	2	0	0	3
TAC ointment 0.1% + Azunol + GRS 2.5 g	0	0	0	1	0	1
DX ointment 0.1% + SRT 3.0 g	0	1	0	0	0	1
DX oint 0.1% + HST 2.5 g	0	0	0	1	5	6
DX oint 0.1% + HST 2.5 g	0	0	1	0	0	1
DX oint 0.1% + GRS 2.5 g	1	0	0	0	3	4
DX oint 0.1%+ Azunol + HST 2.5 g	1	0	0	0	1	2
DX oint 0.1% + Neostelin Green gargle + HST 2.5 g	0	0	0	0	1	1
DX oint 0.1% + Neostelin + GRS 2.5 g	0	0	0	0	1	1
DX oint 0.1%+ Hachiazule gargle 0.1% + GRS 2.5 g	0	2	0	0	0	2
Neostelin green mouthwash + SRT 3 g	0	0	1	0	0	1
Neostelin green mouthwash + HST 2.5 g	0	0	0	0	3	3
Neostelin green mouthwash + GRS 2.5 g + SC 50 µg	0	0	0	0	1	1
Neostelin green mouthwash + BKTN 3 g	0	0	0	1	0	1
Miconazole gel 2% + HST 2.5 g	0	0	1	0	0	1
RACOL-NF Liquid for Enteral Use + HKT 2.5 g	0	0	1	0	0	1
BMZ/Gentamicin oint + Azonol 4% + HST 2.5 g	0	0	0	0	1	1
Loxoprofen tablet 60 mg + HST 2.5 g	0	1	0	0	0	1
Loxoprofen tablet 60 mg + HST 2.5 g + SC 50 µg	0	0	0	0	1	1
Hachiazule gargle 0.1% + BKTN 3 g	0	4	0	0	0	4
White petrolatum + Azunol 4% + HKT 2.5 g	0	0	1	0	0	1

The following is the clinical report of stomatitis patients treated with Hangeshashinto in our hospital, after obtaining the informed consent from the patient, under the condition that the patient is not identified. The patient (female, 29 years old) was subjected to first medical examination on 23 May 2018. She showed the symptoms of stomatitis every few months. Each time, she applied triamcinolone acetonide (Kenalog®, Bristol-Myers Squibb Co., Tokyo, Japan) ointment herself, but got only short-term healing. When stomatitis developed again on early May 2018, Kenalog®did not work. Herpes simplex virus was detected in the oral cavity on 21 May. Administration of acyclovir, a popular anti-HSV agent, did not improved, but rather aggravated her symptom. Upon recommendation by the doctor, she got a close examination by the first author (Y.H.) on 23 May. The pain spread to the entire oral cavity, especially inside the anterior teeth part of the lower lip, and the tongue, feeling of incongruity during meals. There was no swelling or redness in the face. An ulcer suspected of stomatitis is formed in the buccal mucosa and the inner surface of the lips in the oral cavity. There was a tender pain with palpation (Figure 3A).

She was then treated with Hangeshashinto extract granules 2.5 g × 3 packages 14 days, and neostelin green mouthwash 0.2% 40 mL. On 6 June, a new stomatitis was formed in the molar part on the right upper side, and became slightly larger, however, the application of medicines was continued. It then became smaller and disappeared on 10 June. Some redness remained on the buccal gingiva of Upper right 6, but all other parts were healed. On 17 July, there was no mouth sores on the mucosal surface (Figure 3B).

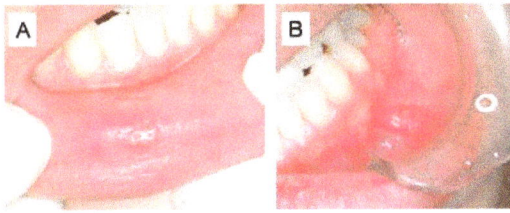

Figure 3. Therapeutic effect of Hangeshashinto on stomatitis. (**A**): Before Hangeshashinto treatment; (**B**): After Hangeshashinto treatment.

3. Data Search for Traditional Medicine for the Treatment of Stomatitis

Stomatitis is a painful oral mucosal disorder, generated from various causes. Especially stomatitis in patients undergoing chemotherapy is severe, sometimes accompanied by eating difficulties. One common stomatitis often encountered is recurrent aphtha (recurrent aphthous stomatitis: RAS). RAS developed at a rate of 5–25% in the stomatitis patients [1], and treatment of RAS with Chinese patent medicines has been reported [8]. More recently, healing effects of Kampo on chemotherapy-induced stomatitis have been published [9,10]. Changes in the number of papers that related to Chinese Traditional Medicine was searched with PubMed (Figure 4A) and Ichushi (Figure 4B) (Figure 4). The publication of TCM appeared in 1980, and increased in the number more dramatically after 2000 in both cases.

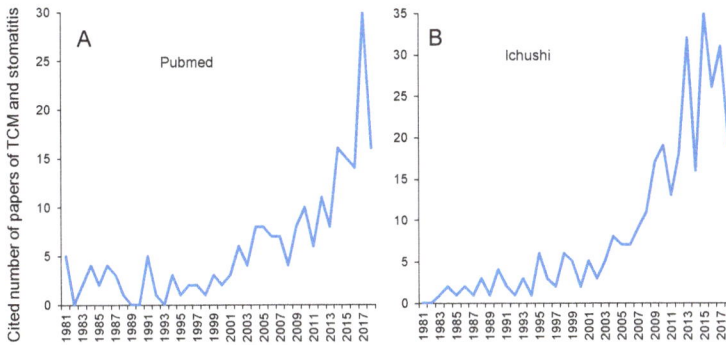

Figure 4. Increase of number of papers that cite TCM and stomatitis. (**A**): Data from Pubmed; (**B**): Data from Ichushi.

The most frequently used drugs for treatment of stomatitis, based on Pubmed search, were steroids (hydrocortisone acetate, triamcinolone acetonide, dexamethasone, beclometasone dipropionate (1 + 51 + 148 + 12 = 212 reports), followed by TCM (53 reports) > Kampo medicine (13 reports) and azunol ointment (main component: dimethyl isopropylazulene) (0 report) (Table 3). When corrected for the total numbers of references in each group, Kampo medicine was found to be the most popular for treating the stomatitis (0.92% of total application), followed by betamethasone (0.80%) > triamcinolone acetonide (0.74%) > beclometasone dipropionate (0.32%) > dexamethasone (0.22%) > hydrocortisone acetate (0.11%) > TCM (0.09%). It should be noted that Kampo medicine has been used for the purpose of treating stomatitis 10 times (= 0.92/0.09) than TCM (Table 3).

Table 3. Medicines used for treatment of stomatitis (data obtained from Pubmed on 16 January 2019).

Medicines	Number of References		%
	Alone A	+ Stomatitis B	(A/B) × 100
Azunol Ointment (Dimethyl Isopropylazulene)	18	0	0
Hydrocortisone Acetate	890	1	0.11
Triamcinolone Acetonide	6891	51	0.74
Dexamethasone	68,125	148	0.22
Betamethasone	8478	68	0.80
Beclometasone	3751	12	0.32
Kampo Medicine	1406	13	0.92
Hangeshashinto	28	10	35.71
Coptis Rhizome	150	1	0.67
Ginger	3264	1	0.03
Ginseng	8868	4	0.05
Glycyrrhiza	3244	17	0.52
Glycyrrhizin	2389	7	0.29
Jujube	802	0	0
Pinellia Tuber	94	0	0
Scutellaria Root	502	2	0.40
Traditional Chinese medicine (TCM)	61,115	53	0.09

A total of 18 Kampo medicines for the treatment of stomatitis are prescribed by hospitals and Rikkosan, Tokishakuyakusan> Kamishoyosan, Orengedokuto, Rikkunshito, Jpractitioners, according to the search with Pubmed and Ichushi. According to Pubmed, Hangeshashinto is the most frequently used [11,12], followed by Hochuekkito, uzentaihoto Unseiin > Shigyakusan, Saikokeishikankyoto, Saikokeishito, Orento, Inchinkoto, San'oshashinto, Goreisan, Keishibukuryogan and Shosaikoto (Figure 5A). The search by Ichushi reported the similar order of administration frequency: Hangeshashinto > Juzentaihoto, Hochuekkito > Rikkunshito > Orengedokuto > Orento > Rikkosan > Goreisan > Shosaikoto > Inchinkoto > Kamishoyosan > Unseiin > Tokishakuyakusan > Saikokeishito > Keishibukuryogan > San'oshashinto > Shigyakusan > Saikokeishikankyoto (Figure 5B).

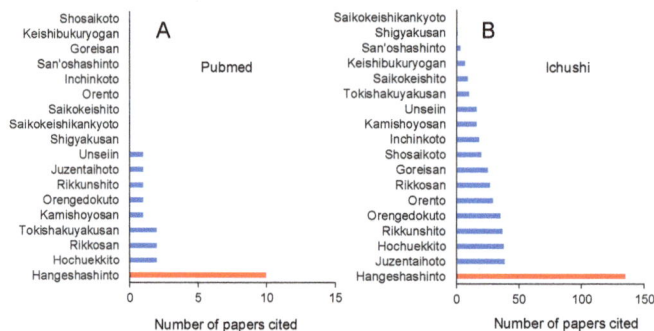

Figure 5. Hangeshashinto is the most popular kampo medicine for the treatment of stomatitis. Data obtained from Pubmed on 16 January 16 2019. (A): Data from pubmed; (B): Data from Ichushi.

Goreisan, known as "hydrostatic modulator" for edema, diarrhea, headache, nausea, and dizziness [13] is used to treat dry mouth. Rikkosan, a negative regulator of IL-1β network [14], plays a supplementary role for stomatitis by relieving the pain. Kamishoyosan (KSS), that enhances peripheral circulation and reduces stress and associated pain [15], and saikokeishikankyoto, that reduces posttraumatic stress [16], are effective to refractory and recurrent stomatitis.

While hangeshashinto is mainly administered to patients with stomatitis at the middle to late stage, orento is used for the early stage of stomatitis, such as acute aphthous stomatitis [17]. This may be due to shorter treatment time of orento required for pain relief and complete cure (2.6 and 6.3 days, respectively), as compared with those of steroid ointment (7.5 and 12.3 days, respectively) [18]. Although orento is used clinically very often, the paper of orento is limited. This may be due to the fact that early stomatitis heals much faster, as compared to intractable, recurrent stomatitis and chemotherapy-induced stomatitis. Most of fundamental and clinical research studies have been focusing on the stomatitis in the patients with head and neck cancer who received chemotherapy or radiation chemotherapy, to keep the patient's QOL and treatment continuity [19,20].

4. Application of Traditional Medicines for Pediatric Population

Kampo medicines and Hangeshashinto have been used for elderly person approximately one order higher rates, as compared with pediatric population (Table 4). Publication of TCM was approximately 44.5-fold (= 61,264/1409) as compared with Kampo medicine. Frequency of the use of TCM for elderly person was again one order higher than that for pediatrics (8494/844 = 10.1) (Table 4). This reflects that Kampo medicine and TCM are used to treat and improve the conditions of patients with many kinds of diseases.

Table 4. Medicines used for treatment of stomatitis (data obtained from Pubmed on 16 January 2019).

Cited by	Number of References	% of Control
Kampo medicine (control)	1409	100.0
Kampo medicine + elderly	242	17.2
Kampo medicine + adult	287	20.0
Kampo medicine + young	43	3.1
Kampo medicine + child	33	2.3
Kampo medicine + pediatric	26	1.8
Hangeshashinto	28	100.0
Hangeshashinto + elderly	6	21.4
Hangeshashinto + adult	6	21.4
Hangeshashinto + young	1	3.6
Hangeshashinto + child	1	3.6
Hangeshashinto + pediatric	0	0.0
TCM	61,264	100.0
TCM + elderly	8494	13.9
TCM + adult	10,349	16.9
TCM + young	2343	3.8
TCM + child	1588	2.6
TCM + pediatric	844	1.4

These traditional medicines have been used to cure the skin diseases and abdominal pain, from long ago, although there are few reports on stomatitis for pediatric population. Licorice is a crude drug prescribed in various herbal formulas in traditional Japanese and Chinese medicines, and also used worldwide as a food natural sweetener [21]. Therefore, licorice makes it easier for medication use in children.

5. Why Hangeshashinto Is So Popular for the Treatment of Stomatitis?

Among seven constitutional plant extracts, glycyrrhiza and glycyrrhizin (the major component of glycyrrhiza) have been cited most frequently as the therapeutics for stomatis (Table 3). Among 53 papers that investigated the biological activity of Hangeshashinto, 26 papers (49%) dealt with its anti-inflammatory activity, followed by mucosal protection (ten papers, 19%), based on the search by PubMed. The most well-known biological activity of glycyrrhizin was again anti-inflammatory activity (Figure 6).

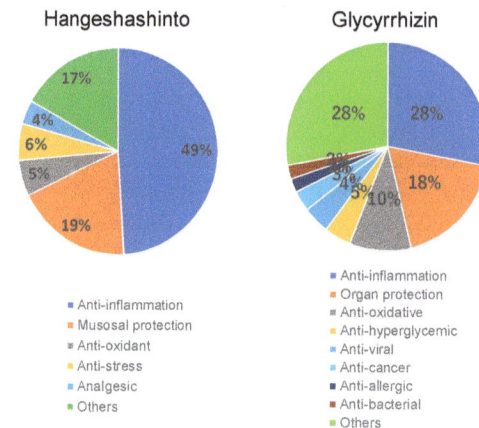

Figure 6. Prominent anti-inflammatory activity of Hangeshashinto.

We have recently reported that Hangeshashinto and Glycyrrhiza inhibited PGE$_2$ production in IL-1-β-stimulated human periodontal ligament fibroblast (selectivity index [SI (CC_{50}/EC_{50}) = 285 and 59, respectively) [22,23]. This suggests that anti-stomatitis activity of Hangeshashinto may be at least in part by Glycyrrhiza.

It has become increasingly apparent that oral health is co-related well with general health. Generally, the anti-HIV activity of Kampo medicine, prepared by hot water extraction, is generally weak [24]. However, alkaline extract of licorice extract [25], green tea, oolong tea and orange flower [26], that contain significant amount of lignin-carbohydrate complex, shows higher anti-viral activity than hot water extract. Supplementation of alkaline extract may further expand the therapeutic ranges of Kampo medicine (Figure 7).

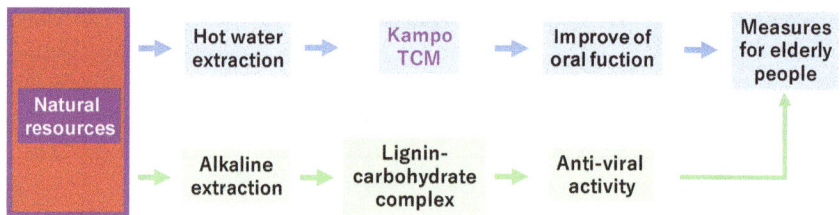

Figure 7. Supplementation of alkaline extract to Kampo prescription extends its therapeutic potential.

6. Conclusions

Literature searches demonstrated that among 18 Kampo medicines, Hangeshashinto is most frequently used in Japan, possibly due to the presence of glycyrrhiza that contains anti-inflammatory glycyrrhizin. It was surprising that Hangeshashinto has not been used in China. Since Kampo medicines are prepared by hot water extraction, they have low levels of lignin–carbohydrate complexes (LCC) that are extracted by alkaline extracts and shows the prominent antiviral activity among three major polyphenols. By adding an alkaline extract rich in LCC to Kampo medicine, its therapeutic potential will become much broader. Up to now, traditional medicines have few cases of adaptation to children, but inclusion of sweet licorice ingredient will make it easier for children to take without resistance. Hangeshashinto is applicable for the treatment of stress gastritis, and seems to be the best Kampo medicine for the treatment of stomatitis, judging from the huge number of publications.

Author Contributions: Y.H., writing the paper; H.S. and T.K. data collection; H.S., writing the paper.

Funding: This work was partially supported by KAKENHI from the Japan Society for the Promotion of Science (JSPS): Sakagami H, 16K11519.

Acknowledgments: The authors acknowledge Tsumura Co. Ltd for the supply of Kampo.

Conflicts of Interest: The authors declare no conflict of interest.

Abbreviations

BKTN	Byakkokaninjinto
BMZ	betamethasone
DX	dexamethasone
GRS	Goreisan
HIV	Human immunodeficiency virus
HKT	Hangekobokuto
HST	Hangeshashinto
LCC	Lignin-carbohydrate complex
SRT	Saireito
SC	Salcoat Capsule for oral spray
TAC	Triamcinolone Acetonide
TCM	Traditional Chinese Medicine

References

1. Edgar, N.R.; Saleh, D.; Miller, R.A. Recurrent aphthous stomatitis: A Review. *J. Clin. Aesthet. Dermatol.* **2017**, *10*, 26–36.
2. Kunikullaya, U.K.; Kumar, M.A.; Ananthakrishnan, V.; Jaisri, G. Stress as a cause of recurrent aphthous stomatitis and its correlation with salivary stress markers. *Chin. J. Physiol.* **2017**, *60*, 226–230. [CrossRef] [PubMed]
3. Tugrul, S.; Koçyiğit, A.; Doğan, R.; Eren, S.B.; Senturk, E.; Ozturan, O.; Ozar, O.F. Total antioxidant status and oxidative stress in recurrent aphthous stomatitis. *Int. J. Dermatol.* **2016**, *55*, e130–e135. [CrossRef]
4. Yoshino, F.; Yoshida, A.; Nakajima, A.; Wada-Takahashi, S.; Takahashi, S.S.; Lee, M.C. Alteration of the redox state with reactive oxygen species for 5-fluorouracil-induced oral mucositis in hamsters. *PLoS ONE* **2013**, *20*, e82834. [CrossRef] [PubMed]
5. Sonis, S.T. Mucositis: The impact, biology and therapeutic opportunities of oral mucositis. *Oral Oncol.* **2009**, *45*, 1015–1020. [CrossRef] [PubMed]
6. Wanga, P.-L.; Kaneko, A. Introduction to Kampo medicine for dental treatment—Oral pharmacotherapy that utilizes the advantages of Western and Kampo medicines. *Jpn. Dent. Sci. Rev.* **2018**, *54*, 197–204. [CrossRef]
7. Kato, S.; Saito, A.; Matsuda, N.; Suzuki, H.; Ujiie, M.; Sato, S.; Miyazaki, K.; Kodama, T.; Satoh, H. Management of afatinib-induced stomatitis. *Mol. Clin. Oncol.* **2017**, *6*, 603–605. [CrossRef]
8. Zhou, P.; Mao, Q.; Hua, H.; Liu, X.; Yan, Z. Efficacy and safety of Chinese patent medicines in the treatment of recurrent aphthous stomatitis: A systematic review. *J. Am. Dent. Assoc.* **2017**, *148*, 17–25. [CrossRef]
9. Takeda, H.; Sadakane, C.; Hattori, T.; Katsurada, T.; Ohkawara, T.; Nagai, K.; Asaka, M. Rikkunshito, an herbal medicine, suppresses cisplatin-induced anorexia in rats via 5-HT2 receptor antagonism. *Gastroenterology* **2008**, *134*, 2004–2013. [CrossRef]
10. Kono, T.; Suzuki, Y.; Mizuno, K.; Miyagi, C.; Omiya, Y.; Sekine, H.; Mizuhara, Y.; Miyano, K.; Kase, Y.; Uezono, Y. Preventive effect of oral goshajinkigan on choronic oxaliplatin-induced hypoesthesia in rats. *Sci. Rep.* **2015**, *5*, 16078. [CrossRef]
11. Kono, T.; Kaneko, A.; Matsumoto, C.; Miyagi, C.; Ohbuchi, K.; Mizuhara, Y.; Miyano, K.; Uezono, Y. Multitargeted effects of hangeshashinto for treatment of chemotherapy-induced oral mucositis on inducible prostaglandin E2 production in human oral keratinocytes. *Integr. Cancer Ther.* **2014**, *13*, 435–445. [CrossRef]
12. Matsumoto, C.; Sekine-Suzuki, E.; Nyui, M.; Ueno, M.; Nakanishi, I.; Omiya, Y.; Fukutake, M.; Kase, Y.; Matsumoto, K. Analysis of the antioxidative function of the radioprotective Japanese traditional (Kampo) medicine, hangeshashinto, in an aqueous phase. *J. Radiat. Res.* **2015**, *56*, 669–677. [CrossRef] [PubMed]
13. Terasawa, K. Evidence-based reconstruction of Kampo medicine: Part II—theconcept of Sho. *Evid. Based Complement. Altern. Med.* **2004**, *1*, 119–123. [CrossRef]

14. Horie, N.; Hashimoto, K.; Hino, S.; Kato, T.; Shimoyama, T.; Kaneko, T.; Kusama, K.; Sakagami, H. Anti-inflammatory potential of Rikkosan based on IL-1β network through macrophages to oral tissue cells. *In Vivo* **2014**, *28*, 563–569. [PubMed]

15. Yamaguchi, K. Traditional Japanese herbal medicines for treatment of odontopathy. *Front. Pharmacol.* **2015**, *6*, 176. [CrossRef]

16. Numata, T.; Gunfan, S.; Takayama, S.; Takahashi, S.; Monma, Y.; Kaneko, S.; Kuroda, H.; Tanaka, J.; Kanemura, S.; Nara, M.; et al. Treatment of posttraumatic stress disorder using the traditional Japanese herbal medicine saikokeishikankyoto: A randomized, observer-blinded, controlled trial in survivors of the great East Japan earthquake and tsunami. *Evid. Based Complement. Altern. Med.* **2014**, *2014*, 683293. [CrossRef]

17. Oka, S. The effects of Oren-to on Stomatitis. *Pharm. Med.* **2007**, *25*, 35–38. (In Japanese)

18. Sunagawa, M.; Yamaguchi, K.; Tsukada, M.; Ebihara, N.; Ikemoto, H.; Hisamitsu, T. Kampo (traditional Japanese herbal) formulae for treatment of stomatitis and oral mucositis. *Medicines (Basel)* **2018**, *5*, 130. [CrossRef] [PubMed]

19. Yamashita, T.; Araki, K.; Tomifuji, M.; Kamide, D.; Tanaka, Y.; Shiotani, A. A traditional Japanese medicine–Hangeshashinto (TJ-14)–alleviates chemoradiation-induced mucositis and improves rates of treatment completion. *Support Care Cancer* **2015**, *23*, 29–35. [CrossRef]

20. Ohnishi, S.; Takeda, H. Herbal medicines for the treatment of cancer chemotherapy-induced side effects. *Front. Pharmacol.* **2015**, *6*, 14. [CrossRef]

21. Sakagami, H. Chapter 1. Introductory chaper: Fugure prespect of licorice, popular crude drug and food sweetener. In *Biological Activities and Action Mechanisms of Licorice Ingredients*; Intech: Houston, TX, USA, 2017; pp. 3–12. ISBN 978-953-51-5195-1.

22. Kato, T.; Segami, N.; Sakagami, H. Anti-inflammatory activity of hangeshashinto in IL-1β-stimulated gingival and periodontal ligament fibroblasts. *In Vivo* **2016**, *30*, 257–264. [PubMed]

23. Ara, T.; Sogawa, N. Effects of shinbuto and ninjinto on prostaglandin E2 production in lipopolysaccharide-treated human gingival fibroblasts. *PeerJ* **2017**, *5*, e4120. [CrossRef]

24. Kato, T.; Horie, N.; Matsuta, T.; Umemura, N.; Shimoyama, T.; Kaneko, T.; Kanamoto, T.; Terakubo, S.; Nakashima, H.; Kusama, K.; et al. Anti-UV/HIV activity of Kampo medicines and constituent plant extracts. *In Vivo* **2012**, *26*, 1007–1013. [PubMed]

25. Ohno, H.; Miyoshi, S.; Araho, D.; Kanamoto, T.; Terakubo, S.; Nakashima, H.; Tsuda, T.; Sunaga, K.; Amano, S.; Ohkoshi, E.; et al. Efficient utilization of licorice root by alkaline extraction. *In Vivo* **2014**, *28*, 785–794. [PubMed]

26. Sakagami, H.; Sheng, H.; Yasui, T.; Fukuchi, K.; Oizumi, T.; Ohno, H.; Yamamoto, M.; Fukuda, T.; Kotohda, K.; Yoshida, H.; et al. Chapter 18. Therapeutic potential of solubilized nanolignin against oral diseases. In *Nanostructures for Oral Medicicne*; Elsevier: New York, NY, USA, 2017; pp. 545–576. ISBN 978-0-323-47720-8.

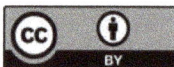

medicines

MDPI

Review

The Biological Efficacy of Natural Products against Acute and Chronic Inflammatory Diseases in the Oral Region

Toshiaki Ara [1], Sachie Nakatani [2], Kenji Kobata [2], Norio Sogawa [1] and Chiharu Sogawa [3,*]

[1]   Department of Dental Pharmacology, Matsumoto Dental University, 1780 Gobara Hirooka,
     Shiojiri 399-0781, Japan; toshiaki.ara@mdu.ac.jp (T.A.); norio.sogawa@mdu.ac.jp (N.S.)
[2]   Faculty of Pharmacy and Pharmaceutical Sciences, Josai University, 1-1 Keyakidai, Sakado,
     Saitama 350-0295, Japan; s-nakata@josai.ac.jp (S.N); kobata@josai.ac.jp (K.K.)
[3]   Department of Dental Pharmacology, Okayama University Graduate School of Medicine, Dentistry and
     Pharmaceutical Sciences, 2-5-1 Shikata-cho, Okayama 700-8525, Japan
*   Correspondence: caoki@md.okayama-u.ac.jp; Tel.: +81-86-235-6661

Received: 26 October 2018; Accepted: 8 November 2018; Published: 13 November 2018

Abstract: The oral inflammatory diseases are divided into two types: acute and chronic inflammatory diseases. In this review, we summarize the biological efficacy of herbal medicine, natural products, and their active ingredients against acute and chronic inflammatory diseases in the oral region, especially stomatitis and periodontitis. We review the effects of herbal medicines and a biscoclaurin alkaloid preparation, cepharamthin, as a therapy against stomatitis, an acute inflammatory disease. We also summarize the effects of herbal medicines and natural products against periodontitis, a chronic inflammatory disease, and one of its clinical conditions, alveolar bone resorption. Recent studies show that several herbal medicines such as kakkonto and ninjinto reduce LPS-induced PGE_2 production by human gingival fibroblasts. Among herbs constituting these herbal medicines, shokyo (*Zingiberis Rhizoma*) and kankyo (*Zingiberis Processsum Rhizoma*) strongly reduce PGE_2 production. Moreover, anti-osteoclast activity has been observed in some natural products with anti-inflammatory effects used against rheumatoid arthritis such as carotenoids, flavonoids, limonoids, and polyphenols. These herbal medicines and natural products could be useful for treating oral inflammatory diseases.

Keywords: inflammatory disease; stomatitis; periodontitis; anti-osteoclast activity; cepharanthin; herbal medicine; natural product; arachidonic acid cascade

1. Introduction

Oral inflammatory disease is a general term for the inflammatory lesions developed in oral mucosa. The pathogenesis of oral inflammatory diseases is non-uniform due to the involvement of various factors—such as external and mechanical stimuli, the presence of microorganisms, and the overall physical conditions—that play a role in the onset of inflammation. There is a wide range of variations in the aspect of oral inflammatory diseases, and the aspect is unequal. Therefore, we construed the oral inflammatory diseases as a symptom of inflammation, and categorized them into acute and chronic inflammatory diseases. In the oral region, the representative example of acute inflammatory diseases is stomatitis (also named as oral mucositis), and that of chronic inflammatory diseases is periodontitis. Several Japanese herbal medicines (also known as kampo medicines) are clinically used for the treatment of inflammatory diseases. Recent reviews have summarized the therapeutic application of herbal medicines for oral diseases such as stomatitis and periodontitis [1]. For example, hangeshashinto (TJ-14) is used for inflammatory diseases such as acute or chronic gastrointestinal catarrh, nervous gastritis and stomatitis.

In this review, we aim to summarize the biological efficacy of herbal medicine, natural products, and their active ingredients against acute and chronic inflammatory diseases in the oral region, especially stomatitis and periodontitis.

2. Biological Efficacy of Natural Products against Acute Inflammatory Disease: Stomatitis

2.1. Stomatitis (Oral Mucositis)

Stomatitis is an inflammatory condition of the oral and oropharyngeal mucosa with both pain and ulcers in severe cases. The causes of stomatitis is classified into (1) bacterial or viral infection, (2) chemotherapy and/or radiation for the treatment of cancers, (3) autoimmune disease (such as lichen planus and pemphigus vulgaris), and (4) unknown (such as recurrent aphthous stomatitis). Recurrent aphthous stomatitis is a common condition characterized by the repeated formation of benign and non-contagious mouth ulcers (aphthae). However, the cause of aphthous stomatitis is still unknown.

2.2. Effect of Hangeshashinto on Stomatitis

Recently, clinical administration of herbal medicine, such as the treatment of recurrent aphthous stomatitis, has been increasing in Japan. Herbal medicines are chosen according to the patient's condition, called "sho" (pattern), for example "excess pattern" or "deficiency pattern." Among the herbal medicines, some products such as hangeshashinto (TJ-14), orengedokuto (TJ-15), orento (TJ-120), inchinkoto (TJ-135), byakkokaninjinto (TJ-34), juzentaihoto (TJ-48), and shosaikoto (TJ-9) are selected in the treatment against oral inflammatory diseases, including recurrent aphthous stomatitis, according to the patient's pattern [2]. In addition, it seems that hangeshashinto is considered effective in the treatment of stomatitis caused by anti-tumor agents and radiation therapy [2].

In a preliminary study, rinsing with hangeshashinto reduced the grade of stomatitis [by Common Terminology Criteria for Adverse Events (CTCAE) version 4.0, National Cancer Institute, Bethesda, MD] [3]. Moreover, in a double-blind, placebo-controlled, random, phase II study, the rinsing of the oral cavity with hangeshashinto showed a trend to reduce the risk of chemotherapy-induced stomatitis in patients with gastric cancer [4]. In this study, hangeshashinto reduced the risk of grade 1 stomatitis but did not reduce those of more than grade 2 [4]. In a retrospective study, rinsing and gargling with hangeshashinto prevented grade 3/4 stomatitis induced by (chemo)radiation in patients with head and neck cancers (odds ratio = 0.21, 95% CI: 0.045–0.780, hangeshashinto: $n = 27$, placebo: $n = 32$) [5]. In addition, hangeshashinto also improved the rates of the treatment of stomatitis [5].

In an animal model, free intake of diet mixed with 2% hangeshashinto prevented radiation-induced mucositis within the buccal mucosa in hamsters [6]. In addition, hangeshashinto inhibited the infiltration of neutrophils and COX-2 expression in irradiated buccal mucosa [6]. Moreover, in an in vitro study using oral keratinocytes, hangeshashinto was suggested to be effective in the treatment of chemotherapy-induced stomatitis [7]. As just described, hangeshashinto is effective for the improvement of stomatitis although there is little evidence in in vivo and in vitro studies.

2.3. Effect of Cepharanthin® on Stomatitis

A biscoclaurin alkaloid preparation, Cepharanthin® (CE), has also been used for the cure of oral mucosal disease, such as recurrent aphthous stomatitis, leukoplakia, and oral lichen planus. CE is a drug product, prepared from extracts of *Stephania cephalantha* Hayata, and has been widely used for several decades to treat a range of acute and chronic diseases in Japan [8,9]. As CE is reported to elicit an anti-inflammatory effect and increase blood stem cell count, immuno-enhancing effects, and anti-allergic properties, it has seen clinical application against inflammatory diseases as well as post-radiation-therapy leukocytopenia, pit viper bite, alopecia areata, and bronchial asthma. Nakase et al. reported that the rate of excellent or moderate efficacy was 100% for aphthous stomatitis and 25.0% for reducing the size of oral lichen planus, and its efficacy for glossodynia was 83.4% by CE treatment with gargle-internal use (15 mg/day) for two weeks [10]. Moreover, Saki et al. also reported—regarding the efficacy of CE against these oral mucosal diseases— that the improvement rate by oral administration of CE (20 mg/day) for 4 weeks or more was 83.3% for aphthous stomatitis, 87.0% for oral lichen planus, 77.8% for glossodynia, and 80.0% for leukoplakia. In this case, they evaluated the clinical response and rated according to the assessment points such as the degrees of pain, ulcer, erosion, and erythema [11]. Taken together, it is considered that CE is beneficial in the cure of aphthous stomatitis, according to previous clinical reports [12].

CE is a biscoclaurin alkaloid preparation, and the main active ingredients are four alkaloids: cepharanthine (26%), isotetrandrine (32%), berbamine (13%), and cycleanine (10%) (Figure 1). Using a mixture of these four active ingredients in CE exhibits almost an equal effect as that of CE [13,14]. Functional mechanisms of CE and its main active ingredients for inflammatory diseases have been reported in previous studies. For example, CE reduced the production of superoxide anion (O_2^-) by neutrophils [15] and by macrophages [16], and decreased the levels of several types of reactive oxygen species (O_2^-, H_2O_2, OH·) by behaving as a reactive oxygen species (ROS) scavenger [17].

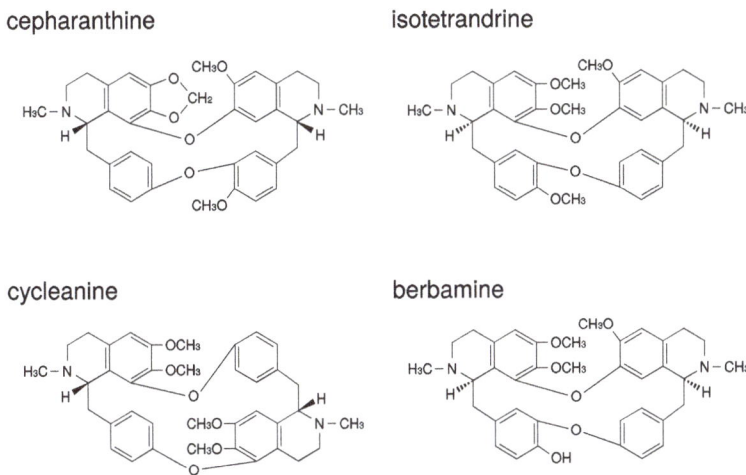

Figure 1. The structures of active ingredients in Cepharanthin®.

According to previous literatures corresponding to the application of the four main active ingredients, cepharanthine was reported to inhibit the synthesis of leukotriene B4 through the reduction of arachidonic acid release [18]. Moreover, each of the four main active ingredients reduced NO production by activated macrophages [19]. However, there was a difference in the efficacy against the O_2^- and TNF-α production among main active ingredients; the efficacy of cepharanthine and isotetrandrine seemed to be more than that of berbamine and cycleanine in the reduction of O_2^- production by neutrophils [20]. It was also reported that cepharanthine, isotetrandrine, and cycleanine, but not berbamine, significantly reduced the level of TNF-α or acute lethal toxicity induced by lipopolysaccharide (LPS) in mice [13,21]. Additionally, Matsuno et al. reported that the decreasing effect of O_2^- production through neutrophil stimulation by arachidonic acid and N-formylmethionine-leucyl-phenylalanine (FMLP) was more evident in cepharanthine than in opsonized zymogen [20]. This finding indicates the cell membrane to be a possible operating point of CE, and this hypothesis is supported in the following study by Sugiyama et al., who reported that cepharanthine could inhibit histamine release from mast cells through the stabilization of the membrane by decreasing membrane fluidity via interaction with the lipid bilayer of the cell membrane [22].

Interestingly, the pharmacological actions of CE on living bodies vary depending on the method of administration. We reported that the single injection of CE reduced the LPS-induced histidine decarboxylase (HDC) activity, although contrastingly, LPS-induced HDC activity in mice spleens increased after consecutive administration of CE [23]. Moreover, it was considered that mast cell was closely associated with this reduction of HDC activity, because LPS-induced HDC activity in mast-cell-deficient mice increased, but decreased in normal mice following a single administration of CE [23]. CE has immuno-enhancing effects as well as anti-inflammatory effects. The inhibition of mast cells may be closely related to the difference of CE action.

Conclusively, CE is considered to be an effective treatment of oral inflammatory diseases, such as recurrent aphthous stomatitis, through the reduction of various function in immunocytes closely related to inflammation.

3. Biological Efficacy of Natural Products against Chronic Inflammatory Disease; Periodontitis

3.1. Periodontitis

Periodontal disease (periodontitis) comprises a group of infections that leads to inflammation of the gingiva and destruction of periodontal tissues, and is accompanied by alveolar bone loss in severe clinical cases. The tissue destruction is the result of activation of the host's immuno-inflammatory response to virulent factors such as LPS and peptidoglycan. In inflammatory responses and tissue degradation, prostaglandin E_2 (PGE_2), interleukin (IL)-6, and IL-8 play important roles. As PGE_2 has several functions in vasodilation, the enhancement of vascular permeability and pain, and osteoclastogenesis induction, PGE_2 participates in inflammatory responses and alveolar bone resorption in periodontitis [24].

Generally, periodontitis is a chronic inflammation, and the elimination of these virulent factors by initial preparation is very important for the treatment of periodontitis. However, during the acute advanced stage, non-steroidal anti-inflammatory drugs (NSAIDs) are administrated to improve gingival inflammation. In fact, many studies have demonstrated that systemic administration of acid NSAIDs prevented gingival inflammation and alveolar bone resorption in animals and humans [25]. However, acid NSAIDs are well known to have side effects such as gastrointestinal dysfunction and bronchoconstriction. Therefore, the usage of alternative agents is necessary for patients with gastrointestinal ulcer or bronchial asthma. Previously, we suggested that several herbal medicines are effective for the improvement of periodontitis. In this review, we focused on the anti-inflammatory effects of herbal medicines on mainly periodontitis —in particular, about the effects on human gingival fibroblasts (HGFs). In addition, we summarized the effects of ingredients in herbs and their mechanism against arachidonic acid cascade.

Here, we will explain the importance of HGFs in the study of periodontitis. (1) HGFs are the most prominent cells in periodontal tissue. LPS-treated HGFs produce inflammatory chemical mediators, such as PGE_2, and inflammatory cytokines such as IL-6 and IL-8. (2) More importantly, unlike macrophages, HGFs continue to produce PGE_2 [26], IL-6, and IL-8 [27] in the presence of LPS. From these findings, the large amount of chemical mediators and cytokines derived from HGFs may be contained in periodontal tissues. Therefore, we believe that examining the effects of pharmaceuticals on HGFs is needed in the study of periodontitis.

3.2. Brief Summary of Arachidonic Acid Cascade

At first, we explain arachidonic acid cascade briefly, focusing on sites of action for herbs and ingredients. PGE_2 is produced by arachidonic acid cascade (Figure 2). Phospholipids in plasma membrane are digested by phospholipase A_2 (PLA_2), producing arachidonic acid. Cyclooxygenases (COXs) convert arachidonic acid into PGH_2, and thereafter PGE synthase converts into PGE_2.

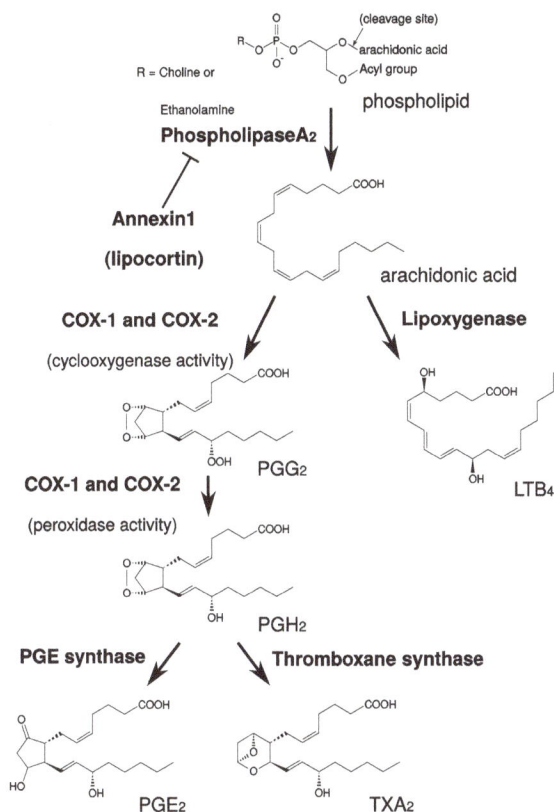

Figure 2. Simplified schema of arachidonic acid cascade.

PLA$_2$ is the most upstream enzyme in the arachidonic acid cascade and releases arachidonic acid from the plasma membrane. PLA$_2$ forms a superfamily and is classified into cytosolic PLA$_2$ (cPLA$_2$), calcium-independent PLA$_2$ (iPLA$_2$), secretory PLA$_2$ (sPLA$_2$), and others [28]. Among these isoforms, cPLA$_2$ is the primary isoform in HGFs from the results using PLA$_2$ inhibitors [29]. cPLA$_2$ activity is directly regulated by extracellular signal-regulated kinase (ERK). The active form of ERK (phosphorylated ERK) phosphorylates Ser505 of cPLA$_2$ and activates cPLA$_2$ [30–32]. Therefore, the suppression of ERK phosphorylation leads to the suppression of cPLA$_2$ activation and the reduction of PGE$_2$ production [30–32]. In contrast, annexin1, also named as lipocortin, is an anti-inflammatory mediator produced by steroidal anti-inflammatory drugs (SAIDs) that inhibits PLA$_2$ activity [33,34].

COX is classified into COX-1 and COX-2. COX-1 is constitutive expressed at low level, and is involved in normal functions such as protection of gastric mucosa. In contrast, COX-2 is induced by the various stimuli such as LPS and peptidoglycan, and involved in inflammatory response. The expression of COX-2 is upregulated by NF-κB. The reduction of PGE$_2$ by anti-inflammatory drugs is one of the important mechanisms. Acid NSAIDs inhibit both COX-1 and COX-2 activities. The inhibition of COX-2 improve inflammatory response, while the inhibition of COX-1 causes gastric irritation. SAIDs also have powerful anti-inflammatory effects, and inhibit NF-κB activity and suppress COX-2 expression.

Recently, protein kinase A (PKA) pathway is reported to regulate LPS-induce PGE$_2$ production in HGFs [35]. PKA inhibitor (H-89) reduced LPS-induced PGE$_2$ production in a concentration-dependent manner. In contrast, PKA activator (dibutyryl cAMP; dbcAMP) and drugs which increased intracellular cAMP (adrenaline and aminophylline) increased LPS-induced PGE$_2$ production in a concentration-dependent manner. However, the effects of PKA pathway on arachidonic acid cascade have not been examined in this report [35].

3.3. Effect of Herbal Medicines on Periosontal Disease

Similar to NSAIDs, several herbal medicines also reduce PGE_2 production. Examples of herbal medicine which have been reported to reduce PGE_2 production in in vitro and/or animal models are shown in Table 1. In particular, we reported that kakkonto (TJ-1), shosaikoto (TJ-9), hangeshashinto (TJ-14), shinbuto (TJ-30), ninjinto (TJ-32), and orento (TJ-120) reduced LPS-induced PGE_2 production using HGFs [36–40]. Other groups have also demonstrated that several herbal medicines reduced PGE_2 production using human periodontal ligament cells [41], human monocytes [42], mouse macrophage RAW264.7 cells [43,44], human oral keratinocytes [7], and animals [45–48].

Table 1. Japanese traditional herbal medicines which are reported to reduce PGE_2 production.

Herbal Medicine	Cells or Animal	References
kakkonto (TJ-1)	HGFs	[36]
shosaikoto (TJ-9)	HGFs	[37]
	human monocytes	[42]
	mouse	[45]
hangeshashinto (TJ-14)	HGFs	[38,41]
	human periodontal ligament cells	[41]
	human oral keratinocytes	[7]
	rat	[46–48]
shinbuto (TJ-30)	HGFs	[39]
ninjinto (TJ-32)	HGFs	[39]
rikkosan (TJ-110)	RAW264.7	[43]
saireito (TJ-114)	RAW264.7	[44]
orento (TJ-120)	HGFs	[40]

We introduce briefly the effects and mechanisms of herbal medicines on periodontitis in clinical, animal, and/or in vitro studies. Moreover, in this section, we will demonstrate the effects of herbal medicines on the reduction of PGE_2 in HGFs. From our data, the mechanisms of these herbal medicines on arachidonic acid cascade are divided into three groups as follows.

- Shosaikoto (TJ-9) inhibited COX-2 activity and suppressed COX-2 expression, but did not alter $cPLA_2$ expression (the effects on annexin1 expression and ERK phosphorylation were not examined) [37]. Hangeshashinto (TJ-14) inhibited both COX-1 and COX-2 activities, and suppressed $cPLA_2$ and COX-2 expressions and ERK phosphorylation [38]. Therefore, these herbal medicines are suggested to inhibit arachidonic acid cascade at multiple points.
- Shinbuto (TJ-30) and ninjinto (TJ-32) enhanced annexin1 expression, but did not alter ERK phosphorylation and COX activity [39]. However, the contribution of enhancement of annexin1 expression is considered to be small because shokyo, which is the main herb in shinbuto to reduce PGE_2 production, did not affect annexin1 expression.
- Kakkonto (TJ-1) suppressed ERK phosphorylation, but neither inhibited COXs activities nor suppressed the expression of molecules in arachidonic acid cascade [36]. In addition, orento (TJ-120) suppressed ERK phosphorylation, but neither inhibited COXs activities nor suppressed the expression of molecules in arachidonic acid cascade, but rather increased COX-2 expression [40]. However, its contribution in the suppression of ERK phosphorylation is considered to be small as described at keihi (*Cinnamomi Cortex*). Indeed, we did not examine the direct effect of herbal medicines on $cPLA_2$ activity. Nevertheless, we consider that these herbal medicines inhibit $cPLA_2$ activity and that this effect is due to shokyo (*Zingiberis Rhizoma*) and kankyo (*Zingiberis Processum Rhizoma*) as described below.

3.4. Effect of Herbs on Arachidonic Acid Cascade

Next, we will demonstrate the experimental results at the herb level. The ingredients in the formula of herbal medicines that were used are shown in Tables 2–7. In our experiments at the herb level, shokyo (*Zingiberis Rhizoma*), kankyo (*Zingiberis Processum Rhizoma*), kanzo (*Glycyrrhizae Radix*), and keihi (*Cinnamomi Cortex*) reduced PGE_2 production (Figures 3 and 4) [29,39]. We summarized major ingredients in herbs and their mechanism against arachidonic acid cascade in Table 8. In addition to these four herbs, ogon (*Scutellariae Radix*), and oren (*Coptidis Rhizoma*) are shown in Table 8 because ogon (included in shosaikoto and hangeshashinto) and oren (included in hangeshashinto and orento) also have several bioactive ingredients such as flavonoids, saponin, and chalcones. We will describe the effects and mechanisms of these herbs, particularly shokyo and kankyo, on arachidonic cascade.

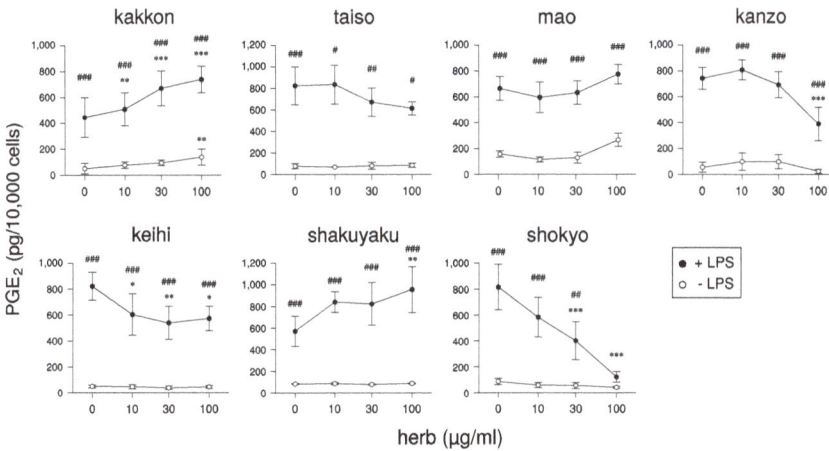

Figure 3. The effect of herbs in kakkonto (TJ-1) on PGE_2 production: This figure is cited from Ara and Sogawa [29] (CC-BY-4.0) and modified for this review.

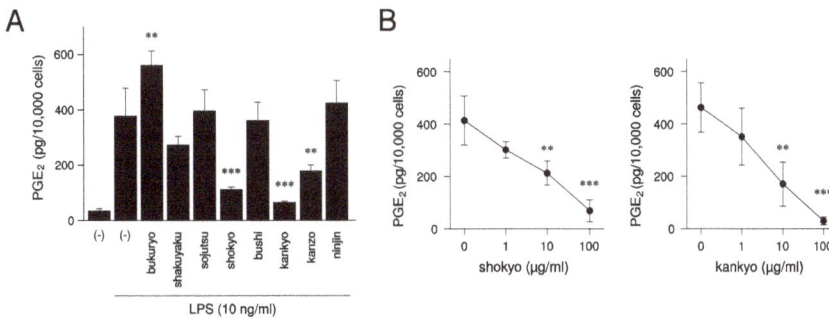

Figure 4. The effect of herbs in shinbuto (TJ-30) and ninjinto (TJ-32) on PGE_2 production: This figure is cited from Ara and Sogawa [39] (CC-BY-4.0) and modified for this review. (**A**): Effect of each herb, (**B**): Concentration-dependent effects of shokyo and kankyo.

Table 2. The ingredients in the kakkonto (TJ-1) formula.

Japanese Name (Latin Name)	Scientific Name	Amount (g)	Amount * (g/g of Product)
kakkon (*Puerariae Radix*)	*Pueraria lobata* Ohwi	4.0	0.111
taiso (*Zizyphi Fructus*)	*Ziziphus jujuba* Miller var. *inermis* Rehder	3.0	0.083
mao (*Ephedrae Herba*)	*Ephedra sinica* Stapf *Ephedra intermedia* Schrenk et C.A.Meyer *Ephedra equisetina* Bunge	3.0	0.083
kanzo (*Glycyrrhizae Radix*)	*Glycyrrhiza uralensis* Fischer *Glycyrrhiza glabra* Linné	2.0	0.056
keihi (*Cinnamomi Cortex*)	*Cinnamomum cassia* Blume	2.0	0.056
shyakuyaku (*Paeoniae Radix*)	*Paeonia lactiflora* Pallas	2.0	0.056
shokyo (*Zingiberis Rhizoma*)	*Zingiber officinale* Roscoe	2.0	0.056
total		18.0	0.500

* 7.5 g of kakkonto product contains 3.75 g of a dried extract of the mixed crude drugs.

Table 3. The ingredients in the shosaikoto (TJ-9) formula.

Japanese Name (Latin Name)	Scientific Name	Amount (g)	Amount * (g/g of Product)
saiko (*Bupleuri Radix*)	*Bupleurum falcatum* Linné	7.0	0.175
hange (*Pinelliae tuber*)	*Pinellia ternata* Breitenbach	5.0	0.125
ogon (*Scutellariae radix*)	*Scutellaria baicalensis* Georgi	3.0	0.075
taiso (*Zizyphi Fructus*)	*Ziziphus jujuba* Miller var. *inermis* Rehder	3.0	0.075
ninjin (*Ginseng Radix*)	*Panax ginseng* C.A. Meyer	3.0	0.075
kanzo (*Glycyrrhizae Radix*)	*Glycyrrhiza uralensis* Fischer *Glycyrrhiza glabra* Linné	2.0	0.050
shokyo (*Zingiberis Rhizoma*)	*Zingiber officinale* Roscoe	1.0	0.025
total		24.0	0.600

* 7.5 g of shosaikoto product contains 4.5 g of a dried extract of the mixed crude drugs.

Table 4. The ingredients in the hangeshashinto (TJ-14) formula.

Japanese Name (Latin Name)	Scientific Name	Amount (g)	Amount * (g/g of Product)
hange (*Pinelliae tuber*)	*Pinellia ternata* Breitenbach	5.0	0.162
ogon (*Scutellariae radix*)	*Scutellaria baicalensis* Georgi	2.5	0.081
kankyo (*Zingiberis Processum Rhizoma*)	*Zingiber officinale* Roscoe	2.5	0.081
kanzo (*Glycyrrhizae Radix*)	*Glycyrrhiza uralensis* Fischer *Glycyrrhiza glabra* Linné	2.5	0.081
taiso (*Zizyphi Fructus*)	*Ziziphus jujuba* Miller var. *inermis* Rehder	2.5	0.081
ninjin (*Ginseng Radix*)	*Panax ginseng* C.A. Meyer	2.5	0.081
oren (*Coptidis rhizoma*)	*Coptis japonica* Makino *Coptis chinensis* Franchet *Coptis deltoidea* C. Y. Cheng et Hsiao *Coptis teeta* Wallich	1.0	0.032
total		18.5	0.600

* 7.5 g of hangeshashinto product contains 4.5 g of a dried extract of the mixed crude drugs.

Table 5. The ingredients in the shinbuto (TJ-30) formula.

Japanese Name (Latin Name)	Scientific Name	Amount (g)	Amount * (g/g of Product)
bukuryo (*Poria Sclerotium*)	*Wolfiporia cocos* Ryvarden et Gilbertson (*Poria cocos* Wolf)	4.0	0.089
shakuyaku (*Paeoniae Radix*)	*Paeonia lactiflora* Pallas	3.0	0.067
sojutsu (*Atractylodis Lanceae Rhizoma*)	*Atractylodes lancea* De Candolle *Atractylodes schinensis* Koidzumi	3.0	0.067
shokyo (*Zingiberis Rhizoma*)	*Zingiber officinale* Roscoe	1.5	0.033
bushi (*Processi Aconiti Radix*)	*Aconitum carmichaeli* Debeaux *Aconitum japonicum* Thunberg	0.5	0.011
total		12.0	0.267

* 7.5 g of shinbuto product contains 2.0 g of a dried extract of the mixed crude drugs.

Table 6. The ingredients in the ninjinto (TJ-32) formula.

Japanese Name (Latin Name)	Scientific Name	Amount (g)	Amount * (g/g of Product)
kankyo (*Zingiberis Processum Rhizoma*)	*Zingiber officinale* Roscoe	3.0	0.083
kanzo (*Glycyrrhizae Radix*)	*Glycyrrhiza uralensis* Fischer *Glycyrrhiza glabra* Linné	3.0	0.083
sojutsu (*Atractylodis Lanceae Rhizoma*)	*Atractylodes lancea* De Candolle *Atractylodes schinensis* Koidzumi	3.0	0.083
ninjin (*Ginseng Radix*)	*Panax ginseng* C.A. Meyer	3.0	0.083
total		12.0	0.333

* 7.5 g of ninjinto product contains 2.5 g of a dried extract of the mixed crude drugs.

Table 7. The ingredients in the orento (TJ-120) formula.

Japanese Name (Latin Name)	Scientific Name	Amount (g)	Amount * (g/g of Product)
hange (*Pinelliae tuber*)	*Pinellia ternata* Breitenbach	6.0	0.133
oren (*Coptidis rhizoma*)	*Coptis japonica* Makino *Coptis chinensis* Franchet *Coptis deltoidea* C. Y. Cheng et Hsiao *Coptis teeta* Wallich	3.0	0.067
kankyo (*Zingiberis Processum Rhizoma*)	*Zingiber officinale* Roscoe	3.0	0.067
kanzo (*Glycyrrhizae Radix*)	*Glycyrrhiza uralensis* Fischer *Glycyrrhiza glabra* Linné	3.0	0.067
keihi (*Cinnamomi Cortex*)	*Cinnamomum cassia* Blume	3.0	0.067
taiso (*Zizyphi Fructus*)	*Ziziphus jujuba* Miller var. *inermis* Rehder	3.0	0.067
ninjin (*Ginseng Radix*)	*Panax ginseng* C.A. Meyer	3.0	0.067
total		24.0	0.533

* 7.5 g of orento product contains 4.0 g of a dried extract of the mixed crude drugs.

Table 8. Major ingredients in herbs and their mechanism against arachidonic acid cascade.

Herb	Ingredients	Mechanisms	References
shokyo/kankyo	gingerol, shogaol	inhibition of COX-2 activity suppression of COX-2 expression suppression of NF-κB activation inhibition of PLA$_2$ activity	[49,50] [7,51–54] [52–56] [57]
kanzo	glycyrrhizin	suppression of COX-2 expression suppression of NF-κB activation inhibition of TLR4 homodimerization	[58–60] [61] [62]
	isoliquiritigenin	suppression of COX-2 expression suppression of NF-κB activation inhibition of TLR4 homodimerization	[58,63,64] [64] [62]
	liquiritin	suppression of COX-2 expression	[58]
keihi	cinnamic aldehyde	suppression of COX-2 expression suppression of NF-κB activation inhibition of COX-activity inhibition of TLR4 oligomerization	[65,66] [67] [68] [69]
ogon	baicalin	suppression of COX-2 expression suppression of NF-κB activation	[7,70] [70]
	baicalein	suppression of COX-2 expression suppression of NF-κB activation	[7,71] [72]
	wogonin	suppression of COX-2 expression suppression of MAPK [a] phosphorylation	[7,73,74] [7]
oren	berberin	suppression of COX-2 expression suppression of NF-κB activation suppression of MAPK [a] phosphorylation enhancement of AMPK [b]	[75] [75] [76–79] [76–78]

[a] MAP kinases; [b] AMP-activated protein kinase.

3.4.1. Shokyo (*Zingiberis Rhizoma*)/Kankyo (*Zingiberis Processum Rhizoma*)

Shokyo is the powdered rhizome of *Zingiber officinale* Roscoe (ginger), and kankyo is the steamed and powdered rhizome of ginger. Both shokyo and kankyo are the aqueous extracts of ginger. Among the herbal medicines shown in Table 1, shokyo is included in kakkonto (TJ-1), shosaikoto (TJ-9), shinbuto (TJ-30), saireito (TJ-114), and orento (TJ-120), and kankyo is included in hangeshashinto (TJ-14) and ninjinto (TJ-32). Many reports have demonstrated that ginger possesses anti-inflammatory effects in human [80,81] and animal models [82–84], and in vitro [85]. Ginger has been widely used in diet and as a treatment for rheumatoid arthritis, fever, emesis, nausea, and migraine headache [80]. A recent systematic review shows that the extracts of ginger including turmeric, ginger, Javanese ginger, and galangal are clinically effective as hypoanalgesic agents [81]. In an animal model, the aqueous extract of ginger significantly reduced serum PGE_2 level by oral or intraperitoneal administration in rats [82]. Moreover, crude hydroalcoholic extract of ginger reduced the serum level of PGE_2, and improved tracheal hyperreactivity and lung inflammation induced by LPS in rats [83]. Ethanol extract of ginger reduced the tissue level of PGE_2, and improved acetic acid-induced ulcerative colitis in rats [84].

Gingerols and shogaols are the major ingredients in ginger. Their structures are indicated in Figure 5. With prolonged storage or heat-treatment of ginger, gingerols are converted to shogaols, which are the dehydrated form of the gingerols [80] (Figure 5). Therefore, kankyo contains a larger amount of shogaols than shokyo although both shokyo and kankyo contain gingerols and shogaols. In in vitro models, gingerols and shogaols have been reported to reduce PGE_2 production by several mechanisms. The effects of gingerols and shogaols on arachidonic acid cascade are briefly summarized in Table 8.

1. Gingerols and shogaols inhibit COX-2 activity. Their IC_{50} values were µM order: 6-gingerol (>50 µM), 8-gingerol (10.0 µM), 10-gingerol (3.7 µM), 6-shogaol (2.1 µM), and 8-shogaol (7.2 µM) in human lung adenocarcinoma A549 cells [49], and 10-gingerol (32.0 µM), 8-shogaol (17.5 µM), 10-shogaol (7.5 µM) in a cell-free assay [50].
2. Gingerols and shogaols suppress COX-2 expression. For example, 6-, 8-, and 10-gingerol suppressed COX-2 expression in LPS-treated human leukemic monocyte lymphoma U937 cells [51]. Similarly, 6-gingerol and 6-shogaol suppressed LPS-induced COX-2 expression in mouse macrophage RAW264.7 cells [52], mouse microglial BV-2 cells [53], and primary rat astrocytes [86]. 6-Gingerol suppressed COX-2 expression in TPA-treated mouse skin in vivo [54].
3. As aforementioned, the expression of COX-2 is regulated by NF-κB. Gingerols and shogaols are reported to suppress NF-κB activation, and to downregulate COX-2 expression. For example, 6-shogaol suppressed LPS-induced NF-κB activation in RAW264.7 cells [52], mouse primary cultured microglia cells [53], and human breast cancer MDA-MB-231 cells [56]. 6-Shogaol suppressed TPA-induced NF-κB activation in mouse skin [54]. Similarly, 6-gingerol suppressed *Vibrio cholerae*-induced NF-κB activation in human intestinal epithelial cells [55]. These results suggest that gingerols and shogaols suppress NF-κB activation directly or indirectly, leading to the inhibition of COX-2 expression.
4. Gingerols and shogaols inhibit PLA_2 activities [57]. In more detail, $iPLA_2$ activity was inhibited by 6-, 8-, and 10-gingerol and 6-, 8-, and 10-shogaol, whereas $cPLA_2$ activity was inhibited by 6-gingerol and 6-, 8-, and 10-shogaol. In particular, IC_{50} values of 10-shogaol against $iPLA_2$ and $cPLA_2$ were 0.7 µM and 3 µM, respectively, in U937 cells.

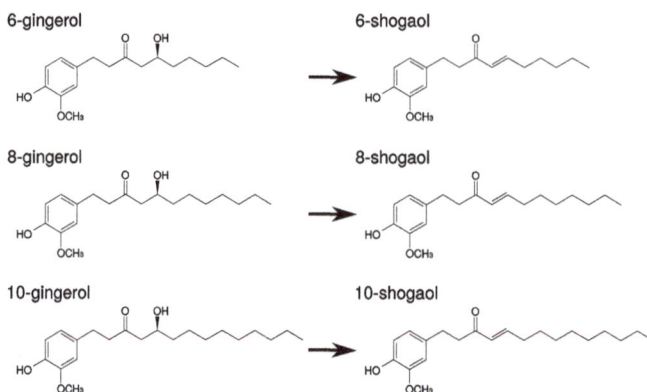

Figure 5. The structures of ingredients in shokyo (*Zingiberis Rhizoma*) and kankyo (*Zingiberis Processum Rhizoma*).

As aforementioned, many reports have examined the effects of ginger. However, there is little report using ginger as "shokyo" and "kankyo." For this reason, we examined the mechanism of the actions of shokyo and kankyo on the reduction of PGE_2 production in HGFs. Shokyo and kankyo concentration-dependently reduced LPS-induced PGE_2 production by HGFs, and the effects of kankyo were slightly stronger than those of shokyo (Figure 4) [39]. The effects of shokyo and kankyo on arachidonic cascade in HGFs are described as follows.

- Both shokyo and kankyo only slightly increased $cPLA_2$ expression, and did not alter annexin1 expression [39].
- Shokyo did not alter LPS-induced ERK phosphorylation in HGFs [29] (but we have not examined the effect of kankyo). Therefore, shokyo (and perhaps kankyo) may have little to no effect on $cPLA_2$ activation, and the subsequent arachidonic acid production.
- Both shokyo and kankyo did not inhibit COX-2 and PGE synthase activities, and did not alter LPS-induced COX-2 expression in HGFs [29,39]. These findings suggest shokyo and kankyo primarily inhibit $cPLA_2$ activity in HGFs. Although we have no direct data to show that shokyo and kankyo inhibit $cPLA_2$ activity, this assumption is consistent with the results that ginger (and gingerols/shogaols) inhibits both $iPLA_2$ and $cPLA_2$ activities [57].

As described above, our data that shokyo did not alter COX-2 activity and COX-2 expression are different from those of gingerols and shogaols in Table 8. Although there is no obvious evidence, the reason may be the preparation method of shokyo and kankyo. Gingerols and shogaols are extremely hydrophobic by their structures. These ingredients were extracted from hydrophobic phase, whereas shokyo and kankyo were prepared by decoction. Therefore, hydrophobic ingredients such as gingerol and shogaol are unlikely to be extracted, and their concentration might be lower than those in previous reports. Quantification of these ingredients is needed to explain these discrepancies.

3.4.2. Kanzo (*Glycyrrhizae Radix*)

Kanzo is the powdered root or stolon of *Glycyrrhiza uralensis* Fischer (licorice). Among the herbal medicines shown in Table 1, kanzo is included in kakkonto (TJ-1), shosaikoto (TJ-9), hangeshashinto (TJ-14), ninjinto (TJ-32), rikkosan (TJ-110), saireito (TJ-114), and orento (TJ-120). Licorice is also known to have anti-inflammatory effects [87] such as inhibition of COX-2 activity [46].

Licorice contains triperpene saponin such as glycyrrhizin (glycyrrhizin acid), and chalcones such as liquiritin and isoliquiritigenin. Their structures are indicated in Figure 6. Glycyrrhizin, liquiritin, and isoliquiritigenin are reported to reduce PGE_2 production. The effects of these ingredients on arachidonic acid cascade are briefly summarized in Table 8.

1. Glycyrrhizin suppressed COX-2 expression in LPS-treated mouse microglial BV2 cells [58] and uterus of ovariectominezed mice [59]. Moreover, orally administrated glycyrrhizin suppressed COX-2 expression in the cerebral cortex of LPS-treated mice [60]. Liquiritin and isoliquiritigenin also suppressed LPS-induced COX-2 expression in RAW264.7 cells [63] and BV2 cells [58].

2. Glycyrrhizin suppressed TNF-α or IL-1β-induced NF-κB activation in human lung epithelial A549 cells [61]. Isoliquiritigenin also suppressed NF-κB activity and suppressed LPS-induced COX-2 expression in RAW264.7 cells [64].

3. Glycyrrhizin and isoliquiritigenin inhibited TLR4 (receptor of LPS) homodimerization and downstream signal pathway [62], resulting in the suppression of COX-2 expression.

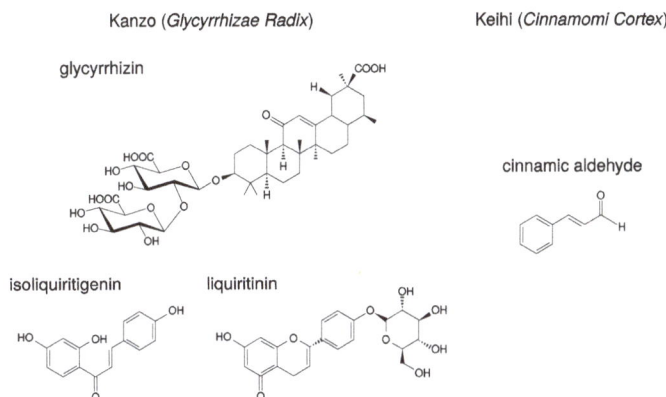

Figure 6. The structures of ingredients in kanzo (*Glycyrrhizae Radix*) and keihi (*Cinnamomi Cortex*).

Indeed, although glycyrrhizin has anti-inflammatory effects, glycyrrhizin is known to show a serious adverse effect, pseudohyperaldosteronism. Excessive dietary intake of licorice can cause a syndrome mimicking hypermineralocorticoidism, characterized by hypertension, hypokalemia, alkalosis, and reduced plasma renin [88–91]. Glycyrrhizin inhibits 11β-hydroxysteroid dehydrogenase type 2 (11β-HSD2), which converts active glucocorticoid cortisol to inactive cortisone [92]. This inhibition results in the activation of renal mineralocorticoid receptors by cortisol, inducing Na^+ reabsorption, K^+ excretion, hypertension, hypokalemia, and metabolic alkalosis. These phenotypes are similar to that of apparent mineralocorticoid excess syndrome. [91,93].

We examined the mechanism of the action of kanzo on the reduction of PGE_2 production in HGFs. However, the effects of kanzo on arachidonic acid cascade in HGFs cannot be explained by those of glycyrrhizin, liquiritin, and isoliquiritigenin.

- As reported previously [46], kanzo inhibited COX-2 activity because kanzo decreased LPS-induced PGE_2 production when arachidonic acid was added [29]. In contrast, kanzo did not inhibit PGE synthase activity because kanzo did not alter LPS-induced PGE_2 production when PGH_2 was added [29].

- Kanzo increased both $cPLA_2$ and annexin1 expressions [29], thus leaving the effect of kanzo on PLA_2 unconcluded.

- Kanzo increased LPS-induced COX-2 expression [29] although glycyrrhizin, liquiritin, and isoliquiritigenin suppressed COX-2 expression [58–60,63,64].
  This result is the same as those observed using orento [40] and saireito [44], which contain kanzo.

Therefore, these effects of kanzo were different from those of glycyrrhizin, liquiritin, and isoliquiritigenin, suggesting that other ingredients may contribute to our findings. In addition, not all herbal medicines which contain kanzo increased annexin1 as kakkonto, hangeshashinto, and orento did not alter annexin1 expression.

3.4.3. Keihi (*Cinnamomi Cortex*)

Keihi is the powdered bark of *Cinnamomum cassia* (cinnamon). Among the herbal medicines shown in Table 1, keihi is included in kakkonto (TJ-1), saireito (TJ-114), and orento (TJ-120). Cinnamon has been widely used for the treatment of fever and inflammation [28]. Cinnamon improves nephritis, purulent dermatitis, and hypertension, and it also enhances wound healing. Cinnamon extracts have been used for the improvement or prevention of common cold, diarrhea, and pain [28]. Ethanol-extract of *C. cassia* reduced LPS-induced PGE$_2$ production by RAW264.7 cells, and it suppressed NF-κB activity and the following COX-2 expression [66].

Keihi contains the ingredients such as cinnamic aldehyde, cinnamic alcohol, cinnamic acid, and coumarin. The structure of cinnamic aldehyde is indicated in Figure 6. Cinnamic aldehyde is reported to reduce PGE$_2$ production. The effects of cinnamic aldehyde on arachidonic acid cascade are briefly summarized in Table 8.

1. Cinnamic aldehyde suppressed carrageenan-induced COX-2 expression and improved footpad edema in mice [65]. Cinnamic aldehyde, but not others, suppressed LPS-induced COX-2 expression and decreased PGE$_2$ production by RAW264.7 cells [65,66].
2. Cinnamic aldehyde suppressed LPS-induced NF-κB activity in RAW264.7 cells and TLR4-expressing HEK293 cells [67].
3. Cinnamic aldehyde inhibited IL-1β-induced COX-2 activity in rat cerebral microvascular endothelial cells although its effect is weak [68].
4. Cinnamic aldehyde inhibited TLR4 oligomerization and downstream signal pathway, which include NF-κB. Sulfhydryl modification is suggested to be an important contributing factor for the regulation of TLR4 activation [69].

We examined the mechanism of action of keihi on the reduction of PGE$_2$ production in HGFs. However, the effects of keihi on arachidonic acid cascade in HGFs cannot be explained by that of cinnamic aldehyde.

- Keihi inhibited COX-2 activity because keihi decreased LPS-induced PGE$_2$ production when arachidonic acid is added [29]. This mechanism is accounted for by that of cinnamic aldehyde. In contrast, keihi did not inhibit PGE synthase activity as well as kanzo.
- As well as kakkonto [81] and orento [40], keihi suppressed ERK phosphorylation in LPS-treated HGFs [29], leading to inhibit cPLA$_2$ activation. However, the contribution of suppression of ERK phosphorylation is considered to be small because the ability of keihi to decrease LPS-induced PGE$_2$ production was weak (Figure 3).
- Keihi increased LPS-induced COX-2 expression.

Therefore, these effects of keihi are different from that of cinnamic aldehyde, suggesting that other ingredients may contribute to our findings.

3.4.4. Ogon (*Scutellariae Radix*)

Ogon is the powdered root of *Scutellaria baicalensis* Georgi. Among the herbal medicines shown in Table 1, ogon is included in shosaikoto (TJ-9), hangeshashinto (TJ-14), and saireito (TJ-114). Among the herbs constituting saireito, ogon is reported to reduce PGE$_2$ production by LPS-treated RAW264.7 cells [44].

The major ingredients of ogon are flavonoids such as baicalin, baicalein, and wogonin. Their structures are indicated in Figure 7. Baicalin is the glucuronide of baicalein and is an inactive form. Administered baicalein is metabolized to baicalin, which is an active form. Baicalin, baicalein, and wogonin reduce PGE$_2$ production in human oral keratinocytes [7] and RAW264.7 cells [94].

1. Wogonin suppressed LPS-induced COX-2 expression in RAW264.7 cells [73,74], whereas baicalin and baicalein did not [73]. Other group demonstrated that baicalein (but not baicalin) suppressed

LPS-induced COX-2 expression in RAW264.7 cells [71]. This discrepancy may be due to the concentrations of LPS and flavonoids among these reports. Moreover, baicalein and wogonin suppressed COX-2 expression in human oral keratinocytes [7].

2. Baicalin [70], baicalein [72], and wogonin [7] suppressed NF-κB activity.
3. Baicalin, baicalein, and wogonin did not inhibit COX-2 activity in RAW264.7 cells [73].

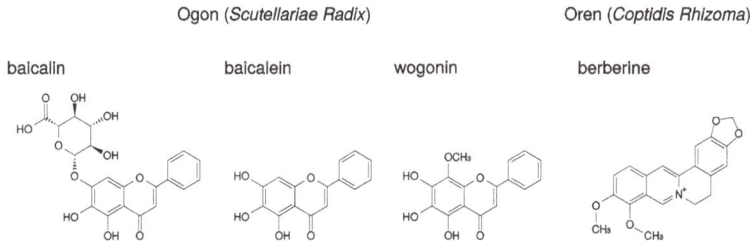

Figure 7. The structures of ingredients in ogon (*Scutellariae Radix*) and oren (*Coptidis Rhizoma*).

Our data indicate that shosaikoto and hangeshashinto, which include ogon, suppressed LPS-induced COX-2 expression in HGFs [37,38]. This mechanism is accounted for by those of baicalin, baicalein, and wogonin.

3.4.5. Oren (*Coptidis Rhizoma*)

Oren is the powdered rhizome of *Coptis japonica* Makino, *Coptis chinensis* Franchet, *Coptis deltoidea* C. Y. Cheng et Hsiao, or *Coptis teeta* Wallich (Ranunculaceae). Among the herbal medicines shown in Table 1, oren is included in hangeshashinto (TJ-14) and orento (TJ-120).

Berberine, one of benzylisoquinoline alkaloid, is the major ingredient of oren. The structure of berberine is indicated in Figure 7. Berberine is reported to reduce PGE$_2$ production. The effects of berberine on arachidonic acid cascade are briefly summarized in Table 8.

1. Berberine suppressed NF-κB activation and COX-2 expression in human leukemia Jurkat cells [75] and oral cancer OC2 and KB cells [95,96].
2. Berberine suppressed MAP kinases phosphorylation (including ERK) and activated AMP-activated protein kinase (AMPK) in peritoneal macrophages and RAW 264.7 cells [76], BV-2 cells [77], and melanoma cells [78]. Therefore, berberine is considered to inhibit cPLA$_2$ activation through suppression of ERK phosphorylation. In addition, because AMPK is reported to suppress NF-κB activation [97], berberine suppressed COX-2 expression due to activation of AMPK.

3.5. Conclusion about Herbal Medicines and Herbs

We have described the effects of herbal medicines, herbs, and their ingredients on arachidonic acid cascade in this review. Several herbal medicines show reduced LPS-induced PGE$_2$ production by HGFs. These results suggest that these herbal medicines may be effective in the improvement of the inflammatory symptoms in periodontitis. Herbal medicines must be properly selected by the patterns of each patient —excess patterns, medium patterns, or deficiency patterns. Among the herbal medicines in our studies, kakkonto (TJ-1) and orento (TJ-120) are used for the patients with excess patterns. Shosaikoto (TJ-9), hangeshashinto (TJ-14), and orento are used for the patients with medium patterns. Shinbuto (TJ-30) and ninjinto (TJ-32) are used for the patients with deficiency patterns. Therefore, it may be possible to use appropriate herbal medicines to patients with any pattern.

As shown in the above-mentioned descriptions, not all effects of herbal medicines are explainable by the effects of herbs constituting herbal medicines. Similarly, not all effects of herbs are explainable by the effects of ingredients contained in herbs. Experiments using "herbal medicines" or "herbs" themselves may be important rather than those using ingredients. The concentrations of these hydrophobic ingredients may also be low because the herbs that we used are water-soluble fractions. Therefore, it is considered that the concentrations of their ingredients need to be measured. Moreover, the unanalyzed ingredients other than those explained in this review are likely to be present. It is to be desired that further analyses reveal the novel ingredients and their action of mechanisms.

4. Anti-Osteoclastogenic Effects of Natural Products

Like periodontitis (PD), rheumatoid arthritis (RA) is a disease associated with inflammation and bone destruction. Although therapeutics of RA have recently advanced with the development of antibody drugs, natural substances displaying anti-inflammatory and anti-osteoclast characteristics against RA are still being used as widely as they have been in the past.

Some studies have revealed a relationship between PD and RA. RA prevalence is increased in patients with PD [98,99]. The presence of PD may contribute to the progression of RA; that is, RA patients with PD receiving non-surgical periodontal treatment resulted in a noteworthy improvement in the clinical outcome for RA [100]. From the aspect of the clinical marker, RA and PD are similar in cytokines and mediators involved in inflammation and bone destruction [101]. For example, TNF-α, receptor activator of nuclear factor-κB ligand (RANKL), and matrix metalloproteinase (MMP) family increase in production in RA and PD [102–106]. Due to these similarities, natural products used for RA are probably effective for PD.

The structures of natural products described in this review are indicated in Figure 8.

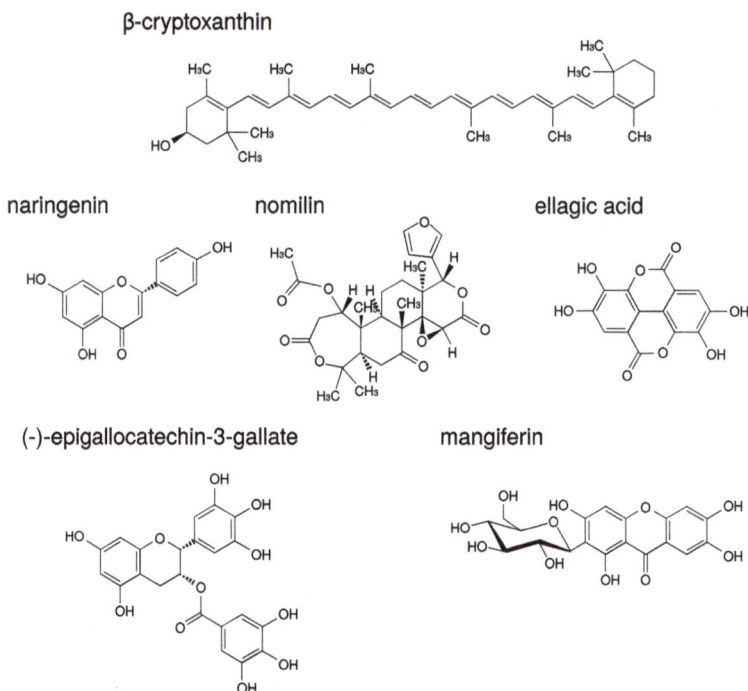

Figure 8. The structures of natural products.

Epidemiological studies have revealed a positive correlation between bone health and increased consumption of fruits and vegetables [107,108]. Some fruits and vegetables contain components that inhibit both inflammation and osteoclast activity.

β-Cryptoxanthin is a carotenoid present in a wide range of citrus fruits and in *Diospyros kaki* Thunb., *Physalis alkekengi* L., etc. β-Cryptoxanthin has a potent inhibitory effect on osteoclast-like cell formation in mouse marrow culture [109]. Moreover, in a mouse model of PD, β-cryptoxanthin suppressed bone resorption in the mandibular alveolar bone in vitro and restored alveolar bone loss induced by LPS in vivo [110].

Naringenin is a flavonoid contained in citrus fruits such as oranges and grapefruits. Accumulating evidence has suggested that naringenin modulates chronic inflammation [111]. In a murine model of collagen-induced arthritis, naringenin inhibited pro-inflammatory cytokine production by decreasing MAPK and NF-κB signaling activation [112]. La et al. showed naringenin thus holds promise as a therapeutic and preventive agent for bone-related diseases such as PD [113]. Thus, there are cases in which components demonstrating anti-osteoclast behavior are demonstrated to be effective against PD. In addition to naringenin, citrus fruits contain components that suppress osteoclast activity via MAPK. Nomilin, a limonoid present in citrus fruits, displays inhibitory effects on osteoclastic differentiation through the suppression of MAPK signaling pathways [114].

Ellagic acid is a polyphenol contained in berries, pomegranates, nuts, etc. Ellagic acid has an anti-inflammatory effect in various organs such as the liver, stomach, small intestine, and skin [115–118]. Moreover, ellagic acid has anti-osteoclast activity and significantly reduced serum levels of pro-inflammatory cytokines, TNF-α, IL-1β, and IL-17 in RA model mice [119]. A recent study supported the traditional use of *Geum urbanum* L. root contained ellagic acid derivatives in cavity inflammation including mucositis, gingivitis, and PD [120].

Additional useful components against both RA and PD have been found in tea. (-)-Epigallocatechin-3-gallate (EGCG) is a major catechin derivative present in green tea. Previous studies have also suggested that EGCG decreases MMP-1, MMP-2, and MMP-3 production by RA synovial fibroblasts, thereby preventing further cartilage and bone destruction [121,122]. Moreover, it has been reported that EGCG selectively inhibited IL-1β-induced IL-6 synthesis in RA synovial fibroblasts and suppressed IL-6 trans-signaling via upregulation of an endogenous inhibitor, a soluble gp130 [123]. Clinical study of EGCG suggested that local drug delivery utilizing green tea extract could be used as an adjunct in the treatment of chronic PD [124].

Traditional medicine in Ayurveda also presents useful teas against RA and PD. *Salacia reticulata* Wight is a plant native to Sri Lanka that has been used for the prevention of RA, gonorrhea, and skin disease. We previously reported that leaf of *S. reticulata* alleviates collagen antibody-induced arthritis in RA model mice [125]. *S. reticulata* contains a polyphenol known as mangiferin that inhibits osteoclastic bone resorption by promoting ERβ mRNA expression in mouse bone marrow macrophage cells [126].

In conclusion, natural products displaying both anti-inflammation and anti-osteoclast characteristics are suggested to be useful for the prevention and treatment of PD.

Author Contributions: C.S. conceived, designed, proved, and edited the whole review manuscript. N.S. and C.S. wrote "Introduction" and the topic of "Biological Efficacy of Natural Products against Acute Inflammatory Disease: Stomatitis", T.A. wrote the topic of "Biological Efficacy of Natural Products against Chronic Inflammatory Disease: Periodontitis", S.N. and K.K. wrote a second half part of the topic "Anti-Osteoclastogenic Effects of Natural Products".

Funding: The work was supported in part by funding from JSPS KAKENHI Grant Number JP16H05144, the Nagano Society for the Promotion of Science, and a Scientific Research Special Grant from Matsumoto Dental University.

Acknowledgments: We would like to thank also to the stuffs of Matsumoto Dental University, Josai University, and Okayama University Graduate School for technical support.

Conflicts of Interest: The authors declare no conflict of interest.

References

1. Veilleux, M.; Moriyama, S.; Yoshioka, M.; Hinode, D.; Grenier, D. A Review of Evidence for a Therapeutic Application of Traditional Japanese Kampo Medicine for Oral Diseases/Disorders. *Medicines* **2018**, *5*, 35. [CrossRef] [PubMed]
2. Wang, P. Kampo medicines for oral disease. *Oral Ther. Pharmacol.* **2012**, *31*, 67–82.
3. Kono, T.; Satomi, M.; Chisato, N.; Ebisawa, Y.; Suno, M.; Asama, T.; Karasaki, H.; Matsubara, K.; Furukawa, H. Topical Application of Hangeshashinto (TJ-14) in the Treatment of Chemotherapy-Induced Oral Mucositis. *World J. Oncol.* **2010**, *1*, 232–235. [PubMed]
4. Aoyama, T.; Nishikawa, K.; Takiguchi, N.; Tanabe, K.; Imano, M.; Fukushima, R.; Sakamoto, J.; Oba, M.; Morita, S.; Kono, T.; et al. Double-blind, placebo-controlled, randomized phase II study of TJ-14 (hangeshashinto) for gastric cancer chemotherapy-induced oral mucositis. *Cancer Chemother. Pharmacol.* **2014**, *73*, 1047–1054. [CrossRef] [PubMed]
5. Yamashita, T.; Araki, K.; Tomifuji, M.; Kamide, D.; Tanaka, Y.; Shiotani, A. A traditional Japanese medicine–Hangeshashinto (TJ-14)–alleviates chemoradiation-induced mucositis and improves rates of treatment completion. *Support Care Cancer* **2015**, *23*, 29–35. [CrossRef] [PubMed]
6. Kamide, D.; Yamashita, T.; Araki, K.; Tomifuji, M.; Shiotani, A. Hangeshashinto (TJ-14) prevents radiation-induced mucositis by suppressing cyclooxygenase-2 expression and chemotaxis of inflammatory cells. *Clin. Transl. Oncol.* **2017**, *19*, 1329–1336. [CrossRef] [PubMed]
7. Kono, T.; Kaneko, A.; Matsumoto, C.; Miyagi, C.; Ohbuchi, K.; Mizuhara, Y.; Miyano, K.; Uezono, Y. Multitargeted effects of hangeshashinto for treatment of chemotherapy-induced oral mucositis on inducible prostaglandin E2 production in human oral keratinocytes. *Integr. Cancer Ther.* **2014**, *13*, 435–445. [CrossRef] [PubMed]
8. Furusawa, S.; Wu, J. The effects of biscoclaurine alkaloid cepharanthine on mammalian cells: Implications for cancer, shock, and inflammatory diseases. *Life Sci.* **2007**, *80*, 1073–1079. [CrossRef] [PubMed]
9. Rogosnitzky, M.; Danks, R. Therapeutic potential of the biscoclaurine alkaloid, cepharanthine. *Pharmacol. Rep.* **2011**, *63*, 337–347. [CrossRef]
10. Nakase, M.; Nomura, J.; Inui, M.; Murata, T.; Kawarada, Y.; Tagawa, T.; Ohsugi, H. Evaluation of clinical efficacy of Cepharanthin® (gargle-internal use) treatment for oral mucosal lesions. *J. Jpn. Oral Muco. Membr.* **1997**, *3*, 76–81. [CrossRef]
11. Saki, H.; Ichihara, H.; Kato, Y.; Ando, M.; Abe, K.; Win, K.; Inoue, T.; Fujitsuka, H.; Hyodo, I.; Sugiyama, T.; et al. Evaluation of clinical efficiency of Cepharanthin® for the treatment of oral mucosal lesions and glossodynia. *J. Jpn. Stomatol. Soc.* **1994**, *43*, 84–89.
12. Saito, Y.; Ikeda, M.; Tanaka, H.; Iijima, J.; Sakata, K. A literatue study of oral therapeutics and pharmacology Report 1; Evidence of off-label use of cepharanthin. *Oral. Ther. Pharmacol.* **2001**, *20*, 110–116.
13. Sogawa, N.; Sogawa, C.; Nakano, M.; Fukuoka, R.; Furuta, H. Effects of propargylglycine on endotoxin-induced acute lethal toxicity and defensive effect of cepharanthin on this toxicity. *J. Okayama Dent. Soc.* **1998**, *17*, 251–259.
14. Sogawa, N.; Sogawa, C.; Furuta, H. A study of active ingredients in Cepharanthin® on enhancement of lipopolysaccharide-induced histidine decarboxylase activities in mice spleens. *Med. Biol.* **2000**, *140*, 69–72.
15. Yokota, T.; Yokota, K.; Matsuura, T.; Shiwa, M. Suppressive effects of Cepharanthin® on the production of superoxide anion by neutrophils during hemodialysis. *J. Jpn. Soc. Dial. Ther.* **1993**, *26*, 1703–1708. [CrossRef]
16. Sawamura, D.; Sato, S.; Suzuki, M.; Nomura, K.; Hanada, K.; Hashimoto, I. Effect of cepharanthin on superoxide anion (O_2^-) production by macrophages. *J. Dermatol.* **1988**, *15*, 304–307. [CrossRef] [PubMed]
17. Akamatsu, H.; Komura, J.; Asada, Y.; Niwa, Y. Effects of cepharanthin on neutrophil chemotaxis, phagocytosis, and reactive oxygen species generation. *J. Dermatol.* **1991**, *18*, 643–648. [CrossRef] [PubMed]
18. Kawada, N.; Mizoguchi, Y.; Kondo, H.; Seki, S.; Kobayashi, K.; Yamamoto, S.; Morisawa, S. Effect of cepharanthine on metabolism of arachidonic acid from rat peritoneal exudate cells. *Jpn. J. Inflamm.* **1988**, *8*, 347–349.
19. Kondo, Y.; Takano, F.; Hojo, H. Inhibitory effect of bisbenzylisoquinoline alkaloids on nitric oxide production in activated macrophages. *Biochem. Pharmacol.* **1993**, *46*, 1887–1892. [CrossRef]

20. Matsuno, T.; Okazoe, Y.; kobayashi, S.; Obuchi, H.; Sato, E.; Edashige, K.; Utsumi, K. Measurement of active oxygen of neutrophils by means of luminol chemiluminescence and their inhibition by biscoclaurine alkaloids. *Igaku Yakugaku* **1989**, *21*, 889–894.

21. Kondo, Y.; Takano, F.; Hojo, H. Suppression of lipopolysaccharide-induced fulminant hepatitis and tumor necrosis factor production by bisbenzylisoquinoline alkaloids in bacillus Calmette-Guerin-treated mice. *Biochem. Pharmacol.* **1993**, *46*, 1861–1863. [CrossRef]

22. Sugiyama, K.; Sasaki, J.; Utsumi, K.; Miyahara, M. Inhibition by cepharanthine of histamine release from rat peritoneal mast cells. *Allergy* **1976**, *25*, 685–690.

23. Sogawa, N.; Aoki-Sogawa, C.; Iwata-Abuku, E.; Inoue, T.; Oda, N.; Kishi, K.; Furuta, H. Opposing pharmacological actions of cepharanthin on lipopolysaccharide-induced histidine decarboxylase activity in mice spleens. *Life Sci.* **2001**, *68*, 1395–1403. [CrossRef]

24. Noguchi, K.; Ishikawa, I. The roles of cyclooxygenase-2 and prostaglandin E_2 in periodontal disease. *Periodontology 2000* **2007**, *43*, 85–101. [CrossRef] [PubMed]

25. Salvi, G.; Lang, N. Host response modulation in the management of periodontal diseases. *J. Clin. Periodontol.* **2005**, *32* (Suppl. 6), 108–129. [CrossRef] [PubMed]

26. Ara, T.; Fujinami, Y.; Imamura, Y.; Wang, P. Lipopolysaccharide-treated human gingival fibroblasts continuously produce PGE_2. *J. Hard Tissue Biol.* **2008**, *17*, 121–124. [CrossRef]

27. Ara, T.; Kurata, K.; Hirai, K.; Uchihashi, T.; Uematsu, T.; Imamura, Y.; Furusawa, K.; Kurihara, S.; Wang, P. Human gingival fibroblasts are critical in sustaining inflammation in periodontal disease. *J. Periodontal. Res.* **2009**, *44*, 21–27. [CrossRef] [PubMed]

28. Burke, J.; Dennis, E. phospholipase A_2 biochemistry. *Cardiovasc Drugs Ther.* **2009**, *23*, 49–59. [CrossRef] [PubMed]

29. Ara, T.; Sogawa, N. Studies on shokyo, kanzo, and keihi in kakkonto medicine on prostaglandin E_2 production in lipopolysaccharide-treated human gingival fibroblasts. *Int. Sch. Res. Notices* **2016**, *2016*, 9351787. [CrossRef] [PubMed]

30. Nemenoff, R.; Winitz, S.; Qian, N.; Van Putten, V.; Johnson, G.; Heasley, L. Phosphorylation and activation of a high molecular weight form of phospholipase A_2 by p42 microtubule-associated protein 2 kinase and protein kinase C. *J. Biol. Chem.* **1993**, *268*, 1960–1964. [PubMed]

31. Lin, L.; Wartmann, M.; Lin, A.; Knopf, J.; Seth, A.; Davis, R. $cPLA_2$ is phosphorylated and activated by MAP kinase. *Cell* **1993**, *72*, 269–278. [CrossRef]

32. Gijón, M.; Spencer, D.; Kaiser, A.; Leslie, C. Role of phosphorylation sites and the C2 domain in regulation of cytosolic phospholipase A_2. *J. Cell. Biol.* **1999**, *145*, 1219–1232. [CrossRef] [PubMed]

33. Gupta, C.; Katsumata, M.; Goldman, A.; Herold, R.; Piddington, R. Glucocorticoid-induced phospholipase A_2-inhibitory proteins mediate glucocorticoid teratogenicity in vitro. *Proc. Natl. Acad. Sci. USA* **1984**, *81*, 1140–1143. [CrossRef] [PubMed]

34. Wallner, B.; Mattaliano, R.; Hession, C.; Cate, R.; Tizard, R.; Sinclair, L.; Foeller, C.; Chow, E.; Browing, J.; Ramachandran, K.; et al. Cloning and expression of human lipocortin, a phospholipase A_2 inhibitor with potential anti-inflammatory activity. *Nature* **1986**, *320*, 77–81. [CrossRef] [PubMed]

35. Ara, T.; Fujinami, Y.; Urano, H.; Hirai, K.; Hattori, T.; Miyazawa, H. Protein kinase A enhances lipopolysaccharide-induced IL-6, IL-8, and PGE_2 production by human gingival fibroblasts. *J. Negat. Results Biomed.* **2012**, *11*, 10. [CrossRef] [PubMed]

36. Kitamura, H.; Urano, H.; Ara, T. Preventive effects of a kampo medicine, kakkonto, on inflammatory responses via the suppression of extracellular signal-regulated kinase phosphorylation in lipopolysaccharide-treated human gingival fibroblasts. *ISRN Pharmacol.* **2014**, *2014*, 784019. [CrossRef] [PubMed]

37. Ara, T.; Maeda, Y.; Fujinami, Y.; Imamura, Y.; Hattori, T.; Wang, P. Preventive effects of a Kampo medicine, Shosaikoto, on inflammatory responses in LPS-treated human gingival fibroblasts. *Biol. Pharm. Bull.* **2008**, *31*, 1141–1144. [CrossRef] [PubMed]

38. Nakazono, Y.; Ara, T.; Fujinami, Y.; Hattori, T.; Wang, P. Preventive effects of a kampo medicine, hangeshashinto on inflammatory responses in lipopolysaccharide-treated human gingival fibroblasts. *J. Hard Tissue Biol.* **2010**, *19*, 43–50. [CrossRef]

39. Ara, T.; Sogawa, N. Effects of shinbuto and ninjinto on prostaglandin E_2 production in lipopolysaccharide-treated human gingival fibroblasts. *PeerJ* **2017**, *5*, e4120. [CrossRef] [PubMed]

40. Ara, T.; Honjo, K.; Fujinami, Y.; Hattori, T.; Imamura, Y.; Wang, P. Preventive effects of a kampo medicine, orento on inflammatory responses in lipopolysaccharide treated human gingival fibroblasts. *Biol. Pharm. Bull.* **2010**, *33*, 611–616. [CrossRef] [PubMed]

41. Kato, T.; Segami, N.; Sakagami, H. Anti-inflammatory activity of hangeshashinto in IL-1β-stimulated gingival and periodontal ligament fibroblasts. *In Vivo* **2016**, *30*, 257–263. [PubMed]

42. Miyamoto, K.; Lange, M.; McKinley, G.; Stavropoulos, C.; Moriya, S.; Matsumoto, H.; Inada, Y. Effects of sho-saiko-to on production of prostaglandin E$_2$ (PGE$_2$), leukotriene B$_4$ (LTB$_4$) and superoxide from peripheral monocytes and polymorphonuclear cells isolated from HIV infected individuals. *Am. J. Chin. Med.* **1996**, *24*, 1–10. [CrossRef] [PubMed]

43. Horie, N.; Hashimoto, K.; Kato, T.; Shimoyama, T.; Kaneko, T.; Kusama, K.; Sakagami, H. COX-2 as possible target for the inhibition of PGE$_2$ production by Rikko-san in activated macrophage. *In Vivo* **2008**, *22*, 333–336. [PubMed]

44. Kaneko, T.; Chiba, H.; Horie, N.; Kato, T.; Hashimoto, K.; Kusama, K.; Sakagami, H. Effect of Sairei-to and its ingredients on prostaglandin E$_2$ production by mouse macrophage-like cells. *In Vivo* **2008**, *22*, 571–575. [PubMed]

45. Inoue, M.; Shen, Y.; Ogihara, Y. Shosaikoto (kampo medicine) protects macrophage function from suppression by hypercholesterolemia. *Biol. Pharm. Bull.* **1996**, *19*, 652–654. [CrossRef] [PubMed]

46. Kase, Y.; Saitoh, K.; Ishige, A.; Komatsu, Y. Mechanisms by which Hange-shashin-to reduces prostaglandin E2 levels. *Biol. Pharm. Bull.* **1998**, *21*, 1277–1281. [CrossRef] [PubMed]

47. Kase, Y.; Hayakawa, T.; Ishige, A.; Aburada, M.; Komatsu, Y. The effects of *Hange-shashin-to* on the content of prostaglandin E$_2$ and water absorption in the large intestine of rats. *Biol. Pharm. Bull.* **1997**, *20*, 954–957. [CrossRef] [PubMed]

48. Kase, Y.; Saitoh, K.; Yuzurihara, M.; Ishige, A.; Komatsu, Y. Effects of *Hange-shashin-to* on cholera toxin-induced fluid secretion in the small intestine of rats. *Biol. Pharm. Bull.* **1998**, *21*, 117–120. [CrossRef] [PubMed]

49. Tjendraputra, E.; Tran, V.; Liu-Brennan, D.; Roufogalis, B.; Duke, C. Effect of ginger constituents and synthetic analogues on cyclooxygenase-2 enzyme in intact cells. *Bioorg. Chem.* **2001**, *29*, 156–163. [CrossRef] [PubMed]

50. van Breemen, R.; Tao, Y.; Li, W. Cyclooxygenase-2 inhibitors in ginger (*Zingiber officinale*). *Fitoterapia* **2011**, *82*, 38–43. [CrossRef] [PubMed]

51. Lantz, R.; Chen, G.; Sarihan, M.; Solyom, A.; Jolad, S.; Timmermann, B. The effect of extracts from ginger rhizome on inflammatory mediator production. *Phytomedicine* **2007**, *14*, 123–128. [CrossRef] [PubMed]

52. Pan, M.; Hsieh, M.; Hsu, P.; Ho, S.; Lai, C.; Wu, H.; Sang, S.; Ho, C. 6-Shogaol suppressed lipopolysaccharide-induced up-expression of iNOS and COX-2 in murine macrophages. *Mol. Nutr. Food Res.* **2008**, *52*, 1467–1477. [CrossRef] [PubMed]

53. Ha, S.; Moon, E.; Ju, M.; Kim, D.; Ryu, J.; Oh, M.; Kim, S. 6-Shogaol, a ginger product, modulates neuroinflammation: A new approach to neuroprotection. *Neuropharmacology* **2012**, *63*, 211–223. [CrossRef] [PubMed]

54. Kim, S.; Kundu, J.; Shin, Y.; Park, J.; Cho, M.; Kim, T.; Surh, Y. [6]-Gingerol inhibits COX-2 expression by blocking the activation of p38 MAP kinase and NF-κB in phorbol ester-stimulated mouse skin. *Oncogene* **2005**, *24*, 2558–2567. [CrossRef] [PubMed]

55. Saha, P.; Katarkar, A.; Das, B.; Bhattacharyya, A.; Chaudhuri, K. 6-Gingerol inhibits *Vibrio cholerae*-induced proinflammatory cytokines in intestinal epithelial cells via modulation of NF-κB. *Pharm. Biol.* **2016**, *54*, 1606–1615. [CrossRef] [PubMed]

56. Ling, H.; Yang, H.; Tan, S.; Chui, W.; Chew, E. 6-Shogaol, an active constituent of ginger, inhibits breast cancer cell invasion by reducing matrix metalloproteinase-9 expression via blockade of nuclear factor-κB activation. *Br. J. Pharmacol.* **2010**, *161*, 1763–1777. [CrossRef] [PubMed]

57. Nievergelt, A.; Marazzi, J.; Schoop, R.; Altmann, K.; Gertsch, J. Ginger phenylpropanoids inhibit IL-1β and prostanoid secretion and disrupt arachidonate-phospholipid remodeling by targeting phospholipases A$_2$. *J. Immunol.* **2011**, *187*, 4140–4150. [CrossRef] [PubMed]

58. Yu, J.; Ha, J.; Kim, K.; Jung, Y.; Jung, J.; Oh, S. Anti-inflammatory activities of licorice extract and its active compounds, glycyrrhizic acid, liquiritin and liquiritigenin, in BV2 cells and mice liver. *Molecules* **2015**, *20*, 13041–13054. [CrossRef] [PubMed]

59. Niwa, K.; Lian, Z.; Onogi, K.; Yun, W.; Tang, L.; Mori, H.; Tamaya, T. Preventive effects of glycyrrhizin on estrogen-related endometrial carcinogenesis in mice. *Oncol. Rep.* **2007**, *17*, 617–622. [CrossRef] [PubMed]

60. Song, J.; Lee, J.; Shim, B.; Lee, C.; Choi, S.; Kang, C.; Sohn, N.; Shin, J. Glycyrrhizin alleviates neuroinflammation and memory deficit induced by systemic lipopolysaccharide treatment in mice. *Molecules* **2013**, *18*, 15788–15803. [CrossRef] [PubMed]

61. Takei, H.; Baba, Y.; Hisatsune, A.; Katsuki, H.; Miyata, T.; Yokomizo, K.; Isohama, Y. Glycyrrhizin inhibits interleukin-8 production and nuclear factor-κB activity in lung epithelial cells, but not through glucocorticoid receptors. *J. Pharmacol. Sci.* **2008**, *106*, 460–468. [CrossRef] [PubMed]

62. Honda, H.; Nagai, Y.; Matsunaga, T.; Saitoh, S.; Akashi-Takamura, S.; Hayashi, H.; Fujii, I.; Miyake, K.; Muraguchi, A.; Takatsu, K. Glycyrrhizin and isoliquiritigenin suppress the LPS sensor toll-like receptor 4/MD-2 complex signaling in a different manner. *J. Leukoc. Biol.* **2012**, *91*, 967–976. [CrossRef] [PubMed]

63. Takahashi, T.; Takasuka, N.; Iigo, M.; Baba, M.; Nishino, H.; Tsuda, H.; Okuyama, T. Isoliquiritigenin, a flavonoid from licorice, reduces prostaglandin E$_2$ and nitric oxide, causes apoptosis, and suppresses aberrant crypt foci development. *Cancer Sci.* **2004**, *95*, 448–453. [CrossRef] [PubMed]

64. Kim, J.; Park, S.; Yun, K.; Cho, Y.; Park, H.; Lee, K. Isoliquiritigenin isolated from the roots of *Glycyrrhiza uralensis* inhibitsLPS-induced iNOS and COX-2 expression via the attenuation of NF-κB in RAW 264.7 macrophages. *Eur. J. Pharmacol.* **2008**, *584*, 175–184. [CrossRef] [PubMed]

65. Liao, J.; Deng, J.; Chiu, C.; Hou, W.; Huang, S.; Shie, P.; Huang, G. Anti-inflammatory activities of *Cinnamomum cassia* constituents in vitro and in vivo. *Evid. Based Complement. Alternat. Med.* **2012**, *2012*, 429320. [CrossRef] [PubMed]

66. Yu, T.; Lee, S.; Yang, W.; Jang, H.; Lee, Y.; Kim, T.; Kim, S.; Lee, J.; Cho, J. The ability of an ethanol extract of *Cinnamomum cassia* to inhibit Src and spleen tyrosine kinase activity contributes to its anti-inflammatory action. *J. Ethnopharmacol.* **2012**, *139*, 566–573. [CrossRef] [PubMed]

67. Kim, B.; Lee, Y.; Lee, J.; Lee, J.; Cho, J. Regulatory effect of cinnamaldehyde on monocyte/macrophage-mediated inflammatory responses. *Mediators Inflamm.* **2010**, *2010*, 529359. [CrossRef] [PubMed]

68. Guo, J.; Huo, H.; Zhao, B.; Liu, H.; Li, L.; Ma, Y.; Guo, S.; Jiang, T. Cinnamaldehyde reduces IL-1β-induced cyclooxygenase-2 activity in rat cerebral microvascular endothelial cells. *Eur. J. Pharmacol.* **2006**, *537*, 174–180. [CrossRef] [PubMed]

69. Youn, H.; Lee, J.; Choi, Y.; Saitoh, S.; Miyake, K.; Hwang, D.; Lee, J. Cinnamaldehyde suppresses toll-like receptor 4 activation mediated through the inhibition of receptor oligomerization. *Biochem. Pharmacol.* **2008**, *75*, 494–502. [CrossRef] [PubMed]

70. Altavilla, D.; Squadrito, F.; Bitto, A.; Polito, F.; Burnett, B.; Di Stefano, V.; Minutoli, L. Flavocoxid, a dual inhibitor of cyclooxygenase and 5-lipoxygenase, blunts pro-inflammatory phenotype activation in endotoxin-stimulated macrophages. *Br. J. Pharmacol.* **2009**, *157*, 1410–1418. [CrossRef] [PubMed]

71. Woo, K.; Lim, J.; Suh, S.; Kwon, Y.; Shin, S.; Kim, S.; Choi, Y.; Park, J.; Kwon, T. Differential inhibitory effects of baicalein and baicalin on LPS-induced cyclooxygenase-2 expression through inhibition of C/EBPβ DNA-binding activity. *Immunobiology* **2006**, *211*, 359–368. [CrossRef] [PubMed]

72. Seo, M.; Lee, S.; Jeon, Y.; Im, J. Inhibition of p65 nuclear translocation by baicalein. *Toxicol. Res.* **2011**, *27*, 71–76. [CrossRef] [PubMed]

73. Chen, Y.; Shen, S.; Chen, L.; Lee, T.; Yang, L. Wogonin, baicalin, and baicalein inhibition of inducible nitric oxide synthase and cyclooxygenase-2 gene expressions induced by nitric oxide synthase inhibitors and lipopolysaccharide. *Biochem. Pharmacol.* **2001**, *61*, 1417–1427. [CrossRef]

74. Pan, M.; Lai, C.; Wang, Y.; Ho, C. Acacetin suppressed LPS-induced up-expression of iNOS and COX-2 in murine macrophages and TPA-induced tumor promotion in mice. *Biochem. Pharmacol.* **2006**, *72*, 1293–1303. [CrossRef] [PubMed]

75. Pandey, M.; Sung, B.; Kunnumakkara, A.; Sethi, G.; Chaturvedi, M.; Aggarwal, B. Berberine modifies cysteine 179 of IκBα kinase, suppresses nuclear factor-κB-regulated antiapoptotic gene products, and potentiates apoptosis. *Cancer Res.* **2008**, *68*, 5370–5379. [CrossRef] [PubMed]

76. Jeong, H.; Hsu, K.; Lee, J.; Ham, M.; Huh, J.; Shin, H.; Kim, W.; Kim, J. Berberine suppresses proinflammatory responses through AMPK activation in macrophages. *Am. J. Physiol. Endocrinol. Metab.* **2009**, *296*, E955–E964. [CrossRef] [PubMed]

77. Lu, D.; Tang, C.; Chen, Y.; Wei, I. Berberine suppresses neuroinflammatory responses through AMP-activated protein kinase activation in BV-2 microglia. *J. Cell. Biochem.* **2010**, *110*, 697–705. [CrossRef] [PubMed]

78. Kim, H.; Kim, M.; Kim, E.; Yang, Y.; Lee, M.; Lim, J. Berberine-induced AMPK activation inhibits the metastatic potential of melanoma cells via reduction of ERK activity and COX-2 protein expression. *Biochem. Pharmacol.* **2012**, *83*, 385–394. [CrossRef] [PubMed]

79. Liang, K.; Ting, C.; Yin, S.; Chen, Y.; Lin, S.; Liao, J.; Hsu, S. Berberine suppresses MEK/ERK-dependent Egr-1 signaling pathway and inhibits vascular smooth muscle cell regrowth after in vitro mechanical injury. *Biochem. Pharmacol.* **2006**, *71*, 806–817. [CrossRef] [PubMed]

80. Afzal, M.; Al-Hadidi, D.; Menon, M.; Pesek, J.; Dhami, M. Ginger: An ethnomedical, chemical and pharmacological review. *Drug Metabol. Drug Interact.* **2001**, *18*, 159–190. [CrossRef] [PubMed]

81. Lakhan, S.; Ford, C.; Tepper, D. *Zingiberaceae* extracts for pain: A systematic review and meta-analysis. *Nutr. J.* **2015**, *14*, 50. [CrossRef] [PubMed]

82. Thomson, M.; Al-Qattan, K.; Al-Sawan, S.; Alnaqeeb, M.; Khan, I.; Ali, M. The use of ginger (*Zingiber officinale* Rosc.) as a potential anti-inflammatory and antithrombotic agent. *Prostaglandins Leukot Essent Fatty Acids* **2002**, *67*, 475–478. [CrossRef] [PubMed]

83. Aimbire, F.; Penna, S.; Rodrigues, M.; Rodrigues, K.; Lopes-Martins, R.; Sertié, J. Effect of hydroalcoholic extract of *Zingiber officinalis* rhizomes on LPS-induced rat airway hyperreactivity and lung inflammation. *Prostaglandins Leukot Essent Fatty Acids* **2007**, *77*, 129–138. [CrossRef] [PubMed]

84. El-Abhar, H.; Hammad, L.; Gawad, H. Modulating effect of ginger extract on rats with ulcerative colitis. *J. Ethnopharmacol.* **2008**, *118*, 367–372. [CrossRef] [PubMed]

85. Podlogar, J.; Verspohl, E. Antiinflammatory effects of ginger and some of its components in human bronchial epithelial (BEAS-2B) cells. *Phytother. Res.* **2012**, *26*, 333–336. [CrossRef] [PubMed]

86. Shim, S.; Kim, S.; Choi, D.; Kwon, Y.; Kwon, J. Anti-inflammatory effects of [6]-shogaol: Potential roles of HDAC inhibition and HSP70 induction. *Food Chem. Toxicol.* **2011**, *49*, 2734–2740. [CrossRef] [PubMed]

87. Shibata, S. A drug over the millennia: Pharmacognosy, chemistry, and pharmacology of licorice. *Yakugaku Zasshi* **2000**, *120*, 849–862. [CrossRef] [PubMed]

88. Farese, R., Jr.; Biglieri, E.; Shackleton, C.; Irony, I.; Gomez-Fontes, R. Licorice-induced hypermineralocorticoidism. *N. Engl. J. Med.* **1991**, *325*, 1223–1227. [CrossRef] [PubMed]

89. Mumoli, N.; Cei, M. Licorice-induced hypokalemia. *Int. J. Cardiol.* **2008**, *124*, e42–44. [CrossRef] [PubMed]

90. Van Uum, S. Liquorice and hypertension. *Neth. J. Med.* **2005**, *63*, 119–120. [PubMed]

91. Palermo, M.; Quinkler, M.; Stewart, P. Apparent mineralocorticoid excess syndrome: An overview. *Arq. Bras. Endocrinol. Metabol.* **2004**, *48*, 687–696. [CrossRef] [PubMed]

92. van Uum, S.; Lenders, J.; Hermus, A. Cortisol, 11β-hydroxysteroid dehydrogenases, and hypertension. *Semin. Vasc. Med.* **2004**, *4*, 121–128. [CrossRef] [PubMed]

93. Walker, B.; Edwards, C. Licorice-induced hypertension and syndromes of apparent mineralocorticoid excess. *Endocrinol. Metab. Clin. N. Am.* **1994**, *23*, 359–377. [CrossRef]

94. Kaneko, T.; Chiba, H.; Horie, N.; Kato, T.; Kobayashi, M.; Hashimoto, K.; Kusama, K.; Sakagami, H. Effect of Scutellariae radix ingredients on prostaglandin E_2 production and COX-2 expression by LPS-activated macrophage. *In Vivo* **2009**, *23*, 577–582. [PubMed]

95. Kuo, C.; Chi, C.; Liu, T. The anti-inflammatory potential of berberine in vitro and in vivo. *Cancer Lett.* **2004**, *203*, 127–137. [CrossRef] [PubMed]

96. Kuo, C.; Chi, C.; Liu, T. Modulation of apoptosis by berberine through inhibition of cyclooxygenase-2 and Mcl-1 expression in oral cancer cells. *In Vivo* **2005**, *19*, 247–252. [PubMed]

97. Liang, Y.; Huang, B.; Song, E.; Bai, B.; Wang, Y. Constitutive activation of AMPK α1 in vascular endothelium promotes high-fat diet-induced fatty liver injury: Role of COX-2 induction. *Br. J. Pharmacol.* **2014**, *171*, 498–508. [CrossRef] [PubMed]

98. Leech, M.; Bartold, P. The association between rheumatoid arthritis and periodontitis. *Best Pract. Res. Clin. Rheumatol.* **2015**, *29*, 189–201. [CrossRef] [PubMed]

99. De Pablo, P.; Dietrich, T.; McAlindon, T. Association of periodontal disease and tooth loss with rheumatoid arthritis in the US population. *J. Rheumatol.* **2008**, *35*, 70–76. [PubMed]

100. Zhao, X.; Liu, Z.; Shu, D.; Xiong, Y.; He, M.; Xu, S.; Si, S.; Guo, B. Association of periodontitis with rheumatoid arthritis and the effect of non-surgical periodontal treatment on disease activity in patients with rheumatoid arthritis. *Med. Sci. Monit.* **2018**, *24*, 5802–5810. [CrossRef] [PubMed]

101. Araújo, V.; Melo, I.; Lima, V. Relationship between periodontitis and rheumatoid arthritis: Review of the literature. *Mediators Inflamm.* **2015**, *2015*, 259074. [CrossRef] [PubMed]

102. Kaur, S.; Bright, R.; Proudman, S.; Bartold, P. Does periodontal treatment influence clinical and biochemical measures for rheumatoid arthritis? A systematic review and meta-analysis. *Semin. Arthritis Rheum.* **2014**, *44*, 113–122. [CrossRef] [PubMed]

103. Javed, F.; Ahmed, H.; Mikami, T.; Almas, K.; Romanos, G.; Al-Hezaimi, K. Cytokine profile in the gingival crevicular fluid of rheumatoid arthritis patients with chronic periodontitis. *J. Investig. Clin. Dent.* **2014**, *5*, 1–8. [CrossRef] [PubMed]

104. Erciyas, K.; Sezer, U.; Ustün, K.; Pehlivan, Y.; Kisacik, B.; Senyurt, S.; Tarakçioğlu, M.; Onat, A. Effects of periodontal therapy on disease activity and systemic inflammation in rheumatoid arthritis patients. *Oral Dis.* **2013**, *19*, 394–400. [CrossRef] [PubMed]

105. Gümüş, P.; Buduneli, E.; Bıyıkoğlu, B.; Aksu, K.; Saraç, F.; Nile, C.; Lappin, D.; Buduneli, N. Gingival crevicular fluid, serum levels of receptor activator of nuclear factor-κB ligand, osteoprotegerin, and interleukin-17 in patients with rheumatoid arthritis and osteoporosis and with periodontal disease. *J. Periodontol.* **2013**, *84*, 1627–1637. [PubMed]

106. Silosi, I.; Cojocaru, M.; Foia, L.; Boldeanu, M.; Petrescu, F.; Surlin, P.; Biciusca, V. Significance of circulating and crevicular matrix metalloproteinase-9 in rheumatoid arthritis-chronic periodontitis association. *J. Immunol. Res.* **2015**, *2015*, 218060. [CrossRef] [PubMed]

107. Li, J.; Huang, Z.; Wang, R.; Ma, X.; Zhang, Z.; Liu, Z.; Chen, Y.; Su, Y. Fruit and vegetable intake and bone mass in Chinese adolescents, young and postmenopausal women. *Public Health Nutr.* **2013**, *16*, 78–86. [CrossRef] [PubMed]

108. Hardcastle, A.; Aucott, L.; Fraser, W.; Reid, D.; Macdonald, H. Dietary patterns, bone resorption and bone mineral density in early post-menopausal Scottish women. *Eur. J. Clin. Nutr.* **2011**, *65*, 378–385. [CrossRef] [PubMed]

109. Uchiyama, S.; Yamaguchi, M. Inhibitory effect of beta-cryptoxanthin on osteoclast-like cell formation in mouse marrow cultures. *Biochem. Pharmacol.* **2004**, *67*, 1297–1305. [CrossRef] [PubMed]

110. Matsumoto, C.; Ashida, N.; Yokoyama, S.; Tominari, T.; Hirata, M.; Ogawa, K.; Sugiura, M.; Yano, M.; Inada, M.; Miyaura, C. The protective effects of β-cryptoxanthin on inflammatory bone resorption in a mouse experimental model of periodontitis. *Mol. Med. Rep.* **2013**, *77*, 860–862. [CrossRef] [PubMed]

111. Zeng, W.; Jin, L.; Zhang, F.; Zhang, C.; Liang, W. Naringenin as a potential immunomodulator in therapeutics. *Pharmacol. Res.* **2018**, *135*, 122–126. [CrossRef] [PubMed]

112. Li, Y.; Chen, D.; Chu, C.; Li, S.; Chen, Y.; Wu, C.; Lin, C. Naringenin inhibits dendritic cell maturation and has therapeutic effects in a murine model of collagen-induced arthritis. *J. Nutr. Biochem.* **2015**, *26*, 1467–1478. [CrossRef] [PubMed]

113. La, V.; Tanabe, S.; Grenier, D. Naringenin inhibits human osteoclastogenesis and osteoclastic bone resorption. *J. Periodontal. Res.* **2009**, *44*, 193–198. [CrossRef] [PubMed]

114. Kimira, Y.; Taniuchi, Y.; Nakatani, S.; Sekiguchi, Y.; Kim, H.; Shimizu, J.; Ebata, M.; Wada, M.; Matsumoto, A.; Mano, H. Citrus limonoid nomilin inhibits osteoclastogenesis in vitro by suppression of NFATc1 and MAPK signaling pathways. *Phytomedicine* **2015**, *22*, 1120–1124. [CrossRef] [PubMed]

115. Gu, L.; Deng, W.; Liu, Y.; Jiang, C.; Sun, L.; Sun, X.; Xu, Q.; Zhou, H. Ellagic acid protects Lipopolysaccharide/ D-galactosamine-induced acute hepatic injury in mice. *Int. Immunopharmacol.* **2014**, *22*, 341–345. [CrossRef] [PubMed]

116. Beserra, A.; Calegari, P.; Souza Mdo, C.; Dos Santos, R.; Lima, J.; Silva, R.; Balogun, S.; Martins, D. Gastroprotective and ulcer-healing mechanisms of ellagic acid in experimental rats. *J. Agric. Food Chem.* **2011**, *59*, 6957–6965. [CrossRef] [PubMed]

117. Marín, M.; María Giner, R.; Ríos, J.; Recio, M. Intestinal anti-inflammatory activity of ellagic acid in the acute and chronic dextrane sulfate sodium models of mice colitis. *J. Ethnopharmacol.* **2013**, *150*, 925–934. [CrossRef] [PubMed]

118. Mo, J.; Panichayupakaranant, P.; Kaewnopparat, N.; Songkro, S.; Reanmongkol, W. Topical anti-inflammatory potential of standardized pomegranate rind extract and ellagic acid in contact dermatitis. *Phytother. Res.* **2014**, *28*, 629–632. [CrossRef] [PubMed]

119. Allam, G.; Mahdi, E.; Alzahrani, A.; Abuelsaad, A. Ellagic acid alleviates adjuvant induced arthritis by modulation of pro- and anti-inflammatory cytokines. *Cent. Eur. J. Immunol.* **2016**, *41*, 339–349. [CrossRef] [PubMed]

120. Granica, S.; Kłębowska, A.; Kosiński, M.; Piwowarski, J.; Dudek, M.; Kaźmierski, S.; Kiss, A. Effects of *Geum urbanum* L. root extracts and its constituents on polymorphonuclear leucocytes functions. Significance in periodontal diseases. *J. Ethnopharmacol.* **2016**, *188*, 1–12. [CrossRef] [PubMed]
121. Ahmed, S.; Pakozdi, A.; Koch, A. Regulation of interleukin-1β-induced chemokine production and matrix metalloproteinase 2 activation by epigallocatechin-3-gallate in rheumatoid arthritis synovial fibroblasts. *Arthritis Rheum.* **2006**, *54*, 2393–3401. [CrossRef] [PubMed]
122. Yun, H.; Yoo, W.; Han, M.; Lee, Y.; Kim, J.; Lee, S. Epigallocatechin-3-gallate suppresses TNF-α-induced production of MMP-1 and -3 in rheumatoid arthritis synovial fibroblasts. *Rheumatol. Int.* **2008**, *29*, 23–29. [CrossRef] [PubMed]
123. Ahmed, S.; Marotte, H.; Kwan, K.; Ruth, J.; Campbell, P.; Rabquer, B.; Pakozdi, A.; Koch, A. Epigallocatechin-3-gallate inhibits IL-6 synthesis and suppresses transsignaling by enhancing soluble gp130 production. *Proc. Natl. Acad. Sci. USA* **2008**, *105*, 14692–14697. [CrossRef] [PubMed]
124. Gadagi, J.; Chava, V.; Reddy, V. Green tea extract as a local drug therapy on periodontitis patients with diabetes mellitus: A randomized case-control study. *J. Indian Soc. Periodontol.* **2013**, *17*, 198–203. [PubMed]
125. Sekiguchi, Y.; Mano, H.; Nakatani, S.; Shimizu, J.; Wada, M. Effects of the Sri Lankan medicinal plant, *Salacia reticulata*, in rheumatoid arthritis. *Genes Nutr.* **2010**, *5*, 89–96. [CrossRef] [PubMed]
126. Sekiguchi, Y.; Mano, H.; Nakatani, S.; Shimizu, J.; Kataoka, A.; Ogura, K.; Kimira, Y.; Ebata, M.; Wada, M. Mangiferin positively regulates osteoblast differentiation and suppresses osteoclast differentiation. *Mol. Med. Rep.* **2017**, *16*, 1328–1332. [CrossRef] [PubMed]

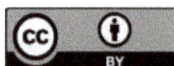

![medicines logo] *medicines*

MDPI

Article

Quercetin Enhances the Thioredoxin Production of Nasal Epithelial Cells In Vitro and In Vivo

Yukako Edo [1], Amane Otaki [2] and Kazuhito Asano [3,*

[1] Graduate School of Health Sciences, Showa University Graduate School, Yokohama 226-8555, Japan;
     yukakoeddy18@gmail.com
[2] Division of Nursing, Showa University School of Nursing and Rehabilitation Sciences, Yokohama 226-8555,
     Japan; aotaki@nr.showa-u.ac.jp
[3] Division of Physiology, Showa University School of Nursing and Rehabilitation Sciences,
     Yokohama 226-8555, Japan
*   Correspondence: asanok@med.showa-u.ac.jp; Tel.: +81-45-985-6538

Received: 17 October 2018; Accepted: 18 November 2018; Published: 21 November 2018

Abstract: Background: Thioredoxin (TRX) acts as both a scavenger of reactive oxygen species (ROS) and an immuno-modulator. Although quercetin has been shown to favorably modify allergic rhinitis (AR) symptoms, its influence on TRX production is not well defined. The present study was designed to examine whether quercetin could favorably modify AR symptoms via the TRX production of nasal epithelial cells in vitro and in vivo. **Methods**: Human nasal epithelial cells (HNEpCs) were stimulated with H_2O_2 in the presence of quercetin. TRX levels in 24-h culture supernatants were examined with ELISA. BALB/c male mice were intraperitoneally sensitized to ovalbumin (OVA) and intranasally challenged with OVA every other day, beginning seven days after the final sensitization. The mice were orally administered quercetin once a day for five consecutive days, beginning seven days after the final sensitization. Nasal symptoms were assessed by counting the number of sneezes and nasal rubbing behaviors during a 10-min period immediately after the challenge. TRX levels in nasal lavage fluids obtained 6 h after the challenge were examined by ELISA. **Results**: Treatment with 1.0 nM quercetin increased H_2O_2-induced TRX levels. The oral administration of 20.0 mg/kg of quercetin significantly inhibited nasal symptoms after the challenge. The same dose of quercetin significantly increased TRX levels in nasal lavage fluids. **Conclusions**: Quercetin's ability to increase TRX production may account, at least in part, for its clinical efficacy toward AR.

Keywords: allergic rhinitis; mice; quercetin; thioredoxin; nasal epithelial cell; production; increase; in vitro; in vivo

---

1. Introduction

Allergic rhinitis (AR) is a well-known type of chronic allergic inflammation that occurs in the nasal mucosa and is characterized by multiple symptoms such as sneezing, itching, and watery rhinorrhea [1,2]. Although AR is not life-threatening, it places a significant burden on patients and society because its symptoms lead to inconveniences in daily life. These clinical symptoms also exert adverse effects on industrial work productivity and school learning performance, resulting in increased medical costs and lower quality of life [1,2].

AR treatment can be divided into three main categories: allergen avoidance, drug therapy, and immunomodulating therapy [3]. Allergen avoidance is the safest mode of treatment, but it is often insufficient to obtain satisfactory results [3]. Although histamine H1 receptor antagonists and topical steroids can significantly ease the associated symptoms, they require repeated treatment sessions over the patient's lifetime [3,4]. Moreover, the currently available therapeutic agents cause adverse effects, including dizziness, dry mouth, and constipation [3,4]. Although immunotherapy induces immunological tolerance through the subcutaneous injection of or sublingual application of allergens, it has several disadvantages: it requires several years of therapy, is expensive, and contains a risk of anaphylaxis [5]. Furthermore, many patients dislike taking daily medication merely for prevention [3]. Therefore, the development of new medications for the treatment of allergic diseases, including AR, is desired.

Quercetin is a dietary flavonoid found in red wine, tea, many fruits, and onions [6]. For many years, the possible healthy biological activities of quercetin have been studied, with anti-pollinosis, anti-diabetic, and anti-viral activity reported [7]. Moreover, quercetin acts as a scavenger of free radicals, which damage cell membranes, tamper with DNA, and even cause cell death [8–10]. Quercetin also plays a role in allergic inflammatory responses by inhibiting mast cells and eosinophils from producing chemical mediators (e.g., histamine and leukotriene) and inflammatory cytokines, which are responsible for the induction and persistence of allergic reactions [11,12]. Furthermore, the oral administration of quercetin can alleviate ocular and nasal symptoms observed in patients with pollinosis [13]. Quercetin's attenuating effect on the clinical symptoms of allergic reactions has also been observed in experimental animal models of allergic asthma and AR [14–16]. Although these reports strongly suggest that quercetin is a good dietary supplement candidate for preventing the development of allergic diseases such as AR, the precise mechanisms by which quercetin modulates the clinical symptoms of allergic diseases remain unknown.

It is currently accepted that inflammatory cells including eosinophils, which are the most important effector cells in the development of inflammatory diseases, produce several types of toxic granule proteins and reactive oxygen species (ROS), such as O_2 and H_2O_2 [17,18]. Although the physiological production of ROS is generally considered essential in host defense and to maintain homeostasis, the overproduction of ROS and their metabolites are harmful and cause oxidative stress responses, which are implicated in the pathogenesis of allergic inflammatory airway diseases, including AR [17,19]. Conversely, under normal physiological conditions, several types of endogenous antioxidants, such as glutathione and superoxide dismutase, prevent the development of oxidative stress responses [19]. Among these, thioredoxin (TRX) has attracted attention as an endogenous antioxidant protein. TRX is a 12-kDa protein with two redox (reduction/oxidation) active half-cysteine residues [20,21]. In addition to its anti-oxidative activity, TRX is reported to exert immunomodulatory effects. The administration of exogenous TRX suppresses airway hyperresponsiveness induced by specific allergens by inhibiting eosinophil accumulation in the airways of asthmatic mouse models [22,23]. TRX has also been reported to augment the production of Th1-type cytokines, such as IL-12 and IFN-γ, which prevent allergic responses. These reports suggest that manipulating TRX production may be a good target for the treatment of chronic airway allergic diseases, including AR [22,23]. However, the influence of quercetin on the production of TRX is currently unclear. Therefore, the present study investigated the influence of quercetin on the TRX system by examining the ability of agents from human nasal epithelial cells (HNEpCs) to affect TRX production in vitro and in vivo.

2. Materials and Methods

2.1. Mice

Specific 5-week-old pathogen-free BALB/c male mice were purchased from CLEA Japan Co., Ltd. (Tokyo, Japan). The mice were maintained in our animal facility at 25 °C ± 2 °C with 55% ± 10% humidity under a 12-h dark/light cycle and were allowed free access to tap water and standard laboratory rodent chow (Oriental Yeast Co., Ltd., Tokyo, Japan) throughout the experiments. Each control and experimental group consisted of five mice. All animal experiments were approved by the Ethics Committee for Animal Experiments of Showa University (Approved No. 54011). Date of approval: 1 April 2018.

2.2. Reagents

Quercetin was purchased from Sigma-Aldrich Co., Ltd. (St. Louis, MO, USA) as a preservative-free pure powder. Quercetin was first dissolved in dimethyl sulfoxide (DMSO) at a concentration of 10.0 mM. This solution was then diluted with Airway Epithelial Cell Growth Media (AECG medium; PromoCell GmbH, Heidelberg, Germany) at appropriate concentrations for the experiments; then, the solution was sterilized by passing through 0.2-μm filters and was stored at 4 °C until use. To assess in vivo use, quercetin was mixed with 5% tragacanth gum solution at a concentration of 7.5 mg/mL [13]. Chicken ovalbumin (OVA; grade V) and $Al(OH)_3$ (alum) were obtained from Sigma-Aldrich Co. Ltd. as preservative-free pure powders.

2.3. Cell Culture

HNEpCs, purchased from PromoCell GmbH, were suspended in AECG medium (PromoCell GmbH) at a concentration of 5×10^5 cells/mL and used as target cells. The HNEpCs (5×10^5 cells/mL) were stimulated with 12.5–100.0 μM H_2O_2 for 24 h in a final volume of 2.0 mL. To examine the influence of quercetin on TRX production, the HNEpCs (5×10^5 cells/mL) were stimulated with 50.0 μM H_2O_2 in the presence of 0.1–10.0 nM quercetin for 24 h in a final volume of 2.0 mL. To examine TRX mRNA expression, the cells were stimulated with 50.0 μM H_2O_2 in the presence of 0.1–10.0 nM quercetin for 12 h. Quercetin was added to the cell cultures 2 h before H_2O_2 stimulation.

2.4. Assay to Assess Cytotoxicity of H_2O_2 and Quercetin

HNEpCs (5×10^5 cells/mL) were cultured with either 12.5–100.0 μM H_2O_2 or 0.1–10.0 nM quercetin for 24 h. The cells were then collected, and cell viability was assessed by the trypan blue dye exclusion test. The dead cells were stained with trypan blue, and the proportion of dead cells was determined by counting 300 total cells.

2.5. Assay to Assess TRX mRNA Expression

TRX mRNA expression was examined by the methods described previously (24). Briefly, Poly A^+ mRNA was extracted from cultured cells with oligo(dT)-coated magnetic micro beads (Milteny Biotec, Bergisch Gladbach, Germany). The first-strand cDNA was synthesized from 1.0 μg of Poly A^+ mRNA using a Superscript cDNA synthesis kit (Invitrogen Corp., Carlsbad, CA, USA) according to the manufacturer's recommendations. Polymerase chain reaction (PCR) was then performed using a GeneAmp 5700 Sequence Detection System (Applied Biosystems, Forster City, CA, USA). The PCR mixture consisted of 2.0 μL of sample cDNA solution (100 ng/μL), 25.0 μL of SYBR-Green Mastermix (Applied Biosystems), 0.3 μL of both sense and antisense primers, and distilled water for a final volume of 50.0 μL. The conditions used for the reaction was as follows: 4 min at 94 °C, followed by 40 cycles of 15 s at 95 °C and 60 s at 60 °C. GAPDH was used as an internal control. TRX mRNA levels were calculated using the comparative parameter threshold cycle and normalized to GAPDH. The primers used for real-time RT-PCR were as follows: 5′-GCCTTGCAAAATGATTCAAGC-3′ (Sense) and 5′-TTGGCTCCAGAAAATTCACC-3′ (Antisense) for TRX [24], and 5′-TGTTGCCATCAATGACCCCTT-3′ (Sense) and 5′-CTCCACGACGTACTCAGCG-3′ (Antisense) for GAPDH [24].

2.6. Sensitization and Treatment of Mice

BALB/c mice were sensitized with an intraperitoneal injection of 20.0 μg/mL OVA in phosphate-buffered saline (PBS) combined with 1.0 mg of alum in a total volume of 200.0 μL on days 0, 7, and 14 [3,4]. On days 21, 23, and 25, the mice were intranasally instilled with 100 μg of OVA (5.0 μL in PBS) [3,4]. The mice were orally administered 10, 15, 20, or 25 mg/kg of quercetin using a stomach tube in a volume not exceeding 0.5 mL once a day for five consecutive days, beginning on day 21 relative to the sensitization.

2.7. Collection of Nasal Lavage Fluids

The mice were anesthetized by intraperitoneal injection with 50.0 mg/kg sodium pentobarbital (Kyoritsu Seiyaku Co., Ltd., Tokyo, Japan) 6 h after the OVA nasal challenge. The trachea was exposed and cannulated to introduce 1.0 mL of PBS [16]. The lavage fluid from the nares was collected and centrifuged at 3000 rpm for 15 min at 4 °C. After measuring IgA levels with ELISA (Bethyl Lab., Inc., Montgomery, TX, USA), the fluids were stored at −40 °C until use [16].

2.8. Assessment of Nasal Symptoms

Nasal allergy symptoms were assessed by counting the number of sneezes and nasal rubbing movements for 10 min immediately after the OVA nasal instillation. The experimental mice were placed into plastic animal cages (35 × 20 × 30 cm) for approximately 10 min to acclimate. After the nasal instillation of 0.1% OVA solution in PBS in a volume of 5.0 µL, the mice were placed into plastic cages (two animals/cage), and the number of sneezes and nasal rubbing movements were counted for 10 min [16].

2.9. TRX Assay

The TRX levels in the culture supernatants and nasal lavage fluids were examined using human and mouse TRX ELISA test kits (CUSABIO TECHNOLOGY LLC., Huston, TX, USA) according to the manufacturer's recommendations. The minimum detectable levels of the ELISA test kits were 1.172 ng/mL and 0.078 ng/mL for humans and mice, respectively.

2.10. Oxidative Stress Assay

The oxidative stress responses in the nasal mucosa were evaluated by measuring lipid peroxide levels in nasal lavage fluids using d-ROM tests (DIACRON, Via Zircone, Italy) according to the manufacturer's recommendations. The results were expressed as mean Carratelli Units (CARR U) ± SE.

2.11. Statistical Analysis

The statistical significance between the control and experimental groups was assessed with an ANOVA followed by Dunette's multiple comparison test. A *P* value of less than 0.05 was considered significant.

3. Results

3.1. Influence of H_2O_2 Stimulation on TRX Production from HNEpCs in Vitro

The first experiments were performed to examine whether H_2O_2 stimulation could increase TRX production from HNEpCs and to determine the optimal concentration of H_2O_2 for stimulation. Thus, the cells were stimulated with various concentrations of H_2O_2 for 24 h, and the TRX levels in the culture supernatants were determined via ELISA. As shown in Figure 1, the stimulation of cells with H_2O_2 caused a significant increase in the ability of cells to produce TRX. As little as 2.5 µM H_2O_2 caused a strong stimulation in TRX production. Maximum production was observed with 25.0–75.0 µM H_2O_2 whereas 100.0 µM H_2O_2 was inhibitory (Figure 1).

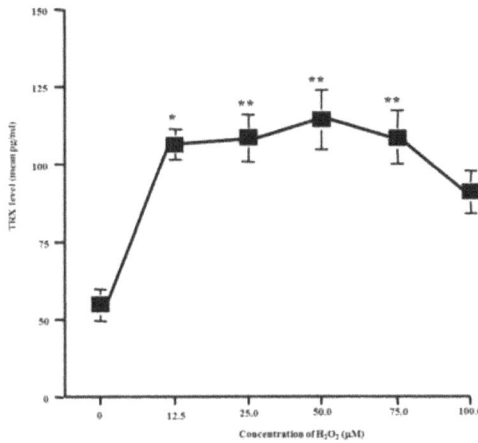

Figure 1. Influence of H_2O_2 on thioredoxin (TRX) production from HNEpCs in vitro. Nasal epithelial cells (5×10^5 cells) were stimulated with various concentrations of H_2O_2. After 24 h, TRX levels in culture supernatants were examined with ELISA. The data are expressed as the mean pg/mL $\pm$ SE of triplicate cultures. One representative experiment of two is shown in this figure. *: $P < 0.05$ versus control (0); **: $P > 0.05$ versus 12.5 μM H_2O_2.

3.2. In Vitro Influence of Quercetin on H_2O_2-Induced TRX Production from HNEpCs

The second set of experiments was designed to examine the influence of quercetin on the TRX production of HNEpCs after H_2O_2 stimulation. The cells were stimulated with 50.0 μM H_2O_2 in the presence or absence of quercetin for 24 h. TRX levels in the culture supernatants were examined by ELISA. As shown in Figure 2, the treatment of cells with quercetin at concentrations of both 0.1 nM and 0.5 nM barely affected the ability of the cells to produce TRX: the TRX levels in the culture supernatants were nearly identical (not significant) to those detected in the controls. At concentrations greater than 1.0 nM, however, quercetin induced significantly increased TRX levels in culture supernatants compared to those levels in the controls.

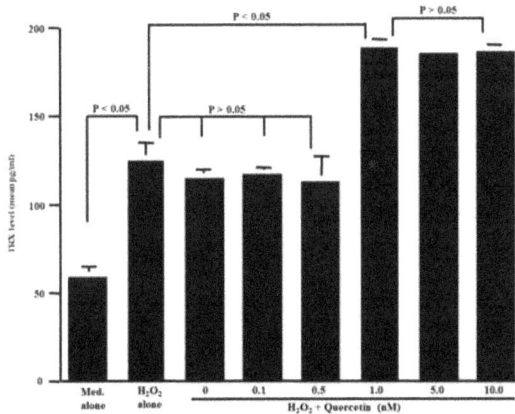

Figure 2. Influence of quercetin on thioredoxin (TRX) production from HNEpCs induced by H_2O_2 stimulation in vitro. Nasal epithelial cells (5×10^5 cells) were stimulated with 50 μM H_2O_2 in the presence of various concentrations of quercetin for 24 h. TRX levels in culture supernatants were examined with ELISA. The data are expressed as the mean pg/mL $\pm$ SE of triplicate cultures. One representative experiment of two is shown in this figure. Med. alone: Medium alone.

3.3. Influence of H₂O₂ and Quercetin on Cell Viability

The third set of experiments was performed to examine the influence of H_2O_2 and quercetin on cell viability. HNEpCs were cultured with either H_2O_2 or quercetin for 24 h, and cell viability was examined via the trypan blue dye exclusion test. Although the cells cultured with H_2O_2 concentrations less than 50.0 μM did not display reduced cell viability, 100.0 nM H_2O_2 caused significant cell death (Figure 3A). We then examined the influence of quercetin on cell viability. Quercetin did not exert cytotoxic effects on HNEpCs; the number of dead cells observed in cells cultured with 100.0 nM quercetin was nearly identical to that observed in controls (Figure 3B).

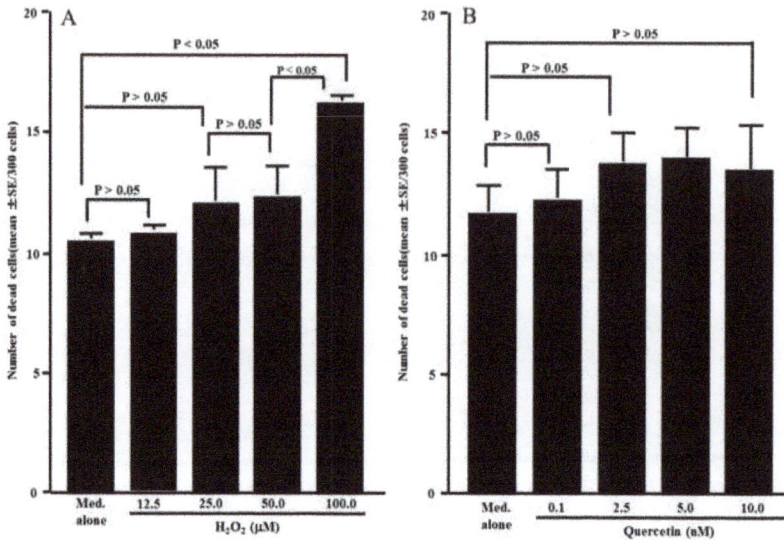

Figure 3. Influence of H_2O_2 (**A**) and quercetin (**B**) on cell viability. Nasal epithelial cells (5×10^5 cells) were stimulated with various concentrations of either H_2O_2 or quercetin for 24 h. The trypan blue exclusion test was performed, and the number of dead cells was counted out of 300 total cells. The data are expressed as the mean number of dead cells ± SE of triplicate cultures. One representative experiment of two is shown in this figure. Med. alone: Medium alone.

3.4. Influence of Quercetin on TRX mRNA Expression

The fourth set of experiments was performed to examine the influence of quercetin on TRX mRNA expression in HNEpCs stimulated with 50.0 μM H_2O_2. The stimulation of HNEpCs with H_2O_2 caused significant increases in TRX mRNA expression compared to the non-stimulated (Med. alone) controls (Figure 4). However, TRX mRNA expression was significantly suppressed in HNEpCs treated with more than 1.0 nM quercetin but not in HNEpCs treated with less than 0.5 nM, whereas TRX mRNA expression was increased by stimulation with H_2O_2 (Figure 4).

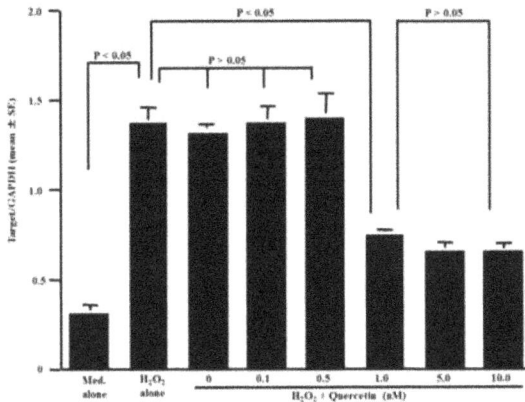

Figure 4. Influence of quercetin on TRX mRNA expression in HNEpCs. Nasal epithelial cells (5×10^5 cells) were stimulated with 50 μM H_2O_2 in the presence or absence of quercetin for 12 h. TRX mRNA levels in the cultured cells were examined by RT-PCR. The data are expressed as the mean Target/GAPD $\pm$ SE of triplicate cultures. One representative experiment of two is shown in this figure. Med. alone: Medium alone.

3.5. Influence of Quercetin on Oxidative Stress Responses in Nasal Mucosa

The fifth set of experiments was performed to examine whether oxidative stress responses were occurred in OVA-sensitized mice and whether quercetin administration into OVA-sensitized mice could modulate oxidative stress responses. Therefore, OVA-sensitized mice were orally administered 10.0–25.0 mg/kg of quercetin at days 21–25 after sensitization. Nasal lavage fluids were obtained 6 h after the final nasal OVA challenge, and lipid peroxide levels in nasal secretions were examined by the d-ROM test. Quercetin treatment significantly decreased lipid peroxide levels in the nasal lavage fluids of the mice, whereas the OVA nasal challenge increased lipid peroxide levels (Figure 5).

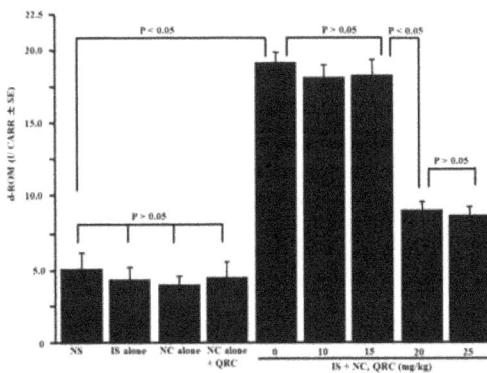

Figure 5. Influence of quercetin on the appearance of lipid peroxide in nasal lavage fluids after ovalbumin (OVA) sensitization in mice. BALB/c mice were sensitized by an intraperitoneal injection of OVA on days 0, 7, and 14. Seven days after the final sensitization, the OVA-sensitized mice were intranasally challenged with OVA on days 21, 23, and 25, and various concentrations of quercetin were administered orally once a day for five consecutive days. Nasal lavage fluids were obtained from mice 6 h after the OVA nasal challenge. Lipid peroxide levels were measured using the d-ROM test. The data are expressed as the mean CARR U $\pm$ SE of five mice. NS: non-sensitized; IS: intraperitoneal sensitization; NC: nasal challenge alone; QRC: quercetin.

3.6. Influence of Quercetin on the Appearance of TRX in Nasal Lavage Fluids

The sixth set of experiments was designed to examine the influence of quercetin on the appearance of TRX in nasal lavage fluids obtained from sensitized mice after the OVA nasal challenge. The OVA-sensitized mice were orally administered 10.0–25.0 mg/kg of quercetin at days 21–25 after sensitization. Nasal lavage fluids were obtained 6 h after the final nasal OVA challenge. As shown in Figure 6, the oral administration of 20.0 and 25.0 mg/kg of quercetin, but not 10.0 and 15.0 mg/kg, could increase TRX levels in nasal lavage fluids.

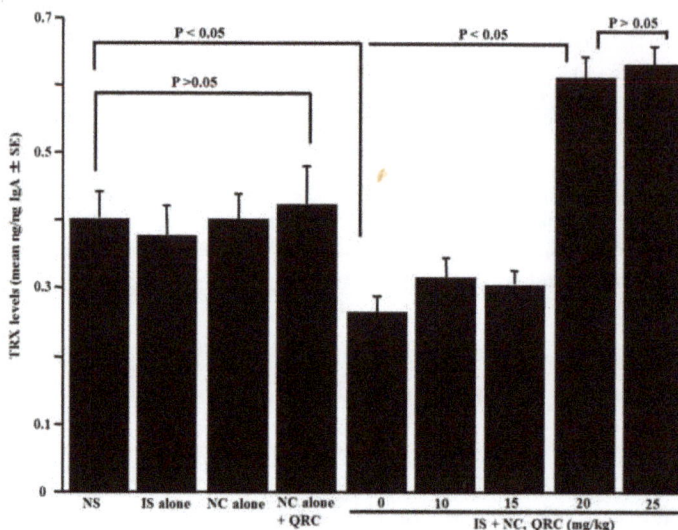

Figure 6. Influence of quercetin on the appearance of thioredoxin (TRX) in nasal lavage fluids obtained from OVA-sensitized mice after the OVA nasal challenge. BALB/c mice were sensitized by an intraperitoneal injection of OVA on days 0, 7, and 14. Seven days after the final sensitization, the OVA-sensitized mice were intranasally challenged with OVA on days 21, 23, and 25, and various concentrations of quercetin were administered orally once a day for five consecutive days. Nasal lavage fluids were obtained from the mice 6 h after the nasal antigenic challenge. TRX levels were examined by an ELISA. The data are expressed as the mean ng/ng IgA ± SE of five mice. NS: non-sensitized; IS: intraperitoneal sensitization; NC: nasal challenge alone; QRC: quercetin.

3.7. Influence of Quercetin on the Development of OVA-Induced Nasal Allergy-Like Symptoms

The final set of experiments was performed to examine whether the oral administration of quercetin in OVA-sensitized mice could inhibit the development of nasal allergy-like symptoms, which were induced by the nasal antigenic challenge. Nasal symptoms were assessed by counting the number of sneezes and nasal rubbing movements for 10 min immediately after the OVA nasal challenge. As shown in Figure 7, treating the OVA-sensitized mice with less than 15.0 mg/kg of quercetin could not inhibit the development of nasal allergy-like symptoms: the number of sneezes and nasal rubbing movements were nearly identical (not significant) to those observed in the non-treated controls. Conversely, the oral administration of more than 20.0 mg/kg of quercetin attenuated the development of nasal allergy-like symptoms, and the number of sneezes and nasal rubbing movements was significantly lower than those observed in the non-treated controls (Figure 7).

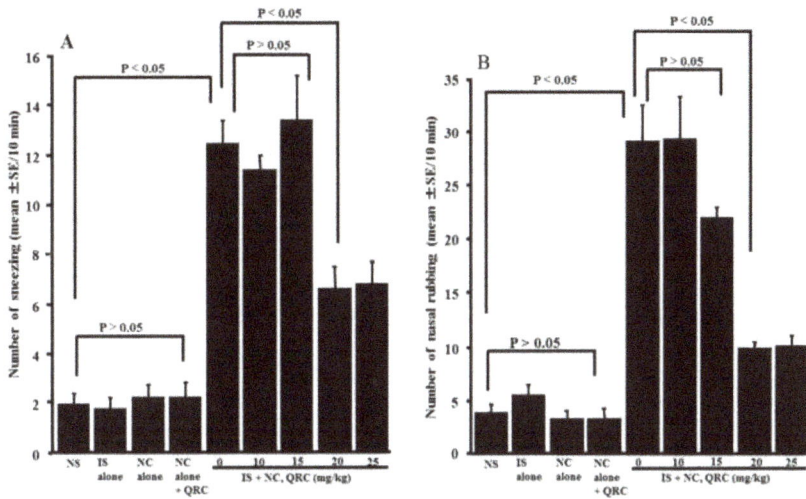

Figure 7. Influence of quercetin on the development of nasal allergy-like symptoms in OVA-sensitized mice after the OVA nasal challenge. BALB/c mice were sensitized by an intraperitoneal injection of OVA on days 0, 7, and 14. Seven days after the final sensitization, the OVA-sensitized mice were intranasally challenged with OVA on days 21, 23, and 25, and various concentrations of quercetin were administered orally once a day for five consecutive days. Nasal allergy-like symptoms, the number of sneezes (**A**), and nasal rubbing behaviors (**B**) were counted for 10 min immediately after the final nasal antigenic challenge. The data are expressed as the mean ± SE of five mice. NS: non-sensitized; IS: intraperitoneal sensitization; NC: nasal challenge alone; QRC: quercetin.

4. Discussion

The results obtained from the in vitro experiments clearly show that quercetin can increase the ability of HNEpCs to produce TRX in response to H_2O_2 stimulation. The minimum concentration that caused a significant increase in TRX production was 1.0 nM.

After the oral administration of 64 mg of quercetin to humans, quercetin plasma levels gradually increased and attained peak at 650 nM, with a half-life elimination of 17–24 h [25]. Although there is no standard recommended dosage of quercetin, a dose of 1200 to 1500 mg per day is commonly used [26] as a supplement. It is also observed that a 1200 mg dose could lead to a plasma concentration of up to 12 µM [25], which is higher than the concentration necessary to induce the increase in the ability of HNEpCs to produce TRX in vitro. Based on these reports, the findings of the present in vitro study may reflect the biological function of quercetin in vivo. At present, we cannot exclude the possibility that the stimulation of thioredoxin production at higher concentrations of hydrogen peroxide and quercetin may be cellular protective mechanism against the cytotoxicity induced by these agents. Further experiments are needed to test this possibility.

AR is defined as an allergic inflammation of the nasal mucosa and is characterized by a symptom complex that consists of any combination of sneezing, nasal congestion, and nasal itching, among others [1,2]. These symptoms are primarily induced by chemical mediators from mast cells, such as histamine, tryptase, and kinin [1,2]. These mediators also recruit other inflammatory cells, including neutrophils and eosinophils, to the mucosa [1]. These polymorphonuclear leukocytes secrete harmful granular proteins and ROS, which cause tissue remodeling and persistent AR [18,27]. Because ROS are necessary for life, the body initiates several mechanisms to decrease ROS-induced tissue damage and to repair damage that occurs, including several enzymes and proteins [19]. Among these mechanisms, TRX attracts attention as not only an important anti-oxidative factor but also as a protective factor in the development of various inflammatory diseases, including AR [22,23]. TRX is reported to suppress eosinophil chemotaxis induced by CC chemokine stimulation through the suppression of both the activation of extracellular signal-regulated kinase 1/2 and p38 mitogen-activated protein kinase pathways [28]. Treating mice with TRX inhibits the development of airway inflammation and the overproduction of macrophage inflammatory protein (MIP)-1, RANTES, IL-4, and IL-5, which are responsible for the development of allergic inflammatory responses [22,23]. Furthermore, airway remodeling and eosinophilic inflammation induced by chronic antigen exposure were prevented in TRX transgenic mice that displayed overproduction of TRX [23]. Together with these reports, the present results obtained in in vivo experiments suggest that quercetin increases TRX production in the nasal mucosa and results in a favorable modification of the clinical conditions of AR. However, before concluding that the oral administration of quercetin in AR patients increases the ability of nasal cells, particularly epithelial cells, to produce TRX and attenuate the development of AR, we must examine the influence of quercetin on TRX production in vivo. Therefore, the second half of the study was performed to examine whether quercetin could also increase the ability of nasal cells to produce TRX after specific allergen inhalation and whether this activity was related to the development of nasal allergy-like symptoms in OVA-sensitized mice. The present in vivo data showed that nasal lavage fluids obtained from sensitized-non-treated mice contained higher levels of lipid peroxide compared to those from non-sensitized mice. Moreover, the oral administration of quercetin decreased lipid peroxide levels and increased TRX levels in nasal lavage fluids. Furthermore, the oral administration of quercetin to OVA-sensitized mice inhibited the development of nasal allergy-like symptoms after the OVA nasal challenge. The minimum concentration that caused significant changes in these parameters was 20 mg/kg. From these results, it can be reasonably interpreted that the actions of quercetin on TRX production may represent a possible mechanism that can explain the favorable effects of quercetin on AR.

The present data clearly show that quercetin enhances the ability of nasal cells to produce TRX in response to stimulation with either H_2O_2 or specific allergens in vitro and in vivo, despite the suppression of TRX mRNA expression. Furthermore, our previous report clearly showed that quercetin inhibited the production of chemokines, such as eotaxin and macrophage inflammatory protein-1beta (MIP-1β), by suppressing the mRNA expression of chemokines in eosinophils after stem cell factor simulation [29]. Furthermore, quercetin exerts suppressive effects on the activation of transcription factors, which are essential for several types of endogenous immune-modulatory proteins [30]. Synthesis of proteins in cells requires two quite different steps: in transcription, the first step, specific mRNA is synthetized from DNA in the nucleus. The newly synthetized mRNA travels through the nuclear membrane into the cytoplasm where it binds to mRNA-binding sites on ribosomes and initiates protein synthesis, which is called translation. From these established concepts, there is a possibility that quercetin increases the translatable activity of TRX mRNA and results in the production and secretion of large amounts of TRX from nasal epithelial cells after stimulation. Although glucocorticoids, which are considered first-line therapeutic agents in the treatment of AR [2], are accepted to exert their immune-modulatory effects by suppressing inflammatory mediator mRNA expression, they can increase the ability of cells to produce an immune-modulatory peptide, uteroglobin, after inflammatory stimulations by enhancing the translation of uteroglobin mRNA [31,32]. These reports support the speculation that the translation of TRX mRNA is enhanced by quercetin and results in the appearance of a large amount of TRX in both culture supernatants and nasal secretions.

Oral allergy syndrome (OAS), also recognized as pollen-food syndrome, is an allergic response in the oral cavity following the ingestion of fruits, vegetables, or nuts. OAS reportedly occurs in approximately 20–70% of patients with AR and atopy [33]. Pollen-specific IgE antibodies in AR patients recognize homologous dietary allergens that share the same epitopes of pollen and trigger the cross-reaction between allergens in pollens and those in foods, resulting in the development of OAS [33]. OAS includes several allergic reactions that occur very rapidly, within minutes of eating a trigger food. The most common symptoms are itchy mouth, scratchy throat, or swelling of the lips, tongue, and throat [33,34]. Although no standard treatment for OAS exists, antihistamines and oral steroids can help relieve symptoms [33], which suggests that quercetin will be a good candidate to supplement the treatment of OAS.

5. Conclusions

The results obtained from the present experiments strongly suggest that quercetin increases the ability of nasal epithelial cells, to produce TRX after stimulation with oxidants or allergens. Moreover, quercetin results in the attenuation of development of the clinical symptoms of AR by suppressing oxidative stress responses in nasal mucosa.

Author Contributions: Cell culture and assay for thioredoxin and lipid peroxide, Y.E.; animal experiments, statistical analysis of the data, and drawing figures, A.O.; conceptualization, study design, and manuscript writing, K.A.

Funding: This research received no external funding.

Conflicts of Interest: All the authors have no conflicts of interest in this study.

References

1. Pawankar, R.; Mori, S.; Ozu, C.; Kimura, S. Overview on the pathomechanisms of allergic rhinitis. *Asia Pac. Allergy* **2011**, *1*, 157–167. [CrossRef] [PubMed]
2. Ramirez-Jimenez, F.; Pavon-Romero, G.; Juarez-Martinez, L.L.; Teran, L.M. Allergic rhinitis. *J. Allergy Ther.* **2012**, *S5*, 006. [CrossRef]
3. Jung, D.; Lee, S.; Hong, S. Effects of acupuncture and moxibustion in a mouse model of allergic rhinitis. *Otolaryngol. Head Neck Surg.* **2011**, *146*, 19–25. [CrossRef] [PubMed]
4. Jeong, K.T.; Kim, S.G.; Lee, J.; Park, Y.N.; Park, H.H.; Parl, N.Y.; Kim, K.J.; Lee, H.; Lee, Y.J. Anti-allergic effect of a Korean traditional medicine, Biyeom-Tang on mast cells and allergic rhinitis. *BMC Comp. Altern. Med.* **2014**, *14*, 54. [CrossRef] [PubMed]
5. Van Cauwenberg, P.; Bachert, C.; Passalacua, G. Consensus statement on the treatment of allergic rhinitis. European Academy of Allergology and Clinical Immunology. *Allergy* **2000**, *55*, 116–134. [CrossRef]
6. Ishizawa, K.; Yoshizumi, M.; Kawai, Y.; Terao, J.; Kihira, Y.; Ikeda, Y.; Tomita, S.; Minakuchi, K.; Tsuchiya, K.; Tamaki, T. Pharmacology in health food: Metabolism of quercetin in vivo and its protective effect against arteriosclerosis. *J. Pharmacol. Sci.* **2011**, *115*, 466–470. [CrossRef] [PubMed]
7. Hattori, M.; Mizuguchi, H.; Baba, Y.; Ono, S.; Nakano, T.; Zhang, Q.; Sasaki, Y.; Kobayashi, M.; Kitamura, Y.; Takeda, N.; et al. Quercetin inhibits transcriptional up-regulation of histamine H1 receptor via suppressing protein kinase C-δ/extracellular signal-regulated kinase/poly (ADP-ribose) polymerase-1 signaling pathway in Hela cells. *Int. Immunopharmacol.* **2013**, *15*, 232–239. [CrossRef] [PubMed]
8. Kawada, N.; Seki, S.; Inoue, M.; Kuroki, T. Effect of antioxidants, resveratrol, quercetin, and N-acetylcysteine, on the functions of cultured rat hapatic stellate cells and kupper cells. *Hepatology* **1998**, *27*, 1265–1274. [CrossRef] [PubMed]
9. Amorati, R.; Baschieri, A.; Cowde, A.; Valgimigli, L. The antioxidant activity of quercetin in water solution. *Biomimetics* **2017**, *2*, 9. [CrossRef]
10. Lesjak, M.; Beara, I.; Simin, N.; Pintac, D.; Majkic, T.; Bekvalac, K.; Orcic, D.; Mimica-Dukic, N. Antioxidant and anti-inflammatory activities of quercetin and its derivatives. *J. Funct. Foods* **2018**, *40*, 68–75. [CrossRef]
11. Middleton, E., Jr. Effect of plant flavonoids on immune and inflammatory cell function. *Adv. Exp. Med. Biol.* **1998**, *439*, 175–182. [PubMed]
12. Min, Y.D.; Choi, C.H.; Bark, H.; Son, H.Y.; Park, H.H.; Lee, S.; Park, J.W.; Park, E.K.; Shin, H.I.; Kim, S.H. Quercetin inhibits expression of inflammatory cytokines through attenuation of NF-kB and P38 MAPK in HMC-1 human mast cell line. *Inflamm. Res.* **2007**, *56*, 210–215. [CrossRef] [PubMed]
13. Hirano, T.; Kawai, M.; Arimitsu, J.; Ogawa, M.; Kuwahara, Y.; Hagihara, K.; Shima, Y.; Narazaki, M.; Ogata, A.; Koyanagi, M.; et al. Preventive effect of a flavonoid, enzymatically modified isoquercetin on ocular symptoms of Japanese cedar pollinosis. *Allergol. Int.* **2009**, *58*, 373–382. [CrossRef] [PubMed]
14. Rogerio, A.P.; Kanashiro, A.; Fontanari, C.; de Silva, E.V.; Lucisano-Valim, Y.M.; Soares, E.G.; Faccioli, L.H. Anti-inflammatory activity of quercetin and isoquercetin in experimental murine allergic asthma. *Inflamm. Res.* **2007**, *56*, 402–408. [CrossRef] [PubMed]

15. Dorsch, W.; Bittinger, M.; Kaas, A.; Muller, A.; Kreher, B.; Wagner, H. Antiasthmatic effects of *Galphimia glauca*, gallic acid, and related compounds prevent allergen- and platelet-activating factor-induced bronchial obstruction as well as bronchial hyperreactivity in guinea pigs. *Int. Arch. Allergy Immunol.* **1992**, *97*, 1–7. [CrossRef] [PubMed]

16. Kashiwabara, M.; Asano, K.; Mizuyoshi, T.; Kobayashi, H. Suppression of neuropeptide production by quercetin in allergic rhinitis model rats. *BMC Comp. Altern. Med.* **2016**, *16*, 132. [CrossRef] [PubMed]

17. Min, A.; Lee, Y.A.; Kim, K.; EI-Benna, J.; Shin, M.H. Nox2-derived ROS-mediated surface translocation of BLT1 is essential for exocytosis in human eosinophils induced by LBT4. *Int. Arch. Allergy Immunol.* **2014**, *165*, 40–51. [CrossRef] [PubMed]

18. Suojalehto, H.; Vehmas, T.; Lindstrom, I.; Kennedy, D.W.; Kilpelainen, M.; Plosila, T.; Savukoski, S.; Sipilä, J.; Varpula, M.; Wolff, H.; et al. Nasal nitric oxide is dependent on sinus obstruction in allergic rhinitis. *Laryngoscope* **2014**, *124*, E231–E238. [CrossRef] [PubMed]

19. Sen, S.; Chakraborty, R.; Sridhar, C.; Reddy, Y.S.R.; De, B. Free radicals, antioxidants, diseases and phytomedicines: Current status and future prospect. *Int. J. Pharm. Sci. Rev. Res.* **2010**, *3*, 91–100.

20. Burke-Gaffney, A.; Callister, M.E.J.; Nakamura, H. Thioredoxin: Friend or foe in human disease. *Trends Pharmacol. Sci.* **2005**, *26*, 398–404. [CrossRef] [PubMed]

21. Holmgren, A.; Lu, J. Thioredoxin and thioredoxin reductase: Current research with special reference to human disease. *Biochem. Biophys. Res. Commun.* **2010**, *396*, 120–124. [CrossRef] [PubMed]

22. Ichiki, H.; Hoshino, T.; Kinoshita, T.; Imaoka, H.; Kato, S.; Inoue, H.; Nakamura, H.; Yodoi, J.; Young, H.A.; Aizawa, H. Thioredoxin suppresses airway hyperresponsiveness and airway inflammation in asthma. *Biochem. Biophys. Res. Commun.* **2005**, *334*, 1141–1148. [CrossRef] [PubMed]

23. Imaoka, H.; Hoshino, T.; Takei, S.; Sakazaki, Y.; Kinoshita, T.; Okamoto, M.; Kawayama, T.; Yodoi, J.; Kato, S.; Iwanaga, T.; et al. Effects of thioredoxin on established airway remodeling in a chronic antigen exposure asthma model. *Biochem. Biophys. Res. Commun.* **2007**, *360*, 525–530. [CrossRef] [PubMed]

24. Suzaki, I.; Asano, K.; Kanei, A.; Suzaki, H. Enhancement of thioredoxin production from nasal epithelial cells by the macrolide antibiotic, Clarithromycin in vitro. *Vivo* **2013**, *27*, 351–356.

25. Hollman, P.C.; vd Gaag, M.; Mengelers, M.J.; van Trijp, J.M.; de Vries, J.H.; Katan, M.B. Absorption and disposition kinetics of the dietary antioxidant quercetin in man. *Free Radic. Biol. Med.* **1996**, *21*, 703–707. [CrossRef]

26. Wadsworth, T.L.; Koop, D.R. Effects of *Ginkgo biloba* extract (EGb 761) and quercetin on lipopolysaccharide-induced release of nitric oxide. *Biochem. Pharmacol.* **2001**, *137*, 43–58. [CrossRef]

27. Imoto, Y.; Yamada, T.; Tsukahara, H.; Kimura, Y.; Kato, Y.; Sakashita, M.; Fujieda, S. Nitrite/nitrate in nasal lavage fluid reflect nasal symptoms after a single nasal allergen provocation in patients with seasonal allergic rhinitis. *J. Investig. Allergol. Clin. Immunol.* **2015**, *25*, 382–384. [PubMed]

28. Sannohe, S.; Adachi, T.; Hamada, K.; Honda, K.; Yamada, Y.; Saito, N.; Cui, C.H.; Kayaba, H.; Ishikawa, K.; Chihara, J. Upregulated response to chemokines in oxidative metabolism of eosinophils in asthma and allergic rhinitis. *Eur. Respir. J.* **2003**, *21*, 925–931. [CrossRef] [PubMed]

29. Sakai-Kashiwabara, M.; Abe, S.; Asano, K. Suppressive activity of quercetin on the production of eosinophil chemoattractants from eosinophils in vitro. *Vivo* **2014**, *28*, 515–522.

30. Irie, S.; Kashiwabara, M.; Yamada, A.; Asano, K. Suppressive activity of quercetin on periostin functions in vitro. *Vivo* **2016**, *30*, 17–25.

31. Lopez, M.S.; Nieto, A. Glucocorticoids induce the expression of the uteroglobin gene in rabbit fetal lung explants cultured in vitro. *Biochem. J.* **1985**, *225*, 255–258. [CrossRef]

32. Fernandez-Renau, D.; Lombardero, M.; Nieto, A. Glucocorticoid-dependent uteroglobin synthesis and uteroglobin mRNA levels in rabbit lung explants cultured in vitro. *Eur. J. Biochem.* **1984**, *144*, 523–527. [CrossRef] [PubMed]

33. Price, A.; Ramachandran, S.; Ramachandran, S.; Smith, G.P.; Stevenson, M.L.; Pomeranz, M.K.; Cohen, D.E. Oral allergy syndrome (Pollen-food allergy syndrome). *Dermatitis* **2015**, *26*, 78–88. [CrossRef] [PubMed]

34. Lessof, M.H. Pollen-food allergy syndrome. *J. Allergy Clin. Immunol.* **1996**, *98*, 239–240. [CrossRef]

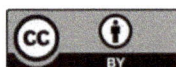

medicines

MDPI

Review

New Functions of Classical Compounds against Orofacial Inflammatory Lesions

Norifumi H. Moritani [1], Emilio Satoshi Hara [2] and Satoshi Kubota [3],*

[1] Department of Oral and Maxillofacial Reconstructive Surgery, Okayama University Graduate School of Medicine, Dentistry and Pharmaceutical Sciences, Okayama 700-8558, Japan; hachi70@md.okayama-u.ac.jp

[2] Department of Biomaterials, Okayama University Graduate School of Medicine, Dentistry and Pharmaceutical Sciences, Okayama 700-8558, Japan; gmd421209@s.okayama-u.ac.jp

[3] Department of Biochemistry and Molecular Dentistry, Okayama University Graduate School of Medicine, Dentistry and Pharmaceutical Sciences, Okayama 700-8558, Japan

* Correspondence: kubota1@md.okayama-u.ac.jp; Tel.: +81-86-235-6645

Received: 13 September 2018; Accepted: 13 October 2018; Published: 1 November 2018

Abstract: Anti-inflammatory agents have been widely used to ameliorate severe inflammatory symptoms of a number of diseases, and such therapeutics are particularly useful for diseases with intolerable pain without significant mortality. A typical example of this is a disease known as stomatitis; although stomatitis itself is not a life-threatening disease, it severely impairs the individual's quality of life, and thus a standard therapeutic strategy for it has already been established. The topical application of a bioactive agent is quite easy, and a strong anti-inflammatory agent can be used without significant adverse effects. In contrast, natural products with relatively mild bioactivity are used for systemic intervention. However, new aspects of classical drugs used in these established therapeutic methods have recently been discovered, which is expanding the utility of these compounds to other oral diseases such as osteoarthritis of temporomandibular joints (TMJ-OA). In this review article, after summarizing the general concept and pathobiology of stomatitis, its established therapeutics are explained. Thereafter, recent advances in the research into related compounds, which is uncovering new biological functions of the agents used therein, are introduced. Indeed, regenerative therapeutics for TMJ-OA may be developed with the classical compounds currently being used.

Keywords: stomatitis; recurrent aphthous stomatitis; oral lichen planus; CCN2; glucocorticoids; alkaloids

1. Introduction

The oral cavity is a biological apparatus that enables the intake of food, drink, and air, thus enabling the intake of the most basic elements needed to support the development, growth, and maintenance of human bodies. Therefore, inflammatory lesions in the oral area are always deleterious to human health, impairing all of the biological activities of the cells constituting an individual. The most common inflammatory diseases in the oral region are those in, or around the teeth. Endodontic inflammation is where there is designated pulpitis, the acute form of which usually yields intolerable pain. However, owing to its poor regeneration potential, recovery of the affected pulp tissue can hardly be expected [1]. As such, a major intervention used to terminate pulpitis is a pulpectomy, which is the removal of the dental pulp under local anesthesia without anti-inflammatory treatment. In contrast, periodontitis is usually chronic and occasionally even asymptomatic. Needless to say, inflammatory responses of the host are critically involved in the etiology of periodontitis [2,3]. However, since periodontitis is based on the infection of a number of oral bacteria, the principal therapeutic methods against periodontitis have been the regulation of bacterial infection. For a better clinical outcome, the utilization of desiccants has recently been proposed [4], and acceleration of periodontal tissue regeneration by laser treatment has also been attempted [5,6]. In addition, the osseous drilling protocol has been regarded as critical for dental implants, rather than inflammation control [7]; therefore, anti-inflammatory molecules are not major agents in the treatment of these dental diseases.

Food intake can be more severely affected by stomatitis as any contact with the affected oral mucosa will cause great pain to the affected individual. Additionally, since it depends on mastication that is performed by the collaborative movement of temporomandibular joints (TMJ), osteoarthritis (OA) of the TMJ strongly restricts its quality and quantity. As will be mentioned in the next section, stomatitis is characterized by prominent inflammatory responses that have no apparent relationship with bacterial infection [8,9]. Notably, in contrast to the dental pulp, the regeneration potential of oral mucosa is quite high; as such, anti-inflammatory compounds have been widely used for the treatment of stomatitis to promptly redeem the individual's food intake ability. In this article, starting from the review of stomatitis and related disorders, established therapeutics using classical compounds are summarized. Then, we report on the recent research topics that unveiled the possible utilities of a few such classical compounds in the treatment of the OA of TMJ for which no fundamental therapeutics have yet to be established. In particular, CCN family protein 2 (CCN2), a profibrotic protein involved in inflammation and tissue regeneration [10], has been found to mediate the novel biological effects therein. As such, we believe that the consideration of CCN2-mediated effects is critical in developing new therapeutic methods against inflammation.

2. Stomatitis and Oral Mucosal Diseases

Stomatitis is a term commonly used to describe the inflammation of oral mucosa. The names of several stomatitis-related conditions are listed in Table 1. Among them, the most commonly recognized type of stomatitis is aphthous stomatitis. Aphthous stomatitis is where there are painful ulcers that are clearly defined as shallow, round, or oval, with a necrotic center covered by yellowish-tan pseudomembranes, and surrounded by an erythematous halo. An example of aphthous stomatitis is shown in Figure 1. The term "aphtha" refers to the clinical condition and is not the name of the disease; the appropriate disease name is recurrent aphthous stomatitis (RAS). As above-mentioned, stomatitis is a generic name for the inflammation of oral mucosa, and is also known as oral mucosal disease.

Table 1. Stomatitis-related conditions.

Disease Names
aphthous stomatitis
recurrent aphthous stomatitis (RAS)
(synonym: recurrent aphthous ulcer)
herpetic stomatitis
catarrhal stomatitis
drug-induced stomatitis
radiation-induced stomatitis
gangrenous stomatitis
nicotinic stomatitis
angular stomatitis
(synonym: angular cheilitis)
denture-related stomatitis

Oral mucosal diseases have numerous conditions such as those listed in Table 1. However, as we cannot present all such diseases, we have at least tried to classify oral mucosal diseases by their clinical manifestations, as shown in Table 2. Furthermore, the classification of the diseases listed in Table 2, according to etiology, is shown in Table 3. The oral mucosal diseases listed in Tables 1–3 pose a number of treatment challenges to clinicians such as: (1) few treatment opportunities being presented at clinics; (2) the cause being largely unknown; (3) symptomatic treatment is the mainstay of treatment, and not causal therapy, where a radical cure is difficult to achieve; and (4) that an efficacious therapy has not yet been established. It is probably recognized that the above-mentioned representative diseases are RAS and oral lichen planus (OLP).

Table 2. Oral mucosal disease; classification by clinical manifestations.

Major Symptoms	Diseases
bulla/vesicle	herpetic stomatitis, herpes zoster, pemphigus, pemphigoid, epidermolysis bullosa hereditaria
erythema, erosion	erythroplakia, drug-induced stomatitis, radiation-induced stomatitis, angular stomatitis, oral candidiasis, OLP
ulcer	RAS, Behçet's disease, gangrenous stomatitis, denture-related stomatitis
white spot/patch	leukoplakia, OLP, nicotinic stomatitis
pigmentation	Peutz–Jeghers syndrome, melanin pigmentation
atrophic disease	glossitis with anemia (e.g., Hunter's glossitis)

RAS, recurrent aphthous stomatitis; OLP, oral lichen planus.

Table 3. Oral mucosal disease; classification by etiology.

Etiology	Diseases
Congenital or developmental anomalies	epidermolysis bullosa hereditaria, Peutz–Jeghers syndrome
Physical or chemical cause	drug-induced stomatitis, radiation-induced stomatitis, nicotinic stomatitis, denture-related stomatitis
Bacterial infection	angular stomatitis, gangrenous stomatitis
Mycotic infection	oral candidiasis, angular stomatitis
Viral infection	herpetic stomatitis, herpes zoster
Allergic disease	drug-induced stomatitis, Quincke's edema
Autoimmune disease	pemphigus, pemphigoid
Precancerous lesion	erythroplakia, leukoplakia
Unidentified or complex cause	RAS, Behçet's disease, OLP

RAS, recurrent aphthous stomatitis; OLP, oral lichen planus.

2.1. Recurrent Aphthous Stomatitis (RAS)

RAS is also known as recurrent aphtha or recurrent aphthous ulcers. RAS occurs as single or multiple recurrences of aphtha occurring irregularly in the oral mucosa (Figure 1). The etiology of RAS is scientifically unclear, but we here show the conditions that are regarded as the etiology of RAS (Table 4). Since the etiology is unknown, its diagnosis is entirely based on history and clinical criteria, and no laboratory procedures exist to confirm the diagnosis.

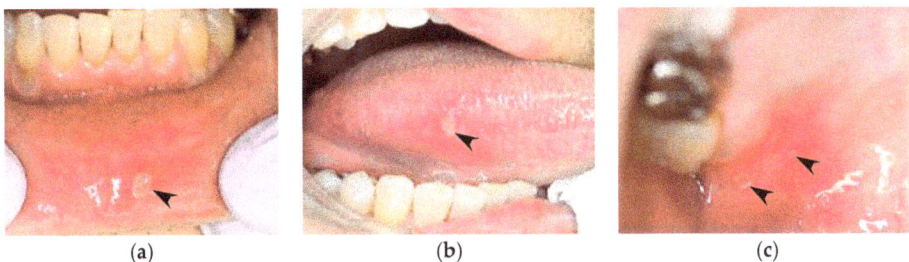

| (a) | (b) | (c) |

Figure 1. Aphthous stomatitis that occurs in a patient with recurrent aphthous stomatitis (RAS). Images are of the same patient and were taken on the same day. (**a**) Lower labial mucosa. (**b**) Right margin of the tongue. (**c**) Right hard palate mucosa (black arrowheads).

Table 4. Proposed etiology of RAS.

Heredity/Genetic Factor
Local trauma such as sharp food and tooth-brushing
Adverse effect of drugs
Deficiency such as iron, zinc, vitamin B12, and folate
Smoking
Virus
Bacteria
Allergy
Hormonal change
Stress
Inflammatory digestive system disease
Immunological abnormality
Cardinal symptom of Behçet's disease
Food hypersensitivity

Generally, the RAS ulcer is resolved spontaneously after a few days or up to 10 days, so the ulcer can be left untreated. However, the RAS ulcer may lead to difficulty in speaking, eating, and swallowing and, thus, may negatively affect the patient's quality of life. As a result, topical therapies for the treatment of ulcers such as steroid ointment or mouthwash are often used. These therapies are directed at palliating symptoms and promoting the rapid healing of the RAS ulcer. However, there is no curative therapy to prevent the recurrence of ulcers, and all available treatment modalities only reduce the frequency or severity of the lesions. Although many causative factors have been proposed, the pathogenesis of RAS is still unknown, and a fundamental treatment for the disease has not been established. RAS is a cardinal symptom of Behçet's disease, which is a systemic inflammatory disorder and is associated with a four-symptom complex of the oral mucosa, genitalia, eyes, and skin [8,9]. RAS occurs in Behçet's disease in all cases and in the whole oral mucosa. Therefore, in the medical examination of patients with RAS, Behçet's disease should be suspected, and a diagnosis to rule it out is necessary.

Behçet's disease has been proposed to be caused by allergy, virus, and autoimmune-related mechanisms, but the exact etiology is still unknown. As for treatment, systemic therapies such as corticosteroid, immunosuppressant, anti-inflammatory, and anti-fibrinolysis medicines are used [11].

2.2. Oral Lichen Planus (OLP)

Oral lichen planus (OLP) is a relatively common diagnosis of oral lesions and has a prevalence of approximately 2% among oral mucosal diseases. OLP presents as reticular or plaque-like white lesions, which are chronic, passing inflammatory lesions with slight hyperkeratosis.

In typical cases, OLP occurs as a reticular white spot at the buccal mucosa (Figure 2). Occasionally, OLP occurs as erythematous lesions with erosion and ulcers. As these symptoms cause discomfort, contact pain, or both in affected subjects, OLP is an intractable disease that may impair the quality of life of patients. The clinical manifestation of OLP varies and presents as white spots that may be reticular, plaque-like, papular, linear, or circular and may occur together with atrophic erythematous, erosive, ulcerative, or rarely bullous-type lesions [12,13]. OLP is diagnosed based on clinical findings such as the previously mentioned pathognomonic gross appearance and the histopathological examination of lesional tissues by biopsy. Pathognomonic histopathological findings are shown in Figure 3. Predisposing factors are not clear yet, but some implicated etiological triggers or aggravating factors of OLP are shown in Table 5 [14–16].

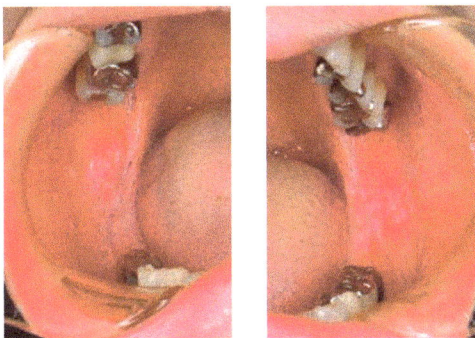

Figure 2. Oral lichen planus (OLP) in a patient, which occurred on both sides of the buccal mucosa with a white and papuloreticular lesion.

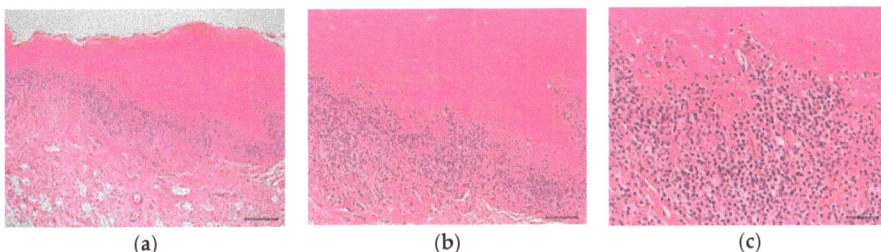

(a) (b) (c)

Figure 3. Hematoxylin and eosin (H&E) staining of an OLP tissue section. (a) Low power photomicrograph. Hyperkeratosis is presented on the surface of the epithelium and a band-like infiltrate of lymphocytes immediately subjacent to the epithelium. Scale bar: 100 µm. (b) Medium power photomicrograph. The rete ridge has a saw-toothed shape. Scale bar: 50 µm. (c) High power photomicrograph. Migration of lymphocytes into the lower epithelium is observed with liquefaction degeneration of the basal layer. The epithelial spinous cell layer directly contacts the infiltrating lymphocytes. Scale bar: 25 µm.

Table 5. Proposed etiology of OLP.

Adverse Drug Reaction
Intraoral dental metal and filler
Intraoral cosmetics including preservatives, aromatic substances
Overwork and stress
Smoking
Hepatitis (hepatitis C in particular)
Oral candidiasis
Herpetic infection
Immunological abnormality

3. Topical or Systemic Therapeutic Agents for RAS and OLP

As the same therapeutic agents are used for RAS and OLP, we mainly describe the medications used in this review (Figure 4). We consider that understanding the mechanism of action of the therapeutic agents for RAS and OLP might contribute to elucidating their etiology.

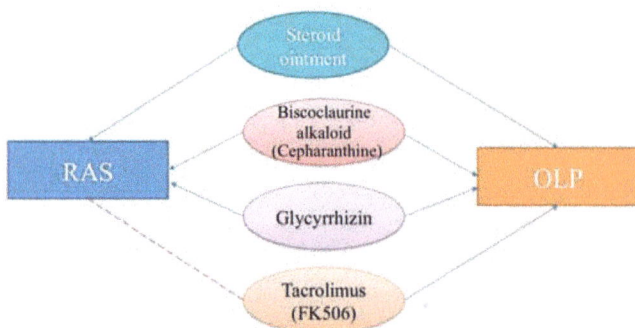

Figure 4. Therapeutic topical and systemic agents for recurrent aphthous stomatitis (RAS) and oral lichen planus (OLP). Blue lines with arrowheads: effective. Red dashed lines: probably effective.

3.1. Glucocorticoids (Topical Use)

In Japan, Dexaltin oral ointment (proprietary name) 1 mg/g or Aphtasolon oral ointment (proprietary name) 0.1% are the major topical therapies used. Dexaltin and Aphtasolon 1.0 g both contain 1.0 mg dexamethasone (Dex), which is the active component. Dex is a corticosteroid glucocorticoid (GCs) and GCs are the most commonly used anti-inflammatory and immunosuppressive drugs. Topical GCs were introduced into medicine approximately 50 years ago. Corticosteroid strength is classified according to their effects in the vasoconstrictor assay and Dex showed the lowest potency in the ranking of a selected group of topical corticosteroid preparations [17]. Therefore, the incidence of associated adverse effects of topical applied steroid is low, and Dex-containing steroid ointments are often used as first choice medications for oral mucosal disease. The molecular mechanisms of the action of steroids include: (1) direct combination of the steroid–steroid receptor complex and DNA sequences called the steroid-responsive element; (2) interactions between the steroid–steroid receptor complex and other transcriptional factors, and (3) non-genomic pathways. The immunosuppressive activity results from the inhibition of neutrophil tissue infiltration, macrophages, eosinophils, and basophils. The anti-inflammatory activity results from both a decrease in the production of inflammatory cytokines and an increase in the production of anti-inflammatory cytokines [18,19]. After entry into the target cells, GCs bind to the GC receptor (GR), which then translocates into the nucleus to directly or indirectly regulate gene transcription. The ligand-activated GR binds as a homodimer to consensus sequences, termed as GC response elements, in the promoter region of GC-sensitive genes to induce the transcription (transactivation) of genes such as tyrosine aminotransferase (*TAT*). An indirect negative regulation of gene expression (transrepression) is achieved by GR-protein interaction. The ligand-activated receptor binds as a monomer to transcription factors such as nuclear factor (NF)-κb and activator protein-1 (AP-1) to inhibit the activity of many proinflammatory transcription factors. This transrepression is considered the key mechanism behind the anti-inflammatory activity of GCs.

3.1.1. RAS

It is generally recognized that topical agents such as steroid ointments are the first treatment choice for RAS. Corticosteroids used in patients with RAS are intended to restrict the inflammatory process associated with the formation of aphthous stomatitis. Corticosteroids may act directly on T lymphocytes in the local environment and alter the response of effector cells to participants of immunopathogenic events. Neutrophils are also found in the surrounding tissue of the RAS ulcers at a marked concentration. The production of oxygen radicals by these neutrophils in RAS has been found to be similar to that in the controls [20].

3.1.2. OLP

The topical use of steroids has been the standard treatment for OLP. In local legion sites of the OLP, oral steroid ointments suppress inflammatory changes and inhibit immune reactions. Therefore, oral steroid ointments are often used as first choice medications for OLP. However, the long-term, repeated application of steroid ointments may be associated with side effects such as candidiasis mainly, which requires attention [21].

3.2. Biscoclaurine Alkaloid (BA) and Cepharanthine (CEP)

Cepharanthine is an alkaloid extracted from the plant *Stephania cepharantha* Hayata, which is naturally found in the woods of southern Formosa, which is now in Taiwan. CEP is a member of a class of compounds known as biscoclaurine alkaloids (BAs). Alkaloids have long attracted the attention of pharmacologists and clinicians owing to their resemblance to polypeptides and their physiological action. It has been widely used in Japan to treat a number of acute and chronic diseases. CEP inhibits tumor necrosis factor (TNF)-α-mediated NF-κB stimulation, plasma membrane lipid peroxidation, and platelet aggregation, and suppresses cytokine production. CEP is recognized to exhibit reactive oxygen species (ROS)-scavenging properties and a protective effect against some of the responses mediated by pro-inflammatory cytokines including TNF-α, interleukin (IL)-1β, and IL-6 [22,23]. In addition, it has been reported that CEP has anti-allergic actions, stabilizes the biological membrane, augments the action of cortical hormones, and improves the peripheral circulation. In Japan, indications for CEP include radiation-induced leukopenia, alopecia areata, and alopecia pityrodes (Cepharanthine package insert, 2018). CEP has not demonstrated significant safety issues, and its side effects have been very rarely reported [22]. In addition, it is available for long-term treatment, and the treatment effect is persistent. Therefore, CEP is often used for OLP.

3.2.1. RAS

RAS has been reported to apparently be related to the excessive generation of ROS including O_2^- [24]. It has been reported that when CEP 3 g (30 mg per day as alkaloid extracted from the plant *S. cepharantha*) was administered daily in three divided doses after each meal for seven cases of RAS patients, the results showed a percent improvement of 71.4% and a response rate of 85.7% [25].

3.2.2. OLP

It has been reported that the administration of BA effectively reduced the generation of O_2^-, one of the most potent reactive oxygen intermediates, and diminished the clinical symptoms of OLP [26]. When CEP was administered to patients with OLP, a significant suppression of O_2^- generation by peripheral blood neutrophils was found as symptoms were improved (such as ulcers, redness, and contact pain of the oral mucosa). Therefore, O_2^- excess generation of the OLP lesion was inhibited by the administration of CEP, and those symptoms were thought to be relieved. Moreover, it has been reported that the rate of plasma inflammatory cytokine production (such as TNF-α, IL-1β, IL-6, and granulocyte-colony stimulating factor (G-CSF)) was unchanged by CEP administration [24,27].

In addition, previous studies have reported improved microcirculation induced by the vasodilatory effect of CEP [28]. Furthermore, in previous studies, CEP 3 g (30 mg/day as the alkaloid extracted from the plant *S. cepharantha*) was administered daily in three divided doses after each meal to 12 patients with OLP [25]. The results indicated a percentage improvement and response rate of 75.0% for each [25]. These reports suggest that the suppression of O_2^- generation by peripheral blood neutrophils may be closely related to the improvement of symptoms of RAS and OLP.

3.3. Glycyrrhizin (GL)

In Japan, glycyrrhizin (GL) is an established treatment for improving liver function in patients with viral hepatitis [29]. GL, which is a triterpenoid saponin isolated from the root of licorice (*Glycyrrhiza glabra*), is a compound consisting of a single glycyrrhetic acid (GA) molecule linked with two glucuronic acid molecules. GL exhibits multiple biological and pharmacological activities such as anti-inflammatory, anti-allergic, and antiviral [e.g., against herpes simplex virus (HSV), Varicella zoster, influenza, hepatitis C virus (HCV), and human immunodeficiency virus (HIV)] effects [30,31]. The mechanism of action of GL is not completely understood. However, a number of recent studies have indicated a number of distinct GL-binding functional proteins (GBFPs) as essential mediators, which are involved in the GL-induced anti-inflammatory effect. These proteins include arachidonate cascade-related enzymes [secretory phospholipase A_2 ($sPLA_2$), 5-lipoxygenase (5-Lox), and cyclooxygenase-2 (Cox-2), inducible nitric oxide synthase (iNOS), and the high mobility group box-1 protein (HMGB1)] [32]. One tablet of glycyron contains 25 mg glycyrrhizic acid as the main ingredient. In Japan, indication for GL includes stomatitis, the improvement of liver function abnormality in chronic hepatitis, eczema, dermatitis, alopecia areata, and strophulus infantum (Glycyron, package insert, 2018).

3.3.1. RAS

Apparently, no previous study has reported the effect of GL on RAS. According to the Glycyron package insert (2018), when glycyron tablets are orally administered at a dose of nine tablets daily for 12 consecutive weeks, it is more than effective at 82.3%. Licorice, the name given to the roots and stolons of Glycyrrhiza species, has been used since ancient times as a traditional herbal remedy [33]. Some reports on the effect of licorice for controlling pain and reducing the healing time of aphthous ulcerations have been published [34–36]. However, these studies suggest that additional research is required to arrive at conclusions on the potential benefits of licorice in RAS [33]. Therefore, it is suggested that GL has a certain effect on RAS because of an effect that occurs in stomatitis (oral mucosal disease).

3.3.2. OLP

Hasizume reported that when glycyron tablets were orally administered at a dose of six tablets daily for almost three consecutive months for OLP affecting the bilateral buccal mucosa with alcoholic chronic hepatitis, the symptoms were remitted [37]. In addition, Glycyrrhizin (GL) was used to treat chronic liver dysfunction in nine patients with OLP who were positive for HCV antibody and HCV RNA. GL was administered intravenously at a dose of 40 mL (0.2% solution) daily for four consecutive weeks, and the results showed that 66.7% of patients with OLP improved clinically [38].

3.4. Tacrolimus (FK506: Topical Use)

Tacrolimus, also called FK506, is a macrolide immunosuppressant produced by *Streptomyces tsukubaensis*, which has similar effects to those of cyclosporin A. It acts by inhibiting calcineurin, a ubiquitous calcium-dependent protein phosphatase that is responsible for immune responses [39]. Tacrolimus was formulated as an ointment for atopic dermatitis that is used commonly and seems effective as a second choice for treating OLP, which is refractory to other standard treatments [40]. Since the relationship between tacrolimus and cancer development has been reported in only a few cases, clinicians must be careful in selecting tacrolimus as a second-line treatment for OLP [41]. In RAS and OLP, immunopathy is regarded as one of the onset triggers. Therefore, if tacrolimus is effective for OLP, it is also expected that there is enough efficacy for RAS. However, tacrolimus is thought to have limited applicability for aphthous treatment as steroidal external preparations have a lower-risk than tacrolimus external preparations.

3.5. Desiccants (Topical Use)

Although not used in Japan, desiccants have been used for the treatment of RAS in the US and other countries. A typical desiccant cocktail contains sulfonic acid and other highly reactive agents, which destroys the attached cells [4]. Destruction of nerve endings results in the prompt relief of pain, which is followed by the regeneration of the destroyed tissue. Thus, the mechanism of action of desiccants can be regarded as the chemical removal of lesions, which is not related to the etiology of RAS. Nowadays, the utility of a desiccant in the treatment of periodontitis is being recognized [4].

4. Role of CCN Family 2 (CCN2) in Inflammation

Steroid hormone derivatives counteract inflammatory responses by inhibiting the action of proinflammatory transcription factors. In addition to this action, these molecules are known to activate the transcription of the *CCN2*, which encodes protein that is critical in wound healing. Therefore, while repressing the inflammatory response, glucocorticoids also promote the last stage of inflammation to reconstruct the damaged tissues.

The protein, CCN2 is a classical member of the CCN family, consisting of six members in mammals. CCN stands for the first letters of the initial names of its three founding members: cysteine-rich 61 (Cyr61/CCN1), connective tissue growth factor (CTGF/CCN2), and nephroblastoma-overexpressed (NOV/CCN3). CCN2 is composed of an insulin-like growth factor binding protein-like (I), von Willebrand factor type C repeat (V), thrompospondin 1 type 1 repeat (T), and C-terminal cystine-knot (C) modules. Multiple interactions via these modules with a variety of biomolecules in the microenvironment yield pleiotropic and context-dependent biological outcomes, which usually induce harmonized tissue development and regeneration [42–44]. Indeed, CCN2 is expressed at particular stages during the development of a variety of tissues and organs. After development and growth, CCN2 is transiently induced upon tissue injury and repair, and the tissue regeneration potential of CCN2 is also indicated [45,46]. CCN2 appears to play a pivotal role to proceed with inflammatory stages.

As illustrated in Figure 5a, *CCN2* expression is differentially regulated by inflammatory mediators. Tumor necrosis factor-α (TNF-α) and nitric oxide repress *CCN2* expression in a variety of cells, whereas histamine contrarily induces it [10]. Moreover, CCN2 itself may enhance the gene expression of inflammatory cytokines in several types of cells. It is indicated that a processed CT module fragment of CCN2 is responsible for its inflammatory actions [47]. Such an apparently complex regulatory network around CCN2 during inflammation suggests that *CCN2* is precisely regulated in order to appear upon the initiation of the last stage of inflammation. Once the CCN2 protein is produced, this molecule starts reconstructing the damaged tissues under the direct interaction with other growth factors and their receptors. As a result, the production of matrix metalloproteinases (MMPs) as well as the extracellular matrix (ECM) components, is enhanced, which are then utilized for tissue reconstruction, as summarized in Figure 5b. Of note, MMP-3 was found to go back into the nuclei of producers to further enhance *CCN2* expression in chondrocytes, representing the collaborative action of CCN2 and MMP-3 [48,49].

After tissue repair, *CCN2* expression should be turned off immediately in order to avoid continuous tissue remodeling and excessive ECM production leading to fibrosis, a typical outcome of chronic inflammation [50–53]. Indeed, *CCN2* overexpression is commonly observed in fibrotic disorders in a variety of organs. Therefore, turning CCN2 production on and off are key for terminating acute and chronic inflammation, respectively. If we could turn on and off the CCN2 production by medication, we would thus be able to successfully control the inflammation and regeneration of affected tissues in a harmonized manner.

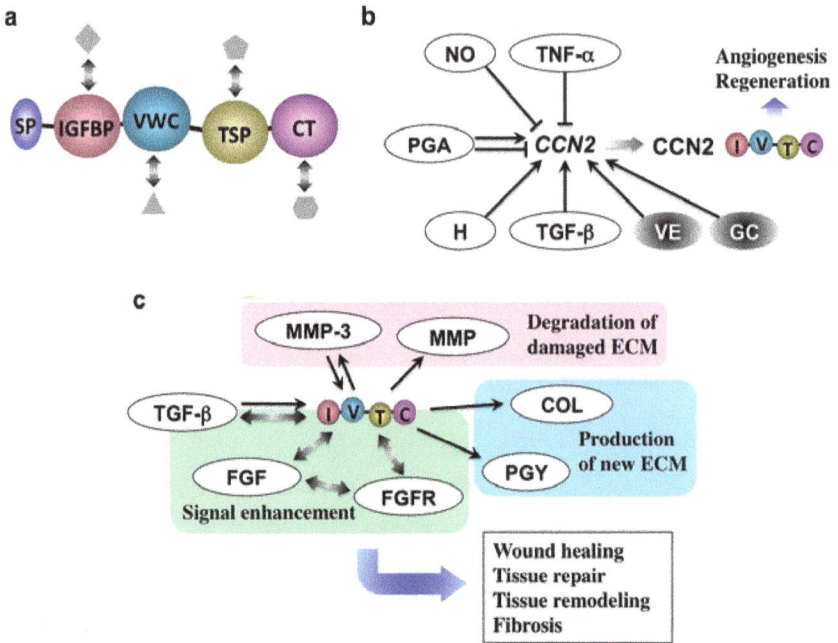

Figure 5. (**a**) Molecular structure of CCN2. Following the signal peptide for secretion (SP), insulin-like growth factor binding protein-like (IGFBP), von Willebrand factor type C repeat (VWC), thrombospondin type I repeat (TSP), and C-terminal cystine knot (CT) modules are connected in tandem. Interaction with multiple co-factors (objects in grey) that support the function of CCN2 is also illustrated. (**b**) CCN2 inducers and repressors. TNF-α, tumor necrosis factor alpha; NO, nitric oxide; PGA, prostaglandin; H, histamine; TGF-β, transforming growth factor beta; VE, vitamin E; GC, glucocorticoid. (**c**) Molecular action of CCN2. MMP, MMPs other than MMP-3; COL, collagen; PGY, proteoglycan; ECM, extracellular matrix; FGFR, fibroblast growth factor receptor; FGF, fibroblast growth factor. Arrows and T-bars indicate induction and repression, respectively. Bidirectional arrows denote direct molecular interactions.

5. Novel Utility of Particular Glucocorticoid and Alkaloid in Orofacial Disorders

5.1. Fluocinolone Acetonide

Due to their enhanced medical utility, most of the ointments used for stomatitis contain synthetic GCs with fluoride introduction at the position of C9 in the steroid nucleus (Figure 6). Dex is the most popular active ingredient, whereas triamcinolone acetonide (TA) is also employed. Another related compound, fluocinolone acetonide (FA) is commonly used in the field of dermatology in the form of an oil or paste, and its effectiveness and safety are also indicated in the treatment of stomatitis [54]. For a long time, the pharmacological effects of these synthetic glucocorticoids were believed to be basically the same. However, surprisingly, screening of the Food and Drug Administration (FDA) of the United States-approved small molecules rediscovered FA as a special molecule with novel biological potential to regenerate cartilage.

Cortisol

Dexamethasone

Triamcinolone (acetonide)

Fluocinolone (acetonide)

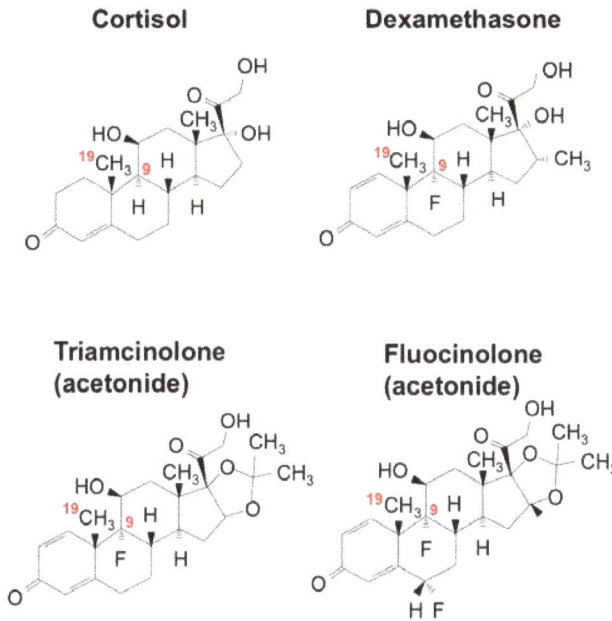

Figure 6. Chemical structures of glucocorticoids. The positions of C9 and C19 are indicated in red.

FA dramatically enhanced the chondrogenesis from mesenchymal stem cells in vitro when it was combined with transforming growth factor (TGF)-β3. Furthermore, analysis in vivo revealed the ability of FA to regenerate damaged articular cartilage in collaboration with TGF-β3 [55]. TGF-β3, as a member of the TGF-β superfamily, is known to enhance extracellular matrix deposition mainly through the canonical signaling pathway mediated by secondary messengers termed Smads. The observed effect of FA was shown to be mediated by the mammalian target of the rapamycin (mTOR)-AKT signaling pathway as well as by the interaction with the Smad pathway and GR activation. This collaboration is highly member-specific, since FA combined with BMP-2, another member of TGF-β superfamily, did not show such an effect. Similarly, articular cartilage regeneration in vivo was not effectively exerted by the combination of TGF-β3 and either TA or Dex. A structural comparison between these three compounds suggests a structural–functional relationship between corticosteroids and the extra functionality to regenerate cartilage in collaboration with TGF-β3 (Figure 7a) [55]. Obviously, the fluoride modification at C16 adds a structural property to enable the unusual collaboration of FA with TGF-β. It should also be noted that FA is able to strongly induce *CCN2* expression in ATDC5 chondrogenic cells, which may result in the modification of TGF-β signaling via direct molecular interaction between these molecules (Figure 7b). Since CCN2 itself regenerates articular cartilage, involvement of this protein in the outcome of FA-TGF-β3 collaboration is strongly suspected (Figure 8).

In the field of orofacial medicine, TMJ dysfunction based on osteoarthritis is one of the major complications that affects proper mastication. However, there are currently no therapeutics for regenerating damaged TMJ cartilage that has been established. However, FA has already been widely approved and is being used in clinics, meaning that its clinical application for recovering damaged TMJ cartilage is now expected, although particular care should be taken to avoid possible side effects as a glucocorticoid.

a

		Dex	TA	FA
Structure	C16 modification	CH$_3$	OH	OH
	C9 modification	-	-	F
Chondrocytic phenotype in vitro		-	↑	↑↑
Chondrogenesis in vitro		-	-	↑↑
Regeneration in vivo		-	-	↑

b

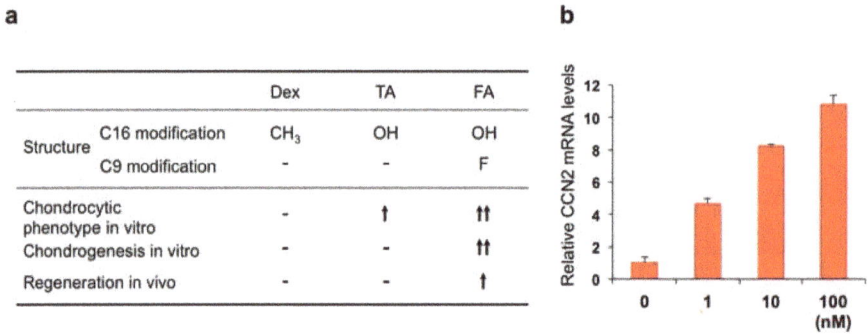

Figure 7. (**a**) Structural–functional relationship of three glucocorticoids. TA, triamcinolone acetonide; FA, fluocinolone acetonide. (**b**) Induction of CCN2 in ATDC5 chondrogenic cells by FA. ATDC5 cells in monolayer culture were treated with different concentrations (1–100 nM: horizontal axis) of FA for 24 h, and analyzed for expression levels of CCN2 mRNA.

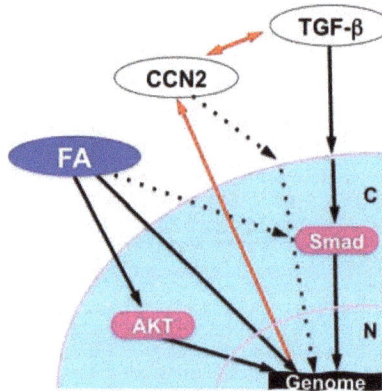

Figure 8. Possible cartilage regeneration mechanism by FA in collaboration with TGF-β. N, Nucleus; C, cytoplasm; FA, fluocinolone acetonide.

5.2. Harmine

As a related attempt to study small molecules that enhance cartilage regeneration, Hara et al. also screened an orphan ligand library based on the ability to induce CCN2 expression. Among the 84 compounds screened, harmine, one of the β-carboline alkaloids, was found to be a potent inducer of CCN2 in the human chondrocytic cell line (Figure 9a). Harmine is a natural product that can be extracted from a plant named *Peganum harmala*, which has been used in folk medicine in a number of countries for thousands of years [56]. Later scientific studies showed an anti-depressant effect of this alkaloid via inhibiting monoamine oxidase activity and its vasorelaxant-like effect by blocking voltage-gated calcium channels. One should take these functions into account upon its clinical application to avoid possible adverse effects. The family of β-carboline alkaloids is composed of several members; however, harmine was confirmed to be the only one that could exert this novel effect to induce CCN2 expression (Figure 9b). Further investigation confirmed harmine's ability to enhance chondrogenesis with the elevated gene expression of chondrocytic marker genes, as well as that of CCN2, in culture. Interestingly, enhanced production of SOX-9, which is a master transcription factor of chondrogenesis, was found to be stronger than that of CCN2. Therefore, harmine enhances chondrogenesis by inducing both CCN2 and SOX-9, which subsequently promotes the production of cartilaginous ECM components [57].

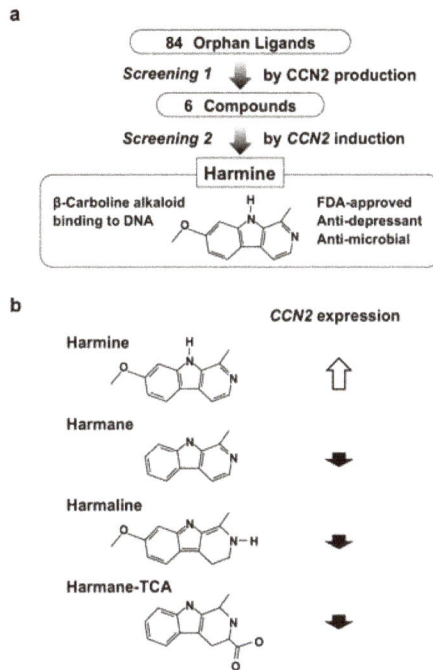

Figure 9. (**a**) Screening procedure employed for the re-discovery of harmine; (**b**) chemical structures and CCN2 inducing the activity of β-carboline alkaloids.

In addition to this novel discovery, the anti-inflammatory effect of this compound was surprisingly also indicated in the same study. Indeed, harmine was shown to protect chondrocytes from the catabolic effects conferred by an inflammatory cytokine, TNF-α (Figure 10) [57]. Therefore, therapeutic use of this compound in OA, including that of TMJ, could well be considered. Also, such a molecular function of this particular alkaloid, counteracting inflammatory response and enhancing regenerative activity, is reminiscent of that of glucocorticoids. Thus, harmine may be an effective agent for the treatment of stomatitis as well, which ought to be examined in future studies.

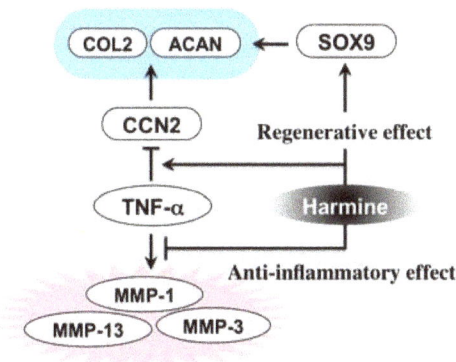

Figure 10. Molecular activity of harmine counteracting the inflammatory degradation of cartilage. COL2, type II collagen; ACAN, aggrecan; MMP, matrix metalloproteinase.

6. Conclusive Remarks

Inflammation in the oral region representative of stomatitis is not typically fatal but is highly painful, and thus strongly impairs an individual's quality of life. Therefore, symptomatic, rather than fundamental treatment has been the major therapeutic strategy for these kinds of diseases. As such, glucocorticoids and alkaloids have commonly been employed to ameliorate local and systemic inflammatory responses for a long time, without significant advances in therapeutics and etiological research. However, recent research on these classical compounds is unveiling their utility in the regenerative therapy of damaged connective tissue, including intractable cartilage defects. These research outcomes also emphasize the close and delicate relationship between inflammation and tissue regeneration, in which CCN2 may be pivotally involved. Further investigation of other classical anti-inflammatory compounds may uncover unexpected molecular functions in those molecules as well, and the research outcome may be of help in exploring novel comprehensive therapeutics to terminate excessive inflammation and promote harmonized tissue regeneration in oral inflammatory lesions.

Author Contributions: N.H.M. and S.K. wrote the paper; E.S.H. contributed the data and proofread the manuscript.

Funding: This work was supported by the Grant-in-Aid for Challenging Research (Exploratory) [JSPS KAKENHI Grant Number 17K19756 (to S.K.)] and for Scientific Research (C) [JSPS KAKENHI Grant Number 18K09743 (to N.H.M.)] sponsored by the Japan Society for the Promotion of Science.

Conflicts of Interest: The authors declare no conflict of interest. The founding sponsors had no role in the writing of the manuscript.

References

1. Hayama, T.; Kamio, N.; Okabe, T.; Muromachi, K.; Matsushima, K. Kallikrein Promotes Inflammation in Human Dental Pulp Cells via Protease-Activated Receptor-1. *J. Cell. Biochem.* **2016**, *117*, 1522–1528. [CrossRef] [PubMed]

2. Takashiba, S.; Naruishi, K.; Murayama, Y. Perspective of cytokine regulation for periodontal treatment: Fibroblast biology. *J. Periodontol.* **2003**, *74*, 103–110. [CrossRef] [PubMed]

3. Yamamoto, T.; Ugawa, Y.; Kawamura, M.; Yamashiro, K.; Kochi, S.; Ideguchi, H.; Takashiba, S. Modulation of microenvironment for controlling the fate of periodontal ligament cells: The role of Rho/ROCK signaling and cytoskeletal dynamics. *J. Cell Commun. Signal.* **2018**, *12*, 369–378. [CrossRef] [PubMed]

4. Isola, G.; Matarese, G.; Williams, R.C.; Siciliano, V.I.; Alibrandi, A.; Cordasco, G.; Ramaglia, L. The effects of a desiccant agent in the treatment of chronic periodontitis: A randomized, controlled clinical trial. *Clin. Oral Investig.* **2018**, *22*, 791–800. [CrossRef] [PubMed]

5. Isola, G.; Matarese, G.; Lo Giudice, G.; Briguglio, F.; Alibrandi, A.; Crupi, A.; Cordasco, G.; Ramaglia, L. A New Approach for the Treatment of Lateral Periodontal Cysts with an 810-nm Diode Laser. *Int. J. Periodontics Restor. Dent.* **2017**, *37*, e120–e129. [CrossRef] [PubMed]

6. Matarese, G.; Ramaglia, L.; Cicciù, M.; Cordasco, G.; Isola, G. The Effects of diode laser therapy as an adjunct to scaling and root planing in the treatment of aggressive periodontitis: A 1-Year randomized controlled clinical trial. *Photomed. Laser Surg.* **2017**, *35*, 702–709. [CrossRef] [PubMed]

7. Marheineke, N.; Scherer, U.; Rücker, M.; von See, C.; Rahlf, B.; Gellrich, N.C.; Stoetzer, M. Evaluation of accuracy in implant site preparation performed in single- or multi-step drilling procedures. *Clin. Oral Investig.* **2018**, *22*, 2057–2067. [CrossRef] [PubMed]

8. Natah, S.S.; Konttinen, Y.T.; Enattah, N.S.; Ashammakhi, N.; Sharkey, K.A.; Hayrinen-Immonen, R. Recurrent aphthous ulcers today: A review of the growing knowledge. *Int. J. Oral Maxillofac. Surg.* **2004**, *33*, 221–234. [CrossRef] [PubMed]

9. Femiano, F.; Lanza, A.; Buonaiuto, C.; Gombos, F.; Nunziata, M.; Piccolo, S.; Cirillo, N. Guidelines for diagnosis and management of aphthous stomatitis. *Pediatr. Infect. Dis. J.* **2007**, *26*, 728–732. [CrossRef] [PubMed]

10. Kular, L.; Pakradouni, J.; Kitabgi, P.; Laurent, M.; Martinerie, C. The CCN family: A new class of inflammation modulators? *Biochimie* **2011**, *93*, 377–388. [CrossRef] [PubMed]

11. Mat, M.C.; Sevim, A.; Fresko, I.; Tuzun, Y. Behcet's disease as a systemic disease. *Clin. Dermatol.* **2014**, *32*, 435–442. [CrossRef] [PubMed]
12. Kovac-Kovacic, M.; Skaleric, U. The prevalence of oral mucosal lesions in a population in Ljubljana, Slovenia. *J. Oral Pathol. Med.* **2000**, *29*, 331–335. [CrossRef] [PubMed]
13. Pentenero, M.; Broccoletti, R.; Carbone, M.; Conrotto, D.; Gandolfo, S. The prevalence of oral mucosal lesions in adults from the Turin area. *Oral Dis.* **2008**, *14*, 356–366. [CrossRef] [PubMed]
14. Ismail, S.B.; Kumar, S.K.; Zain, R.B. Oral lichen planus and lichenoid reactions: Etiopathogenesis, diagnosis, management and malignant transformation. *J. Oral Sci.* **2007**, *49*, 89–106. [CrossRef] [PubMed]
15. Gupta, S.; Jawanda, M.K. Oral Lichen Planus: An Update on Etiology, Pathogenesis, Clinical Presentation, Diagnosis and Management. *Indian J. Dermatol.* **2015**, *60*, 222–229. [CrossRef] [PubMed]
16. Alrashdan, M.S.; Cirillo, N.; McCullough, M. Oral lichen planus: A literature review and update. *Arch. Dermatol. Res.* **2016**, *308*, 539–551. [CrossRef] [PubMed]
17. Schäcke, H.; Schottelius, A.; Döcke, W.D.; Strehlke, P.; Jaroch, S.; Schmees, N.; Rehwinkel, H.; Hennekes, H.; Asadullah, K. Dissociation of transactivation from transrepression by a selective glucocorticoid receptor agonist leads to separation of therapeutic effects from side effects. *Proc. Natl. Acad. Sci. USA* **2004**, *101*, 227–232. [CrossRef] [PubMed]
18. Lowenberg, M.; Stahn, C.; Hommes, D.W.; Buttgereit, F. Novel insights into mechanisms of glucocorticoid action and the development of new glucocorticoid receptor ligands. *Steroids* **2008**, *73*, 1025–1029. [CrossRef] [PubMed]
19. Stahn, C.; Lowenberg, M.; Hommes, D.W.; Buttgereit, F. Molecular mechanisms of glucocorticoid action and selective glucocorticoid receptor agonists. *Mol. Cell. Endocrinol.* **2007**, *275*, 71–78. [CrossRef] [PubMed]
20. Ueta, E.; Umazume, M.; Yamamoto, T.; Osaki, T. Leukocyte dysfunction in oral mucous membrane diseases. *J. Oral Pathol. Med.* **1993**, *22*, 120–125. [CrossRef] [PubMed]
21. Thongprasom, K.; Dhanuthai, K. Steriods in the treatment of lichen planus: A review. *J. Oral Sci.* **2008**, *50*, 377–385. [CrossRef] [PubMed]
22. Rogosnitzky, M.; Danks, R. Therapeutic potential of the biscoclaurine alkaloid, cepharanthine, for a range of clinical conditions. *Pharmacol. Rep.* **2011**, *63*, 337–347. [CrossRef]
23. Akamatsu, H.; Komura, J.; Asada, Y.; Niwa, Y. Effects of cepharanthin on neutrophil chemotaxis, phagocytosis, and reactive oxygen species generation. *J. Dermatol.* **1991**, *18*, 643–648. [CrossRef] [PubMed]
24. Harada, T.; Kingetsu, A.; Nariai, Y.; Yoshimura, H. Effects of biscoclaurine alkaloids on clinical symptoms and superoxide anion generation from peripheral blood neutrophils in patients with oral lichen planus. *Asian J. Oral Maxillofac. Surg.* **2001**, *13*, 117–124.
25. Shinnoki, S.; Morita, N.; Sumiyoshi, M.; Kawashima, N.; Wada, T.; Miyata, K.; Sakamoto, T. Effect of Cepharanthin on intractable oral mucosal disease (oral lichen planus, recurrent aphthous stomatitis). *Dent. Outlook* **1992**, *80*, 1223–1234.
26. Harada, T.; Mishima, K.; Obara, S.; Yoshimura, Y. Effects of radiation therapy on superoxide anion generation from peripheral blood neutrophils in oromaxillary cancer patients: A preliminary report of radiation-induced oral mucositis. *Asian J. Oral Maxillofac. Surg.* **1996**, *8*, 9–14.
27. Harada, T.; Nariai, Y.; Yoshimura, Y. Effects of biscoclaurine alkaloids (Cepharanthin) on patients with oral lichen planus. Study on superoxide anion generation from peripheral blood neutrophils and plasma cytokine levels in patients. *Oral. Ther. Pharm.* **2004**, *23*, 46–53.
28. Asano, M.; Ohkubo, C.; Sasaki, A.; Sawanobori, K.; Nagano, H. Vasodilator effects of cepharanthine, a biscoclaurine alkaloid, on cutaneous microcirculation in the rabbit. *J. Ethnopharmacol.* **1987**, *20*, 107–120. [PubMed]
29. Abe, N.; Ebina, T.; Ishida, N. Interferon induction by glycyrrhizin and glycyrrhetinic acid in mice. *Microbiol. Immunol.* **1982**, *26*, 535–539. [CrossRef] [PubMed]
30. Pompei, R.; Laconi, S.; Ingianni, A. Antiviral properties of glycyrrhizic acid and its semisynthetic derivatives. *Mini Rev. Med. Chem.* **2009**, *9*, 996–1001. [CrossRef] [PubMed]
31. Patrick, L. Hepatitis C: Epidemiology and review of complementary/alternative medicine treatments. *Altern. Med. Rev.* **1999**, *4*, 220–238. [PubMed]
32. Ohtsuki, K. The anti-inflammatory molecular mechanism of glycyrrhizin. *Minophagen Med. Rev.* **2010**, *55*, 95–118.

33. Messier, C.; Epifano, F.; Genovese, S.; Grenier, D. Licorice and its potential beneficial effects in common oro-dental diseases. *Oral Dis.* **2012**, *18*, 32–39. [CrossRef] [PubMed]

34. Moghadamnia, A.A.; Motallebnejad, M.; Khanian, M. The efficacy of the bioadhesive patches containing licorice extract in the management of recurrent aphthous stomatitis. *Phytother. Res.* **2009**, *23*, 246–250. [CrossRef] [PubMed]

35. Martin, M.D.; Sherman, J.; van der Ven, P.; Burgess, J. A controlled trial of a dissolving oral patch concerning glycyrrhiza (licorice) herbal extract for the treatment of aphthous ulcers. *Gen. Dent.* **2008**, *56*, 206–210. [PubMed]

36. Das, S.K.; Das, V.; Gulati, A.K.; Singh, V.P. Deglycyrrhizinated liquorice in aphthous ulcers. *J. Assoc. Phys. India* **1989**, *37*, 647.

37. Hashizume, K. A case of the oral lichen planus with alcoholic chronic hepatitis patients improved by glycyron tablets. *Minophagen Med. Rev.* **2007**, *52*, 352–354.

38. Nagao, Y.; Sata, M.; Suzuki, H.; Tanikawa, K.; Itoh, K.; Kameyama, T. Effectiveness of glycyrrhizin for oral lichen planus in patients with chronic HCV infection. *J. Gastroenterol.* **1996**, *31*, 691–695. [CrossRef] [PubMed]

39. Graef, I.A.; Mermelstein, P.G.; Stankunas, K.; Neilson, J.R.; Deisseroth, K.; Tsien, R.W.; Crabtree, G.R. L-type calcium channels and GSK-3 regulate the activity of NF-ATc4 in hippocampal neurons. *Nature* **1999**, *401*, 703–708. [CrossRef] [PubMed]

40. Shichinohe, R.; Shibaki, A.; Nishie, W.; Tateishi, Y.; Shimizu, H. Successful treatment of severe recalcitrant erosive oral lichen planus with topical tacrolimus. *J. Eur. Acad. Dermatol. Venereol.* **2006**, *20*, 66–68. [CrossRef] [PubMed]

41. Morita, M.; Asoda, S.; Tsunoda, K.; Soma, T.; Nakagawa, T.; Shirakawa, M.; Shoji, H.; Yagishita, H.; Nishikawa, T.; Kawana, H. The onset risk of carcinoma in patients continuing tacrolimus topical treatment for oral lichen planus: A case report. *Odontology* **2017**, *105*, 262–266. [CrossRef] [PubMed]

42. Jun, J.I.; Lau, L.F. Taking aim at the extracellular matrix: CCN proteins as emerging therapeutic targets. *Nat. Rev. Drug Discov.* **2011**, *10*, 945–963. [CrossRef] [PubMed]

43. Kubota, S.; Takigawa, M. The CCN family acting throughout the body: Recent research developments. *Biomol. Concepts* **2013**, *4*, 477–494. [CrossRef] [PubMed]

44. Perbal, B. The concept of the CCN protein family revisited: A centralized coordination network. *J. Cell Commun. Signal.* **2018**, *12*, 3–12. [CrossRef] [PubMed]

45. Kubota, S.; Takigawa, M. The role of CCN2 in cartilage and bone development. *J. Cell Commun. Signal.* **2011**, *5*, 209–217. [CrossRef] [PubMed]

46. Abd El Kader, T.; Kubota, S.; Nishida, T.; Hattori, T.; Aoyama, E.; Janune, D.; Hara, E.S.; Ono, M.; Tabata, Y.; Kuboki, T.; et al. The regenerative effects of CCN2 independent modules on chondrocytes in vitro and osteoarthritis models in vivo. *Bone* **2014**, *59*, 180–188. [CrossRef] [PubMed]

47. Rodrigues-Díez, R.; Rodrigues-Díez, R.R.; Rayego-Mateos, S.; Suarez-Alvarez, B.; Lavoz, C.; Stark Aroeira, L.; Sánchez-López, E.; Orejudo, M.; Alique, M.; Lopez-Larrea, C.; et al. The C-terminal module IV of connective tissue growth factor is a novel immune modulator of the Th17 response. *Lab. Investig.* **2013**, *93*, 812–824. [CrossRef] [PubMed]

48. Eguchi, T.; Kubota, S.; Kawata, K.; Mukudai, Y.; Uehara, J.; Ohgawara, T.; Ibaragi, S.; Sasaki, A.; Kuboki, T.; Takigawa, M. Novel transcription-factor-like function of human matrix metalloproteinase 3 regulating the CTGF/CCN2 gene. *Mol. Cell. Biol.* **2008**, *28*, 2391–2413. [CrossRef] [PubMed]

49. Muromachi, K.; Kamio, N.; Narita, T.; Annen-Kamio, M.; Sugiya, H.; Matsushima, K. MMP-3 provokes CTGF/CCN2 production independently of protease activity and dependently on dynamin-related endocytosis, which contributes to human dental pulp cell migration. *J. Cell. Biochem.* **2012**, *113*, 1348–1358. [CrossRef] [PubMed]

50. Leask, A. CCN2: A bona fide target for anti-fibrotic drug intervention. *J. Cell Commun. Signal.* **2011**, *5*, 131–133. [CrossRef] [PubMed]

51. Abd El Kader, T.; Kubota, S.; Janune, D.; Nishida, T.; Hattori, T.; Aoyama, E.; Perbal, B.; Kuboki, T.; Takigawa, M. Anti-fibrotic effect of CCN3 accompanied by altered gene expression profile of the CCN family. *J. Cell Commun. Signal.* **2013**, *7*, 11–18. [CrossRef] [PubMed]

52. Kubota, S.; Takigawa, M. Cellular and molecular actions of CCN2/CTGF and its role under physiological and pathological conditions. *Clin. Sci.* **2015**, *128*, 181–196. [CrossRef] [PubMed]

53. Toda, N.; Mori, K.; Kasahara, M.; Koga, K.; Ishii, A.; Mori, K.P.; Osaki, K.; Mukoyama, M.; Yanagita, M.; Yokoi, H. Deletion of connective tissue growth factor ameliorates peritoneal fibrosis by inhibiting angiogenesis and inflammation. *Nephrol. Dial. Transplant.* **2018**, *33*, 943–953. [CrossRef] [PubMed]

54. Buajeeb, W.; Pobrurksa, C.; Kraivaphan, P. Efficacy of fluocinolone acetonide gel in the treatment of oral lichen planus. *Oral Surg. Oral Med. Oral Pathol. Oral Radiol. Endodontol.* **2000**, *89*, 42–45. [CrossRef]

55. Hara, E.S.; Ono, M.; Pham, H.T.; Sonoyama, W.; Kubota, S.; Takigawa, M.; Matsumoto, T.; Young, M.F.; Olsen, B.R.; Kuboki, T. Fluocinolone Acetonide Is a Potent Synergistic Factor of TGF-β3-Associated Chondrogenesis of Bone Marrow-Derived Mesenchymal Stem Cells for Articular Surface Regeneration. *J. Bone Miner. Res.* **2015**, *30*, 1585–1596. [CrossRef] [PubMed]

56. Moloudizargari, M.; Mikaili, P.; Aghajanshakeri, S.; Asghari, M.H.; Shayegh, J. Pharmacological and therapeutic effects of *Peganum harmala* and its main alkaloids. *Pharmacogn. Rev.* **2013**, *7*, 199–212. [CrossRef] [PubMed]

57. Hara, E.S.; Ono, M.; Kubota, S.; Sonoyama, W.; Oida, Y.; Hattori, T.; Nishida, T.; Furumatsu, T.; Ozaki, T.; Takigawa, M.; et al. Novel chondrogenic and chondroprotective effects of the natural compound harmine. *Biochimie* **2013**, *95*, 374–381. [CrossRef] [PubMed]

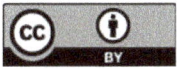

medicines

MDPI

Article

Changes in Metabolic Profiles of Human Oral Cells by Benzylidene Ascorbates and Eugenol

Hiroshi Sakagami [1,*], Masahiro Sugimoto [2,3,4], Yumiko Kanda [5], Yukio Murakami [6], Osamu Amano [7], Junko Saitoh [8] and Atsuko Kochi [8]

1   Meikai University Research Institute of Odontology (M-RIO), 1-1 Keyakidai, Sakado, Saitama 350-0283, Japan
2   Institute for Advanced Biosciences, Keio University, Tsuruoka 997-0052, Japan; msugi@sfc.keio.ac.jp
3   Health Promotion and Preemptive Medicine, Research and Development Center for Minimally Invasive Therapies, Tokyo Medical University, Shinjuku, Tokyo 160-0022, Japan
4   Research and Development Center for Precision Medicine, University of Tsukuba, Tukuba, Ibaraki 305-8550, Japan
5   Department of Microscope, Meikai University School of Dentistry, 1-1 Keyakidai, Sakado, Saitama 350-0283, Japan; k-yumiko@dent.meikai.ac.jp
6   Division of Oral Diagnosis and General Dentistry, Meikai University School of Dentistry, 1-1 Keyakidai, Sakado, Saitama 350-0283, Japan; ymura@dent.meikai.ac.jp
7   Division of Anatomy, Meikai University School of Dentistry, 1-1 Keyakidai, Sakado, Saitama 350-0283, Japan; oamano@dent.meikai.ac.jp
8   Ichijokai Hospital, 4-26-1 Kitakokubu, Ichikawa, Chiba 272-0836, Japan; junchan@kve.biglobe.ne.jp (J.S.); ichi-1@ya2.so-net.ne.jp (A.K.)
*   Correspondence: sakagami@dent.meikai.ac.jp; Tel.: +81-492-792-758

Received: 21 September 2018; Accepted: 24 October 2018; Published: 31 October 2018

Abstract: Background: Sodium-5,6-benzylidene-L-ascorbate (SBA), and its component units, benzaldehyde (BA) and sodium ascorbate (SA), are known to exert antitumor activity, while eugenol exerts anti-inflammatory activity. To narrow down their intracellular targets, metabolomic analysis was performed. **Methods:** Viable cell number was determined by the 3-(4,5-dimethylthiazol-2-yl)-2,5-diphenyltetrazolium bromide (MTT) method. Fine cell structures were observed under transmission electron microscope. Cellular metabolites were extracted with methanol and subjected to capillary electrophoresis-mass spectrometry (CE-MS) for quantification of intracellular metabolites. **Results:** SBA was cleaved into BA and SA under acidic condition. Among these three compounds, BA showed the highest-tumor specificity in vitro against human oral squamous cell carcinoma (OSCC) cell line. BA did not induce the vacuolization in HSC-2 OSCC cells, and its cytotoxicity was not inhibited by catalase, in contrast to SBA and SA. Only BA suppressed the tricarboxylic acid (TCA) cycle at early stage of cytotoxicity induction. Eugenol more rapidly induced the vacuolization and suppressed the TCA cycle in three human normal oral cells (gingival fibroblast, periodontal ligament fibroblast, pulp cell). Neither BA nor eugenol affected the ATP utilization, further supporting that they do not induce apoptosis. **Conclusions:** The present study demonstrated for the first time that both BA and eugenol suppressed the TCA cycle in tumor cells and normal cells, respectively. It is crucial to design methodology that enhances the antitumor potential of BA and reduces the cytotoxicity of eugenol to allow for safe clinical application.

Keywords: metabolomics; oral cell; benzaldehyde; eugenol; inflammation; cytotoxicity

---

1. Introduction

Benzaldehyde (BA) is an antitumor principle of the volatile fraction of figs [1]. Several BA derivatives have been prepared for clinical application. Oral administration of β-cyclodextrin benzaldehyde inclusion compound [2] and intravenous administration of 4,6-benzylidene-α-D-glucose [3] or sodium-5,6-benzylidene-L-ascorbate (SBA) [4,5] to patients with advanced, inoperable carcinoma induced remarkable necrotic changes of the tumor, although they showed weak or no antitumor activity against implanted tumors in mice. SBA had no apparent host immunopotentiation activity such as stimulation of cytokine action or production; activation of monocyte or polymorphonuclear cells; or modulation of poly (ADP-ribose) glycohydrolase activity, suggesting the antitumor activity of SBA might be produced by direct action of authentic SBA or its metabolized form(s) [5]. Using a newly established high-performance liquid chromatography (HPLC) separation technique [6], we demonstrated that under acidic condition the acetal linkage in SBA is hydrolyzed, producing benzaldehyde (BA) and sodium ascorbate (SA) [7] (Figure 1A). However, BA level was not changed during incubation for 48 h in culture medium [7].

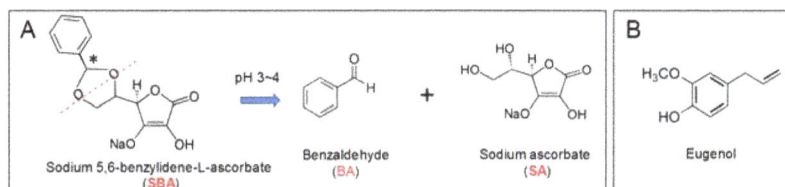

Figure 1. Chemical structure of sodium 5,6-benzylidene-L-ascorbate (SBA) and its hydrolyzed products (benzaldehyde (BA), sodium ascorbate (SA)) (**A**) and eugenol (**B**). SBA has two diastereomers (S and R configurations at stereogenic center indicated by asterisk in A) present at 31% and 69% (determined by chromato-integrator), respectively [6,7].

In vitro study with human oral squamous cell carcinoma (OSCC) cell lines (HSC-2, HSC-3, and HSC-4) and human normal oral cells (gingival fibroblast (HGF), periodontal ligament fibroblast (HPLF), and pulp cell (HPC)) demonstrated that tumor-specificity of BA (TS = 8.8) was four times higher than that of SBA (TS = 2.0), and that neither compounds induced apoptosis (internucleosomal DNA fragmentation, caspase-3, caspase-8, and caspase-9 activation) in OSCC cell line (HSC-2) [8,9], in contrast to HL-60 human promyelocytic leukemic cells [10]. SBA and SA showed common biological properties such as apoptosis induction of HL-60 cells [10], cytotoxicity augmentation with cupper ions, radical generation, and prooxidant action (oxidation potential, hydrogen peroxide production, and methionine oxidation) but showed different properties such as a propensity to react with iron and cysteine analog and catalase sensitivity [11–15] (Table 1). However, to our knowledge, comparative metabolomic study of SBA or SA with BA has not been reported.

Table 1. Biological activities of SBA and its cleaved products, BA and SA.

Biological Activities	SBA	SA	BA	Ref.
Antitumor activity (in vivo)	Yes	No	Yes	[5]
Tumor-specificity (TS = CC_{50} (normal)/CC_{50} (tumor))	2	2.5	8.8	[8,9]
Apoptosis-induction in HSC-2 cells	No	N.D.	No	[8,9]
Apoptosis-induction in HL-60 cells	Yes	Yes	No	[10]
Cytotoxicity by addition of copper	Increase	Increase	N.D.	[11,12]
Cytotoxicity by addition of iron, cysteine analog, catalase	Not clear	Decrease	N.D.	[11–13]
Radical generation	Yes	Yes	N.D.	[11,12]
Oxidation potential, H_2O_2 production, methionine oxidation	Yes	Yes	N.D.	[11–15]

N.D., not determined.

In dentistry, zinc oxide-eugenol formulations have been used for many years as bases, liners, cements, and temporary restorative materials [16], and were previously considered as the preferred material for root canal fillings [17]. However, zinc oxide-eugenol released cytotoxic concentrations of eugenol (Figure 1B) [18], and induced chronic inflammation, without healing the pulp, nor forming the dentin bridge up to 12 weeks postoperatively [19]. However, due to the lack of randomized clinical trials, long-term follow-up studies, and proper coronal sealing, whether eugenol is the best root canal filling material for endodontically treated deciduous teeth is still questionable [20,21]. Eugenol induced very rapid and irreversible cell death [22,23] in both human OSCC cell lines (HSC-2, HSC-4, Ca9-22) and normal oral cells (HGF, HPLF, and HCP) to comparable extents [23]. Eugenol induced apoptotic cell death in human promyelocytic leukemia [24], colon cancer [25], and breast cancer cells [26], but not in human normal oral cells and OSCC cell lines [23].

Apoptosis and non-apoptosis are two alternative forms of cell death, with well-defined morphological and biochemical differences [27]. One crucial physiological difference between apoptotic and non-apoptotic cells is the intracellular ATP level. Since apoptosis is an energy-dependent process, a decrease in ATP to below critical levels may impede the execution of apoptosis and promote necrosis [28,29]. This was supported by our findings that sodium fluoride (NaF), which induced apoptosis in HSC-2 cells [30,31], increased the ATP utilization (assessed by AMP/ATP ratio) [32], whereas eugenol, which induced non-apoptosis [19], did not significantly change the ATP utilization in OSCC cells [33]. However, to our knowledge, the effect of eugenol on cellular metabolites of human normal oral cells has not been investigated.

In the present study, we investigated which metabolic pathways are mostly affected by short treatment with SBA-related compounds and eugenol. To accomplish this, we first determined the minimum exposure time required for the irreversible cell death induction, and then performed the metabolomic analysis. The present study demonstrated for the first time that BA shows several properties distinct from those of SBA and SA, and that both BA and eugenol targeted the tricarboxylic acid (TCA) cycle at early stage of cell death induction.

2. Materials and Methods

2.1. Materials

The following chemicals and materials were obtained from the indicated companies: Dulbecco's modified Eagle's medium (DMEM) from Gibco BRL, Grand Island, NY, USA; fetal bovine serum (FBS), benzaldehyde (MW = 106) (purity: >98%), sodium ascorbate (MW = 198), eugenol (MW = 164) (purity: >98%), NaF, D-mannitol, 20% glutaraldehyde solution, dimethylsulfoxide (DMSO) from Wako Pure Chemical, Osaka, Japan; doxorubicin, catalase (EC1.11.1.6, from bovine liver, 41,000 unit/mg protein) from Sigma-Aldrich Inc., St. Louis, MO, USA; mitomycin C from Merck KGaA, Darmstadt, Germany; 5-fluorouracil (5-FU) from Kyowa, Tokyo, Japan; methotrexate from Nacalai Tesque, Inc., Kyoto, Japan; docetaxel from Toronto Research Chemicals, New York, NY, USA; gefitinib from LC Laboratories®, PKC Pharmaceuticals, Inc., Woburn, MA, USA; SBA (MW = 286) from ChemiScience, Tokyo, Japan; culture plastic dishes and plates (96-well) from Becton Dickinson Labware, Franklin Lakes, NJ, USA. Eugenol was dissolved in DMSO at 400 mM before use, and diluted with medium. As a control, cells treated with 0.5% DMSO were used.

2.2. Cytotoxic Assay

Human OSCC cell line (HSC-2), purchased from Riken Cell Bank (Ibaragi, Japan), and human oral normal cells (HGF, HPLF, and HPC), established from the first premolar tooth extracted from the lower jaw of a 12-year-old girl [34], were cultured in DMEM supplemented with 10% heat-inactivated FBS. Cells were inoculated at 2×10^3 cells per each well of 96-microwell plate. After 48 h, cells were treated with SBA, BA, or SA, as described below. The viable cell number was then determined by MTT method as described previously [8,9,23].

2.3. Fine Cell Structure

HSC-2 cells (2×10^5 cells) were inoculated into 8.4-cm (inner diameter) dish. After 48 h, cells were incubated with 0, 1.25, 2.5, 5, or 10 mM SBA, BA, or SA for 3 h, 3 h, or 30 min, respectively.

Near confluent HPC (19 population doubling level (PDL)), HPLF (15 PDL), and HGF (20 PDL) cells were incubated with 2 mM eugenol for 0, 20, or 40 min (HPLF, HGF) or 0, 30, or 60 min (HPC). Aliquots of the cells were washed three times with 5 mL of cold phosphate-buffered saline without calcium and magnesium (PBS (−)) and then fixed for 1 h with 2% glutaraldehyde in 0.1 M cacodylate buffer (pH 7.4) at 4 °C. The cells were scraped with a rubber policemen, pelleted by centrifugation, post-fixed for 90 min with 1% osmium tetraoxide-0.1 M cacodylate buffer (pH 7.4), dehydrated, and embedded in Araldite M (CIBA-GEIGY Swiss; NISSHIN EN Co., Ltd., Tokyo, Japan). Thin sections were stained with uranyl acetate and lead citrate and were then observed under a JEM-1210 transmission electron microscope, Japan Electron Optics Laboratory (JEOL, Co., Ltd., Tokyo, Japan) (magnification: ×3000 or ×5000) at an accelerating voltage of 100 kV [8,9,35].

2.4. Processing for Metabolomic Analysis

The cells ($2\sim5 \times 10^5$) were inoculated on a 8.4-cm (inner diameter) dish and grown to near confluency. After replacing medium with fresh culture medium, cells were treated for each sample. Experiments were performed twice. The following conditions of incubation time and concentrations were used.

Exp. I: HSC-2 cells were treated for 60 min with 0, 0.625, 1.25, 2.5, 5, or 10 mM SBA for 90 min with 0, 1.25, 2.5, 5, 10, or 20 mM BA or for 30 min with 0, 0.625, 1.25, 2.5, 5, or 10 mM SA. Aliquots of the cells were trypsinized for counting the viable cell number with hemocytometer after staining with trypan blue. The cell numbers recovered from the dishes ranged between $2.65\sim3.03 \times 10^6$ cells (SBA), $1.55\sim1.84 \times 10^6$ cells (BA), and $2.75\sim3.10 \times 10^6$ cells (SA) at the time of cell harvest, respectively.

Exp. II: HSC-2 cells were treated for 70 min without (control), or with 4 or 8 mM SBA, or with 8 or 16 mM BA. HGF (19 PDL), HPLF (15 PDL), and HPC (17 PDL) cells were treated with 2 mM eugenol for 0, 20, 40, 60, or 80 min (HGF, HPLF) or for 0, 30, 60, 80, or 100 min (HPC). The cell numbers recovered from the dishes at the time of cell harvest ranged between $3.83\sim4.22 \times 10^6$ cells (HSC-2), $0.195\sim0.322 \times 10^6$ cells (HGF), $0.280\sim0.495 \times 10^6$ cells (HPLF), and $0.640\sim0.873 \times 10^6$ cells (HPC), respectively.

Aliquots of cells were washed twice with 10 mL of ice-cold 5% D-mannitol and then immersed for 10 min with 1 mL methanol containing internal standard (25 μmol/L each of methionine sulfone, 2-[*N*-morpholino]-ethanesulfonic acid and D-camphor-10-sulfonic acid). The supernatant (methanol extract) was collected. To 400 μL of the dissolved samples, 400 μL of chloroform and 200 μL of Milli-Q water were added and the mixture was centrifuged at $10,000\times g$ for 3 min at 4 °C. The aqueous layer was filtered to remove large molecules by centrifugation through a 5-kDa cut-off filter (Millipore, Billerica, MA) at $9100\times g$ for 2.0 h at 4 °C. Three hundred and twenty microliters of the filtrate was concentrated by freeze drying and dissolved in 50 μL of Milli-Q water containing reference compounds (200 μM each of 3-aminopyrrolidine and trimesate) immediately before capillary electrophoresis (CE)-time-of-flight (TOF)-mass spectrometry (MS) analysis [33,35,36].

2.5. CE-MS Analysis

The instrumentation and measurement conditions used for CE-TOF-MS were described previously [37,38] with slight modification [36].

For cationic metabolite analysis using CE-TOF-MS, a sample was prepared in fused silica capillaries filled with 1 mol/L formic acid as the reference electrolyte [32]. The capillary was flushed with formic acid. Sample solutions (3 nL) were injected at 50 mbar for 5 s and a voltage of 30 kV was applied. The capillary temperature was maintained at 20 °C and the temperature of the sample tray was kept below 5 °C. The sheath liquid was delivered at 10 μL/min. Electrospray ionization (ESI)-TOF-MS was conducted in the positive ion mode. The capillary voltage was set at 4 kV and the flow rate of nitrogen gas (heater temperature = 300 °C) was set at 7 psig. In TOF-MS, the fragmentor, skimmer, and OCT RF voltages were 75, 50, and 125 V, respectively. Automatic recalibration of each acquired spectrum was performed using reference standards. Mass spectra were acquired at a rate of 1.5 cycles/s over a *m/z* range of 50–1000.

For anionic metabolite analysis using CE-TOF-MS, a commercially available COSMO (+) capillary, chemically coated with a cationic polymer, was used for separation. Ammonium acetate solution (50 mmol/L; pH 8.5) was used as the electrolyte for separation. Before the first use, the new capillary was flushed successively with the running electrolyte (pH 8.5), 50 mmol/L acetic acid (pH 3.4), and then the electrolyte again for 10 min each. Before each injection, the capillary was equilibrated for 2 min by flushing with 50 mM acetic acid (pH 3.4) and then with the running electrolyte for 5 min [32]. A sample solution (30 nL) was injected at 50 mbar for 30 s, and a voltage of −30 kV was applied. The capillary temperature was maintained at 20 °C and the sample tray was cooled below 5 °C. An Agilent 1100 series pump equipped with a 1:100 splitter was used to deliver 10 μL/min of 5 mM ammonium acetate in 50% (*v/v*) methanol/water, containing 0.1 μM Hexakis, to the CE interface. Here, it was used as a sheath liquid surrounding the CE capillary to provide a stable electrical connection between the tip of the capillary and the grounded electrospray needle. ESI-TOF-MS was conducted in the negative ionization mode at a capillary voltage of 3.5 kV. For TOF-MS, the fragmentor, skimmer, and OCT RF voltages were set at 100, 50, and 200 V, respectively. The flow rate of the drying nitrogen gas (heater temperature = 300 °C) was maintained at 7 psig. Automatic recalibration of each acquired spectrum was performed using reference standards ([13C isotopic ion of deprotonated acetic acid dimer (2 CH3COOH–H)]$^-$, *m/z* 120.03841), and ([Hexakis + deprotonated acetic acid (M + CH3COOH–H)]$^-$, *m/z* 680.03554). Exact mass data were acquired at a rate of 1.5 spectra/s over a *m/z* range of 50–1000.

Cation analysis was performed using an Agilent CE capillary electrophoresis system, an Agilent G6220A LC/MSD TOF system, an Agilent 1100 series isocratic HPLC pump, a G1603A Agilent CEMS adapter kit, and a G1607A Agilent CE-ESI-MS sprayer kit [35]. Anion analysis was performed using an Agilent CE capillary electrophoresis system, an Agilent G6220A LC/MSD TOF system, an Agilent 1200 series isocratic HPLC pump, a G1603A Agilent CE-MS adapter kit, and a G7100A Agilent CE-electrospray ionization (ESI) source-MS sprayer kit [35].

2.6. Statistical Analysis

Data are expressed as the mean ± standard deviation (S.D.). Raw data of metabolomics analysis were analyzed using our proprietary software, MasterHands [39,40]. Concentrations were calculated using external standards based on relative area (i.e., the area divided by the area of the internal standards). Overall metabolomic profiles were accessed by principal component (PC) analysis (PCA). XLstat (Ver. 2014.1.04, Addinsoft, Paris, France) GraphPad Prism (Version 5.04, GraphPad Software, San Diego, CA, USA), and MeV (Version 4.9.0, http://mev.tm4.org/, Center for Cancer Computational Biology, Dana-Farber Cancer Institute, Boston, MA, USA) were used for PCA and other statistical tests. Differences were considered significant at *p* < 0.05.

3. Results

3.1. Distinct Biological Properties of BA from SBA and SA

3.1.1. Catalase Sensitivity

The addition of catalase (3000 unit/mL) reduced the cytotoxicity of SBA and SA up to >6.4-fold and >24.6-fold, respectively, confirming our previous finding [13]. On the other hand, the cytotoxicity of BA was not affected by the addition of catalase (Figure 2). This suggests that extracellularly released hydrogen peroxide may not be involved in BA-induced cytotoxicity.

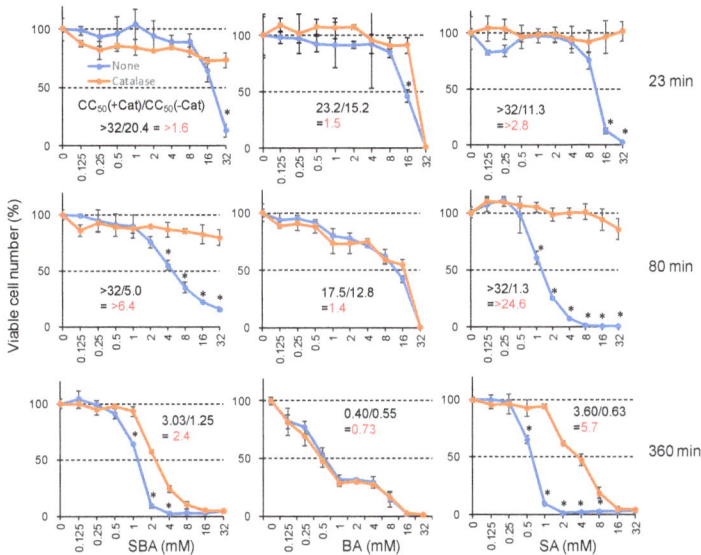

Figure 2. Involvement of extracellularly released hydrogen peroxide in the cytotoxicity induced by SA and SBA, but not BA. HSC-2 cells were incubated for 23, 80, or 360 min with the indicated concentrations of each compound in the presence or absence of catalase (3000 units/mL), and then replaced with fresh medium and incubated for a total of 48 h. Viable cell number was determined by MTT method, and expressed as % of control (drug-free, catalase-free). Each value represents mean ± S.D. of triplicate assays. * Significant difference from control $p < 0.05$.

3.1.2. Minimum Exposure Time Required for Irreversible Cell Death Induction

In order to detect the initial event that leads to irreversible cell death, we first determined the minimum exposure time. HSC-2 cells were incubated for various times, and then medium was replaced with drug-free medium and cells were incubated for up to 48 h. Viable cell number was reduced dose- and time-dependently after treatment with any drugs tested. Cytotoxic action of SA was the fastest, reaching the plateau phase of viable cell number reduction after only 2 h. Cytotoxic action of SBA was slightly slower, requiring 3~6 h to reach the bottom. Cytotoxic action of BA was much slower, requiring 8 h to reach the bottom (Figure 3).

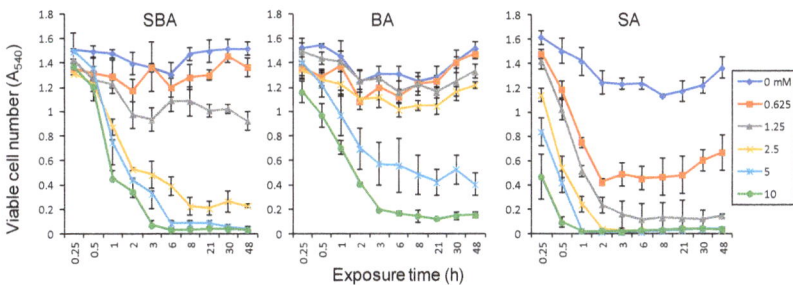

Figure 3. Minimum exposure time required for cytotoxicity induction by SBA, BA, and SA. HSC-2 cells were incubated for the indicated times without (control) or with 0, 0.625, 1.25, 2.5, 5, or 10 mM for each compound, and replaced with fresh drug-free medium. Cells were incubated for a total of 48 h and viable cell number was determined by MTT methods. Each value represents the mean ± S.D. of triplicate assays.

3.1.3. Induction of Mitochondrial Vacuolization

When HSC-2 cells were treated for 3 h with SBA and SA at 2.5 mM or higher concentrations, mitochondrial vacuolization and multivesicular bodies appeared (indicated by red box). On the other hand, BA did not induce such morphological changes (Figure 4).

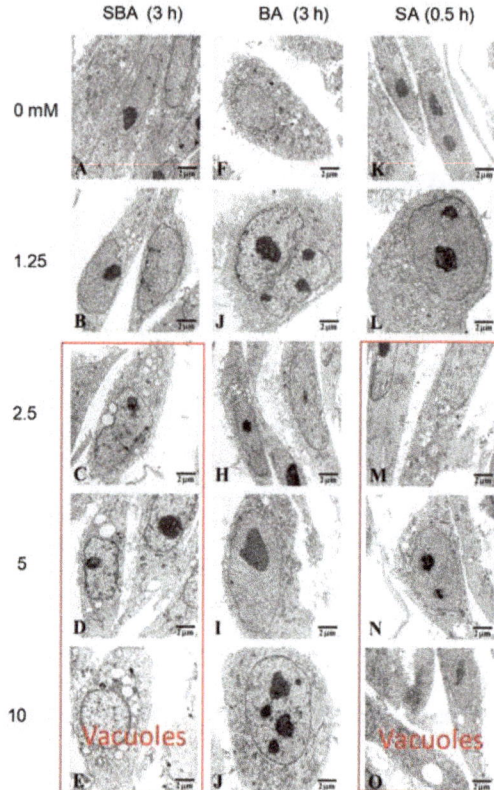

Figure 4. TEM analysis of fine cell structure of HSC-2 cells treated by the indicated concentrations of SBA (**A–E**), benzaldehyde (**F–J**), and sodium ascorbate (**K–O**). Images magnified at ×5000.

3.1.4. Effect on TCA Cycle Metabolites

In order to detect early metabolic changes, HSC-2 cells were incubated for only 60, 90, and 30 min with increasing concentrations of SBA, BA, or SA, respectively, and subjected to metabolomic analysis. We found dramatic changes in the TCA cycle after treatment of BA (Figure 5).

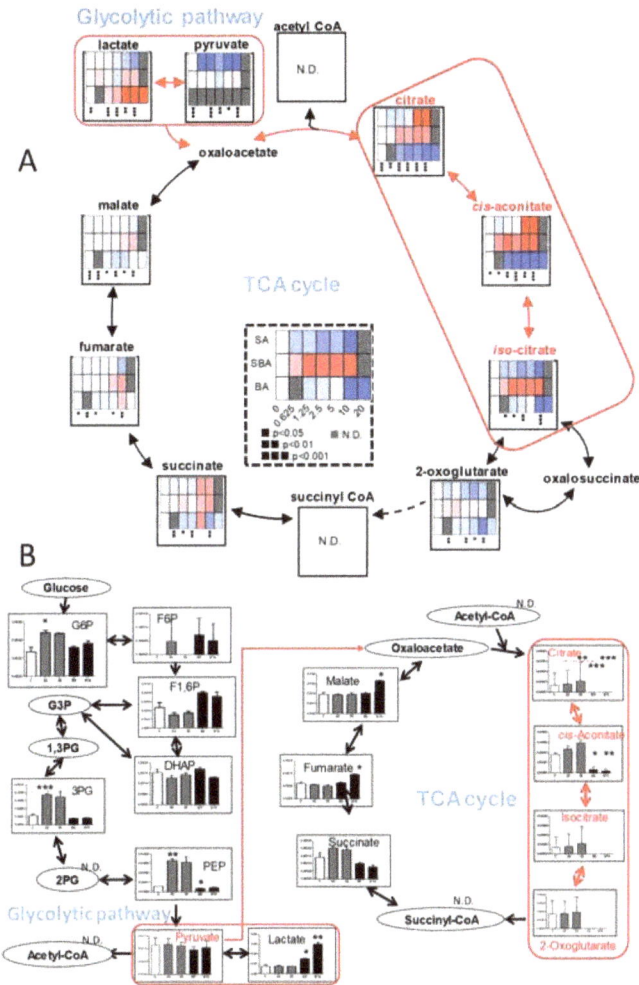

Figure 5. BA, but not SAB nor SA, inhibits the tricarboxylic acid (TCA) cycle. (**A**). Dose-response of SBA (60 min), BA (90 min), SA (30 min). HSC-2 cells were treated as Exp. I in Materials and Methods. Averaged values of quantified metabolites (amol/cell) were calculated by triplicate. To visualize the data in heat maps, each of the values were divided by those of 0 mM, i.e. fold changes were visualized and colored. Blue, white, and red were assigned for the fold changes of 0, 1, and 2, respectively. For the treatments of 0.626 mM, Student's *t*-tests were used, and for those of 20 mM, no statistical test was conducted. Not detected (N.D.) was colored in gray. One-way ANOVAs were conducted and black boxes were assigned below each heat map. (**B**). Dose-response of SBA and BA. HSC-2 cells were treated as Exp. II in Materials and Methods..Horizontal axis from left to right: C, S4, S8, B8, and B16 represent control, 4 and 8 mM SBA, 8 and 16 mM BA, respectively. Treatment time: 70 min. Control and each group were analyzed using Welch's test (both tail) and *p*-values were adjusted by Bonferroni correction. * $p < 0.05$, ** $p < 0.01$, and *** $p < 0.001$. Error bar indicates standard deviation of triplicates.

Within 90 min exposure to BA, intracellular concentrations of citrate, *cis*-aconitate, and *iso*-citrate declined to base-line level in HSC-2 cells, whereas that of succinate, fumarate, and malate maintained almost constant levels, indicating the rapid suppression of TCA cycle progression. In contrast, we could not detect such dramatic changes in other pathways (including pyrimidine metabolism, purine metabolism, glycolysis, pentose phosphate pathway, arginine, proline metabolism and urea cycle, glycine, serine and threonine metabolism, alanine, asparagine and aspartate metabolism, lysine metabolism, beta-alanine biosynthesis and metabolism, methionine and cysteine metabolism, histidine metabolism, tryptophan metabolism, phenylalanine, tyrosine metabolism, valine, leucine and isoleucine metabolism, γ-aminobutyric acid (GABA) biosynthesis and metabolism and glutamine metabolism) (Figure S1, Table S1). We checked the reproducibility of the finding (Table S2). The repeated experiment again showed that citrate, *cis*-aconitate, isocitrate, and 2-oxoglutarate were depleted by 8 or 16 mM BA (Figure 5B).

We next investigated which pathway may be involved in suppressing the TCA cycle. We found that BA increased lactate production, maintaining nearly constant levels of pyruvic acid, suggesting that BA may have reduced the amount of pyruvate that enters the TCA cycle (Figure 5A). We confirmed this finding by repeating the experiment (Figure 5B). BA reduced β-alanine, L-aspartic acid, and adenylosuccinate (Figure 6), which may directly or indirectly reduce the production of citrate.

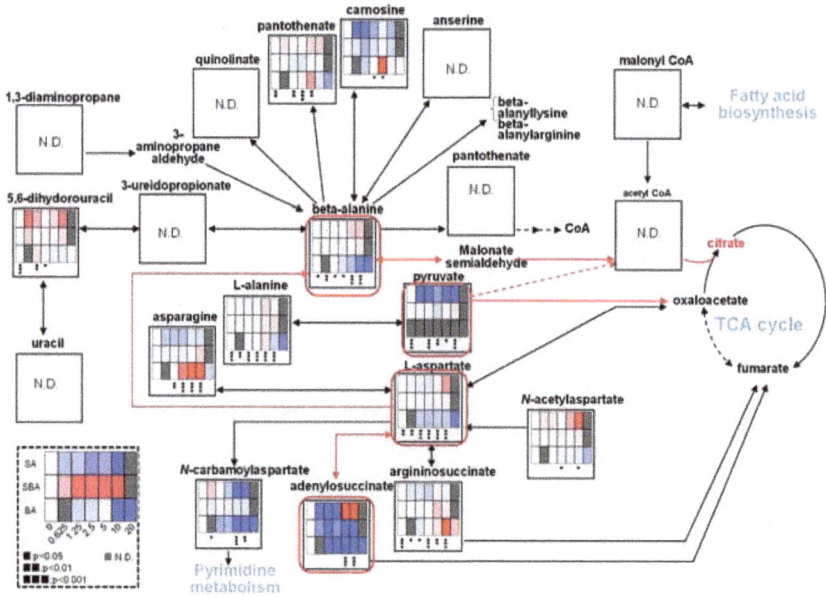

Figure 6. Possible pathway that reduces the supply of citrate by BA. SBA (60 min), BA (90 min), SA (30 min). The procedures used to produce heat maps and statistical analyses were described in Figure 5A.

We next investigated the effect on ATP utilization (Figure 7). BA treatment reproducibly reduced the AMP to less than half of the control level while it maintained a nearly constant ATP level, indicating the reduction of ATP utilization (Figure 7A). SBA treatment slightly elevated ATP but reduced AMP to one-third of the control level, again indicating the reduction of ATP utilization. On the other hand, SA increased the AMP at higher concentration (5 and 10 mM), suggesting the enhancement of ATP utilization (Figure 7A). We checked the reproducibility that both SAB and BA reduced the AMP utilization (Figure 7B). These data suggest that BA may not induce apoptosis in HSC-2 cells, in accord with our previous report [4,5].

We also investigated the changes in redox and amino acids (Figure S1). SBA, BA, and SA increased methionine sulfoxide and oxidized glutathione (GSSG) but reduced Glutathione (GSH) only slightly at higher concentration, suggesting that these compounds showed some minor prooxidant action. It was unexpected that BA dose-dependently reduced GABA, while glutamate was not changed significantly. However, the biological significance of this finding is unclear at present. Glutamine level was kept constant except for at the highest concentration of BA, negating the possibility that BA-induced cell death is not mediated by the deletion of glutamine, one of the energy sources for cell survival.

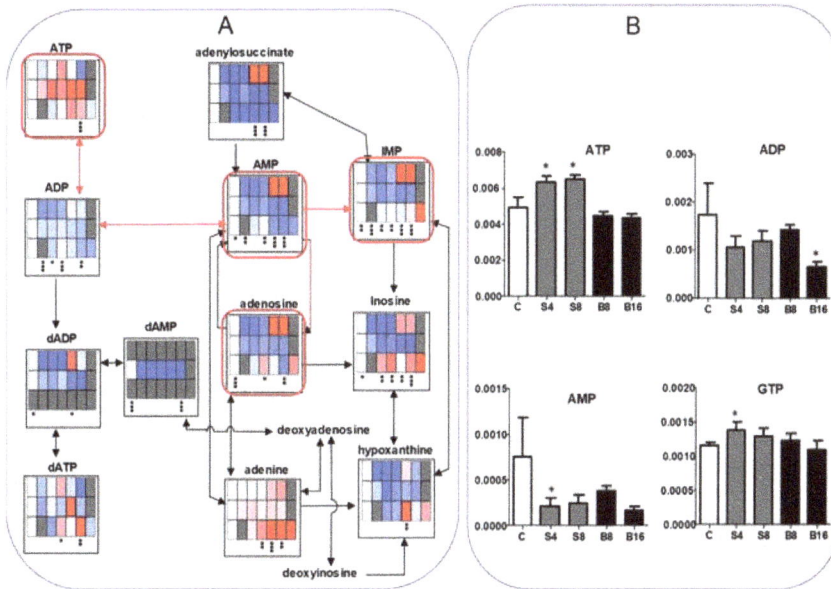

Figure 7. BA as well as SBA, but not, SA, reduce the ATP utilization. (**A**). SBA (60 min), BA (90 min), SA (30 min). HSC-2 cells were treated as Exp. I in Materials and Methods. (**B**). Horizontal axis from left to right: C, S4, S8, B8, and B16 represent control, 4 and 8 mM SBA, 8 and 16 mM BA, respectively. HSC-2 cells were treated as Exp. II in Materials and Methods. Vertical axis, μmol/cell. Each value represents mean ± S.D. (n = 3). The procedures used to produce heat maps and statistical analyses were described in the legend of Figure 5. * $p < 0.05$.

Overall metabolomic profiles were accessed by principal component (PC) analysis (PCA) (Figure 8). Plots of SA, SBA, and BA were separated into non-overlapped clusters with each other. Along with the first PC, SBA was clustered at slightly higher values (−2~5) than SA (−8~−4), and BA was clustered at much higher values (2~23) with the exception of two plots. Along with the second PC, SA (−2~13) and SBA (2~6) distributed into an overlapped region, whereas BA distributed at much lower values (0~−17). This indicates that the changes in the intracellular metabolites induced by SBA are more close to those induced by SA, as compared with those induced by BA.

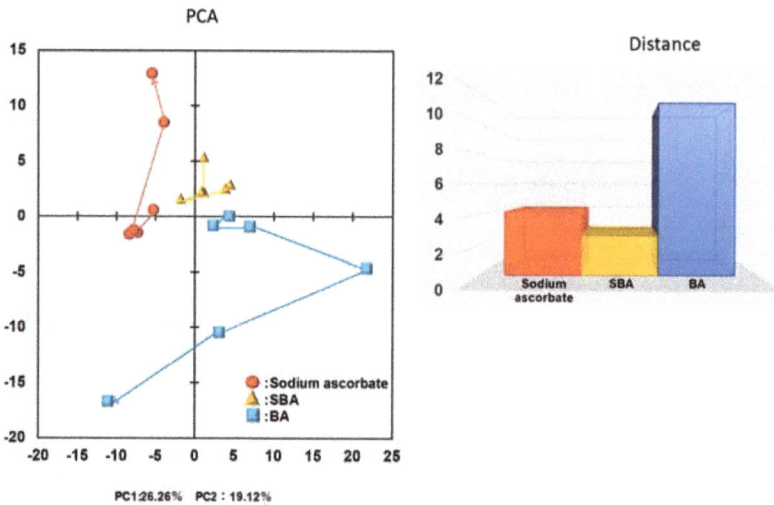

Figure 8. Principal component analysis (PCA) analysis of closeness between SBA related compounds.

3.2. Changes of Metabolic Profiles in Normal Oral Cells Induced by Eugenol

3.2.1. Eugenol Induced Rapid Collapse in Mitochondria

We have previously reported that four dental compounds, hydroquinone, benzoquinone, eugenol, and phtharal, induced irreversible cell death in human oral squamous cell carcinoma (OSCC) cell lines (HSC-2, HSC-4, Ca9-22) and normal human oral cells (HGF, HPLF, HPC) and skin keratinocytes within 4 h, without induction of apoptotic markers. The 50% cytotoxic concentration (CC_{50}) of eugenol was about 0.70~0.82 mM for tumor cells, and 0.75~0.79 mM for normal cells, yielding very low tumor-specificity (TS = 0.4–1.3), as compared with anticancer drugs (5-FU, melphalan, peplomycin) (TS = 4.1–9.7) [23]. Based on this finding, three human normal oral cells were exposed to 2 mM eugenol for up to 100 min.

Exposure of human normal oral cells (HPC, HPLF, HPC) to eugenol for only 20~60 min produced changes in mitochondria and endoplasmic reticulum, inducing mitochondrial collapse, vacuolization, and secondary lysosome (Figure 9).

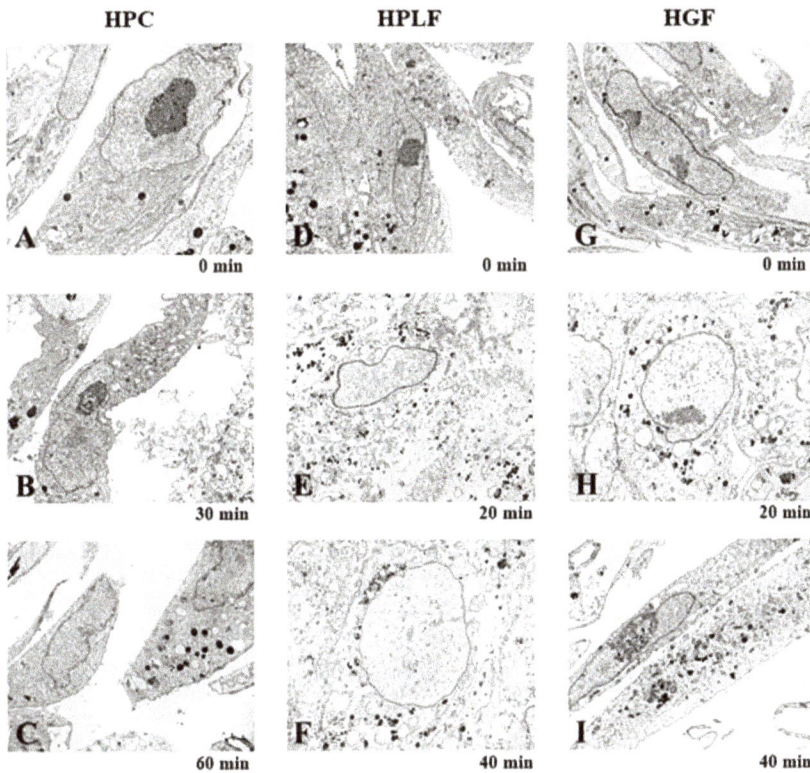

Figure 9. Rapid changes in the mitochondria and endoplasmic reticulum in normal oral cells by eugenol. Human normal oral HCP (**A–C**), HPLF (**D–F**), and HGF (**G–I**) cells were exposed to eugenol (2 mM) for the indicated times, and then subjected to TEM analysis. Images magnified at ×3000.

3.2.2. Eugenol Rapidly Suppressed TCA Cycle

The most dramatic changes to the TCA cycle were observed after treatment with eugenol (Figure 10). Within 20 min exposure to eugenol, intracellular concentrations of citrate, *cis*-aconitate, isocitrate, and 2-oxoglutarate rapidly declined in all three cells, whereas that of succinate, fumarate, and malate maintained almost constant levels over 80~100 min, indicating the rapid suppression of TCA cycle progression. On the other hand, eugenol treatment did not reduce, but rather slightly increased, the intracellular concentration of glycolytic metabolites (G6P, F6P, F1,6P, DHAP, 3PG, PEP, acetyl CoA, pyruvate, lactate) (Figure 10).

Eugenol treatment did not apparently affect the intracellular concentration of ATP in all three cells (Figure 11). Conversion of ATP to ADP was approximately 10%, and that of ADP to AMP was approximately 10% in all cells, indicating the very low incidence of ATP utilization (AMP/ATP = 0.01).

Similarly, eugenol treatment slightly increased the intracellular concentration of 19 amino acids, except for cysteine, which was undetectable in all cells (Table S2).

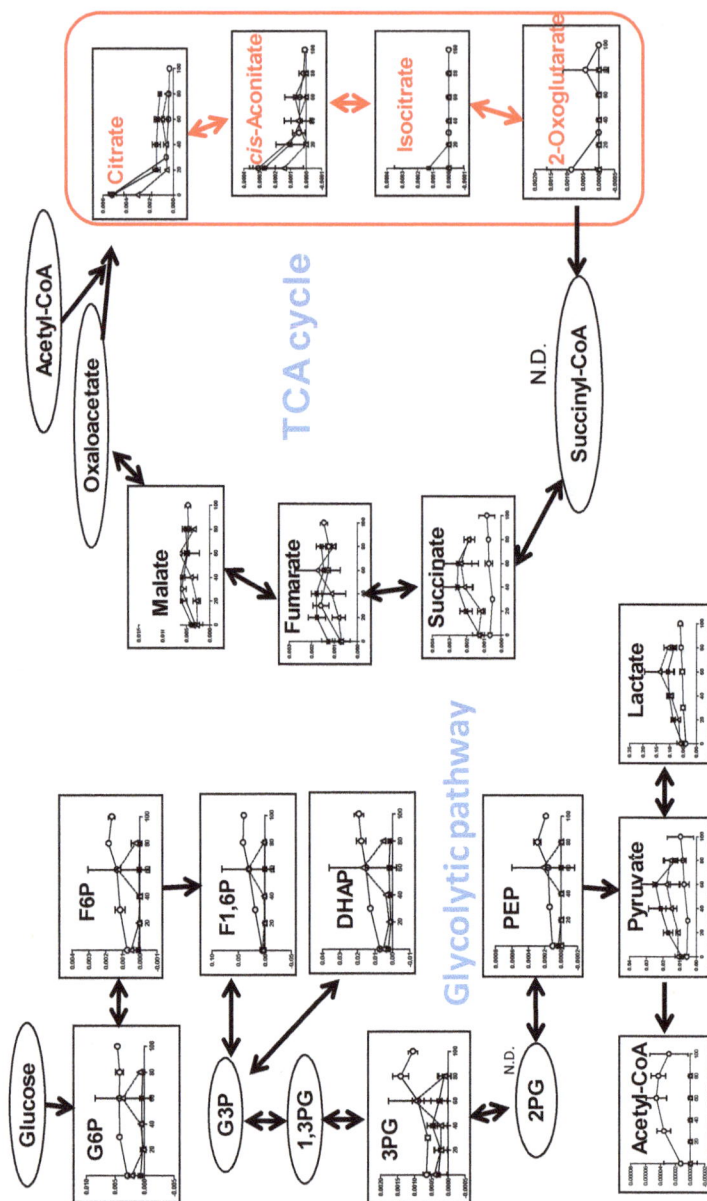

Figure 10. Eugenol suppressed the TCA cycle. HPC (○), HPLF (■), HGF (△). Vertical axis, μmol/cell. Three groups were compared by one-way ANOVA (no post test).

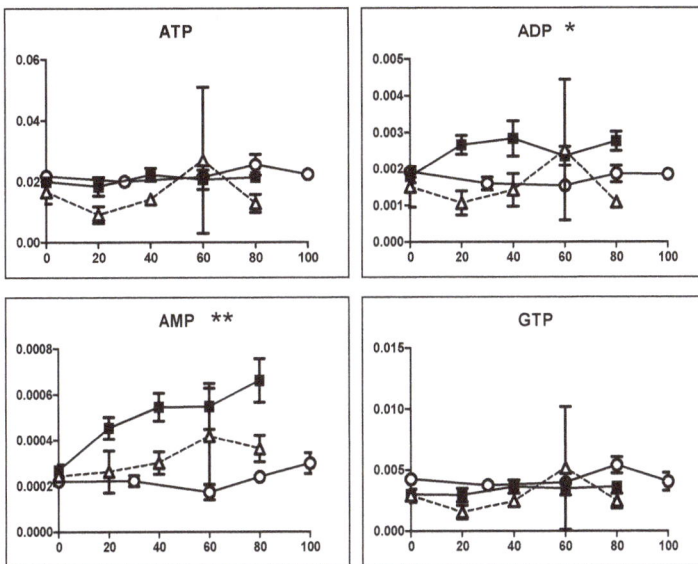

Figure 11. Eugenol generally does not affect the ATP concentrations. HPC (○), HPLF (■), HGF (△). Vertical axis, μmol/cell. Three groups were compared by one-way ANOVA (no post test). * $p < 0.05$, ** $p < 0.01$.

4. Discussion

4.1. Inhibition of TCA Cycle by Benzaldehyde (BA) in Malignant Cells

The present study demonstrated that among three SBA-related compounds (SBA, BA, SA), BA showed the following three distinct properties from others. First, in terms of catalase-sensitivity, the cytotoxicity of BA against human OSCC cell line (HSC-2) was not affected by the addition of catalase, whereas that of SBA and SA was considerably reduced by catalase. This suggests that the release of hydrogen peroxide into the extracellular milieu is important for the cell death induction by SBA and SA, but not so in the cell death induced by BA. Since catalase does not penetrate inside the cells, the possibility that intracellular hydrogen oxide may play a role in the BA-induced cytotoxicity cannot be excluded at present. Second, BA showed an inability to induce vacuolization. Third, BA was shown to inhibit the TCA cycle, possibly due to the poor supply of pyruvate or β-alanine (and their precursors). The reduction of ATP utilization (as assessed by the ratio of AMP/ATP) further supports the non-apoptosis induction by BA [9]. Since BA showed the highest tumor-specificity among three SBA-related compounds, the inhibition of TCA cycle may be the target of anti-cancer therapy.

A closer look at the dose-response of SA revealed its biphasic effect. Lower concentrations (0.625, 1.25, 2.5 mM) of SA increased the intracellular ATP level, while higher concentrations (5, 10 mM) of SA reduced the ATP level. On the other hand, lower concentrations (0.625, 1.25, 2.5 mM) of SA reduced the intracellular concentration of AMP, adenosine, IMP, and inosine, while higher concentrations (5, 10 mM) of SA elevated their concentrations (Figure 7). This further supports the bi-phasic action of SA [12]. We have previously reported that millimolar concentrations of SA (which is a popular reducing agent) produced hydrogen peroxide, reduced intracellular GSH levels, and induced apoptosis in HL-60 human promyelocytic leukemia, in a Ca^{2+}-dependent manner [13].

4.2. Inhibition of TCA Cycle by Eugenol in Non-Malignant Cells

We also found that eugenol (2 mM) induced the rapid suppression of the TCA cycle in all three human normal oral cells (HGF, HPLF, HPC). This was in nice contrast to our previous finding that eugenol slightly elevated the intracellular concentration of isocitrate and did not significantly change that of 2-oxoglutarate [33]. This demonstrated that eugenol reduced the TCA cycle only in normal oral cells, but not in OSCC cells. The present study further confirmed that eugenol induced non-apoptotic cell death, since eugenol did not affect ATP utilization except in HPLF cells (Figure 10). At present, what type of cell death eugenol has induced is yet to be determined. Considering the induction of vacuolization by eugenol, paraptosis (which causes cytoplasmic vacuolization and mitochondria enlargement [41]) may have been induced. Alternatively, considering the pro-inflammatory action of eugenol reported against HGF [42], pyroptosis (called cell inflammatory necrosis), characterized by swelling of the cell, the release of cell contents, and pro-inflammatory cytokines [43] may also be involved. Since natural products can modulate many types of cell death against cancer, such as paraptosis, necroptosis, mitotic catastrophe, and so on [44], further studies are necessary to identify the type of cell death that eugenol induces in normal oral cells. The narrow therapeutic range of eugenol suggests the importance of careful monitoring of its cytotoxicity against oral normal cells during dental treatment.

4.3. Combination Experiments with Anticancer Drugs

We have started the search for anticancer drugs that enhance the cytotoxicity of BA against human OSCC cell line HSC-2 cells. We have previously reported the mean value of CC_{50} of several anticancer drugs against four human OSCC cell lines (Ca9-22, HSC-2, HSC-3, and HSC-4) and their tumor-specificity (TS), which was determined by the ratio of the mean value of CC_{50} against three normal human oral cells (HGF, HPC, and HPC) divided by the mean value of CC_{50} against four OSCC cell lines. The anticancer drugs that we tested for their CC_{50} and TS values are doxorubicin (CC_{50} = 0.09 µM, TS = 70), mitomycin C (CC_{50} = 1.3 µM, TS = 31), methotrexate (CC_{50} < 2.4 µM, TS > 170), 5-FU (CC_{50} = 99 µM, TS = 10), docetaxel (CC_{50} < 0.032 µM, TS > 2708), and gefitinib (CC_{50} = 17 µM, TS = 4) [45]. We found that simultaneous addition of doxorubicin, mitomycin C, methotrexate, 5-FU, docetaxel and gefitinib, and dental medicines such as sodium fluoride and eugenol did not show synergistic augmentation of the cytotoxicity of BA and SBA against HSC-2 cells (Figure 12). Further study is needed to find the optimal condition for enhancing the cytotoxicity of BA against OSCC cells.

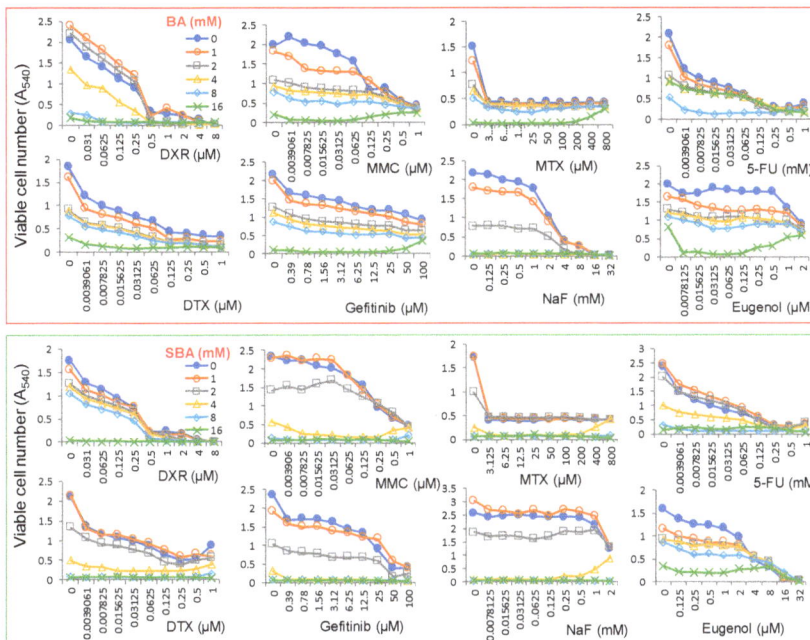

Figure 12. Combination effects of anticancer drugs and dental medicines on the augmentation of the cytotoxicity of BA (upper column) and SBA (lower column). HSC-2 cells were incubated for 48 h with the indicated concentrations of drugs in the presence of 0, 1, 2, 4, 8, or 16 mM BA or SBA, and the viable cell number was determined by MTT methods. Each value represents mean ± S.D. of triplicate assays. DXR, doxorubicin; MMC, mitomycin C; MTX, methotrexate; 5-FU, 5-fluorouracil; DTX, docetaxel; NaF, sodium fluoride.

In conclusion, both BA and eugenol suppressed the TCA cycle at the early stage of non-apoptotic cell death. As compared with eugenol, BA did not induce vacuolization, inhibited growth more slowly, and had higher tumor-specificity. Further studies are needed to design a methodology that enhances the antitumor potential of BA and reduces the cytotoxicity of eugenol in order to allow for safe clinical application. Also, the in vivo metabolic fate of SBA should be monitored for its clinical use.

Supplementary Materials: The following are available online at http://www.mdpi.com/2305-6320/5/4/116/s1, Figure S1: Effect of SBA, BA and SA on Pyrimidine metabolism (A), puring metabolism (B), glycolysis (C), TCA cycle (D), pentose phosphate pathway (E), arginine, proline metabolism and urea cycle (F), glycine, serine and threonine metabolism (G), alanine, asparagine and aspartic acid metabolism, β-alanine biosynthesis and metabolism (H), lysine metabolisum (I), methionine and cysteine metabolism (G), histidine metabolism (K), tryptophane metabolism (L), phenylalanine, tyrosine metabolism (M), valine, leucine and isoleucine metabolism (N) and GABA biosynthesis and metabolism, glutamine metabolism (O) in HSC-2 cells. Table S1: Metabolic changes induced by SBA, BA and SA (A). 171 compounds were detected. Each value represents amol/cell, and can be seen by magnifier. Table S2: Metabolic changes induced by SBA, BA in HSC-2 cells (Exp. I), and by eugenol in HGF, HPC and HPLF cells (Exp. II). 188 compounds were detected. Each value represents amol/cell, and can be seen by magnifier.

Author Contributions: H.S. designed the experiment, performed the cytotoxicity assay, and wrote the paper; M.S. designed and analyzed the metabolomic study; Y.K. performed the TEM analysis; Y.M. contributed the eugenol experiment; O.A. interpreted the TEM data; J.S. and A.K. contributed in the set up for the experiment with SBA and BA.

Funding: This research was funded by Ichijokai hospital, Chiba, Japan, and partially supported by KAKENHI from the Japan Society for the Promotion of Science (JSPS): Sakagami H, 16K11519.

Acknowledgments: The authors acknowledge the intramural support for from Meikai University School of Dentistry.

Conflicts of Interest: One of the authors (H.S.) received financial support from the research fund from Ichijokai hospital, Chiba, Japan. The authors wish to confirm that such financial support has not influenced the outcome the experimental data.

References

1. Takeuchi, S.; Kochi, M.; Sakaguchi, K.; Nakagawa, K.; Mizutani, T. Benzaldehyde as a carcinostatic principle in figs. *Agric. Biol. Chem.* **1978**, *42*, 1449–1451. [CrossRef]
2. Kochi, M.; Takeuchi, S.; Mizutani, T.; Mochizuki, K.; Matsumoto, Y.; Saito, Y. Antitumor activity of benzaldehyde. *Cancer Treat. Rep.* **1980**, *64*, 21–23.
3. Kochi, M.; Isono, N.; Niwayama, M.; Shirakabe, K. Antitumor activity of a benzaldehyde derivative. *Cancer Treat. Rep.* **1985**, *69*, 533–537. [PubMed]
4. Kochi, M.; Ueda, S.; Hagiwara, T. Antitumor activity of sodium benzylidenascorbate. In *Progress in Cancer Research and Therapy 35: Hormones and Cancer 3*; Bresciani, F., King, R.J.B., Eds.; Raven Press: New York, NY, USA, 1988; pp. 338–343.
5. Sakagami, H.; Asano, K.; Fukuchi, K.; Gomi, K.; Ota, H.; Kazama, K.; Tanuma, S.; Kochi, M. Induction of tumor degeneration by sodium benzylideneascorbate. *Anticancer Res.* **1991**, *11*, 1533–1538. [PubMed]
6. Sakagami, H.; Sakagami, T.; Takeda, M.; Iwaki, K.; Takeda, K. Determination of sodium 5,6-benzylidene-l-ascorbate and related compounds by high-performance liquid chromatography. *J. Chromatogr. Coruña* **1993**, *653*, 37–43. [CrossRef]
7. Sakagami, H.; Sakagami, T.; Yamamura, M.; Takahashi, H.; Shibuya, I.; Takeda, M. Stability of sodium 5,6-benzylidene-L-ascorbate. *Anticancer Res.* **1995**, *15*, 1269–1274. [PubMed]
8. Kishino, K.; Hashimoto, K.; Amano, O.; Kochi, M.; Sakagami, H. Tumor-specific cytotoxicity and type of cell death induced by sodium 5,6-benzylidene-L-ascorbate. *Anticancer Res.* **2008**, *28*, 2577–2584. [PubMed]
9. Ariyoshi-Kishino, K.; Hashimoto, K.; Amano, O.; Kochi, M.; Sakagami, H. Tumor-specific cytotoxicity and type of cell death induced by benzaldehyde. *Anticancer Res.* **2010**, *30*, 5069–5076. [PubMed]
10. Kuribayashi, N.; Sakagami, H.; Sakagami, T.; Niimi, E.; Shiokawa, D.; Ikekita, M.; Takeda, M.; Tanuma, S. Induction of DNA fragmentation in human myelogenous leukemic cell lines by sodium 5,6-benzylidene-L-ascorbate and its related compounds. *Anticancer Res.* **1994**, *14*, 969–976. [PubMed]
11. Sakagami, H.; Satoh, K.; Kochi, M. Comparative study of the antitumor action between sodium 5,6-bnzylidene-L-ascorbate and sodium ascorbate (Minireview). *Anticancer Res.* **1997**, *17*, 4451–4452. [PubMed]
12. Sakagami, H.; Satoh, K.; Hakeda, Y.; Kumegawa, M. Apoptosis-inducing activity of vitamin C and vitamin K. *Cell Mol. Biol.* **2000**, *46*, 129–143. [PubMed]
13. Sakagami, H.; Kuribayashi, N.; Iida, M.; Hagiwara, T.; Takahashi, H.; Yoshida, H.; Shiota, F.; Ohata, H.; Momose, K.; Takeda, M. The requirement for and mobilization of calcium during induction by sodium ascorbate and by hydrogen peroxide of cell death. *Life Sci.* **1996**, *58*, 1131–1138. [CrossRef]
14. Sakagami, H.; Satoh, K.; Kadofuku, T.; Takeda, M. Methionine oxidation and apoptosis induction by ascorbate, gallate and hydrogen peroxide. *Anticancer Res.* **1997**, *17*, 2565–2570. [PubMed]
15. Sakagami, H.; Hosaka, M.; Arakawa, H.; Maeda, M.; Satoh, K.; Ida, Y.; Asano, K.; Hisamitsu, T.; Takimoto, M.; Ota, H.; et al. Role of hydrogen peroxide in antitumor activity induction by sodium 5,6-benzylidene-L-ascorbate. *Anticancer Res.* **1998**, *18*, 2519–2524. [PubMed]
16. Sweet, C. Procedure for treatment of exposed and pulpless deciduous teeth. *J. Am. Dent. Assoc.* **1930**, *17*, 1150–1153.
17. Primosch, R.E. Primary tooth pulp therapy as taught in predoctoral pediatric dental programs in the United States. *Pediatr. Dent.* **1997**, *19*, 118–122. [PubMed]
18. Hume, W. An analysis of the release and the diffusion through dentin of eugenol from zinc oxide-eugenol mixtures. *J. Dent. Res.* **1984**, *63*, 881–884. [CrossRef] [PubMed]
19. Glass, R.; Zander, H. Pulp healing. *J. Dent. Res.* **1949**, *28*, 97–107. [CrossRef] [PubMed]
20. Barja-Fidalgo, F.; Moutinho-Ribeiro, M.; Oliveira, M.A.A.; de Oliveira, B.H. A systematic review of root canal filling materials for deciduous teeth: Is there an alternative for zinc oxide-eugenol? *ISRN Dent.* **2011**, *2011*, 1–7. [CrossRef] [PubMed]

21. Hilton, T.J. Keys to clinical success with pulp capping: A review of the literature. *Oper. Dent.* **2009**, *34*, 615–625. [CrossRef] [PubMed]
22. Hume, W.R. Effect of eugenol on respiration and division in human pulp, mouse fibroblasts, and liver cells in vitro. *J. Dent. Res.* **1984**, *63*, 1262–1265. [CrossRef] [PubMed]
23. Koh, T.; Machino, M.; Murakami, Y.; Umemura, N.; Sakagami, H. Cytotoxicity of dental compounds against human oral squamous cell carcinoma and normal oral cells. *In Vivo* **2013**, *27*, 85–96. [PubMed]
24. Atsumi, T.; Fujisawa, S.; Satoh, K.; Sakagami, H.; Iwakura, I.; Ueha, T.; Sugita, Y.; Yokoe, I. Cytotoxicity and radical intensity of eugenol, isoeugenol or related dimers. *Anticancer Res.* **2000**, *20*, 2519–2524. [PubMed]
25. Jaqanathan, S.K.; Mazumdar, A.; Mondhe, D.; Mandal, M. Apoptotic effect of eugenol in human colon cancer cell lines. *Cell Biol. Int.* **2011**, *35*, 607–615. [CrossRef] [PubMed]
26. Vidhya, N.; Devaraj, S.N. Induction of apoptosis by eugenol in human breast cancer cells. *Indian J. Exp. Biol.* **2011**, *49*, 871–878. [PubMed]
27. Majno, G.; Joris, I. Apoptosis, oncosis, and necrosis. An overview of cell death. *Am. J. Pathol.* **1995**, *146*, 3–15. [PubMed]
28. Halestrap, A.P.; Clarke, S.J.; Javadov, S.A. Mitochondrial permeability transition pore opening during myocardial reperfusion—A target for cardioprotection. *Cardiovasc. Res.* **2004**, *61*, 372–385. [CrossRef]
29. Halestrap, A. Biochemistry: A pore way to die. *Nature* **2005**, *434*, 578–579. [CrossRef] [PubMed]
30. Otsuki, S.; Morshed, S.R.M.; Chowdhury, S.A.; Takayama, F.; Satoh, T.; Hashimoto, K.; Sugiyama, K.; Amano, O.; Yasui, T.; Yokote, Y.; et al. Possible link between glycolysis and apoptosis induced by sodium fluoride. *J. Dent. Res.* **2005**, *84*, 919–923. [CrossRef] [PubMed]
31. Otsuki, S.; Sugiyama, K.; Amano, O.; Yasui, T.; Sakagami, H. Negative regulation of NaF-induced apoptosis by Bad-CAII complex. *Toxicology* **2011**, *287*, 131–136. [CrossRef] [PubMed]
32. Sakagami, H.; Sugimoto, M.; Tanaka, S.; Onuma, H.; Ota, S.; Kaneko, M.; Soga, T.; Tomita, M. Metabolomic profiling of sodium fluoride-induced cytotoxicity in an oral squamous cell carcinoma cell line. *Metabolomics* **2014**, *10*, 270–279. [CrossRef]
33. Koh, T.; Murakami, Y.; Tanaka, S.; Machino, M.; Onuma, H.; Kaneko, M.; Sugimoto, M.; Soga, T.; Tomita, M.; Sakagami, H. Changes of metabolic profiles in an oral squamous cell carcinoma cell line induced by eugenol. *In Vivo* **2013**, *27*, 233–244. [PubMed]
34. Kantoh, K.; Ono, M.; Nakamura, Y.; Nakamura, Y.; Hashimoto, K.; Sakagami, H.; Wakabayashi, H. Hormetic and anti-radiation effects of tropolone-related compounds. *In Vivo* **2010**, *24*, 843–852. [PubMed]
35. Sakagami, H.; Shimada, C.; Kanda, Y.; Amano, O.; Sugimoto, M.; Ota, S.; Soga, T.; Tomita, M.; Sato, A.; Tanuma, S.; et al. Effects of 3-styrylchromones on metabolic profiles and cell death in oral squamous cell carcinoma cells. *Toxicol. Rep.* **2015**, *2*, 1281–1290. [CrossRef] [PubMed]
36. Garcia-Contreras1, R.; Sugimoto, M.; Umemura, N.; Kaneko, M.; Hatakeyama, Y.; Soga, T.; Tomita, M.; Scougall-Vilchis, R.J.; Contreras-Bulnes, R.; Nakajima, H.; et al. Alteration of metabolomic profiles by titanium dioxide nanoparticles in human gingivitis model. *Biomaterials* **2015**, *57*, 33–40. [CrossRef] [PubMed]
37. Soga, T.; Baran, R.; Suematsu, M.; Ueno, Y.; Ikeda, S.; Sakurakawa, T.; Kakazu, Y.; Ishikawa, T.; Robert, T.; Nishioka, T.; et al. Differential metabolomics reveals ophthalmic acid as an oxidative stress biomarker indicating hepatic glutathione consumption. *J. Biol. Chem.* **2006**, *281*, 16768–16776. [CrossRef] [PubMed]
38. Sugimoto, M.; Sakagami, H.; Yokote, Y.; Onuma, H.; Kaneko, M.; Mori, M.; Sakaguchi, Y.; Soga, T.; Tomita, M. Non-targeted metabolite profiling in activated macrophage secretion. *Metabolomics* **2012**, *8*, 624–633. [CrossRef]
39. Sugimoto, M.; Wong, D.T.; Hirayama, A.; Soga, T.; Tomita, M. Capillary electrophoresis mass spectrometry-based saliva metabolomics identified oral, breast and pancreatic cancer-specific profiles. *Metabolomics* **2010**, *6*, 78–95. [CrossRef] [PubMed]
40. Sugimoto, M.; Kawakami, M.; Robert, M.; Soga, T.; Tomita, M. Bioinformatics tools for mass spectroscopy-based metabolomic data processing and analysis. *Curr. Bioinform.* **2012**, *7*, 96–108. [CrossRef] [PubMed]
41. Sugimori, N.; Espinoza, J.L.; Trung, L.Q.; Takami, A.; Kondo, Y.; An, D.T.; Sasaki, M.; Wakayama, T.; Nakao, S. Paraptosis cell death induction by the thiamine analog benfotiamine in leukemia cells. *PLoS ONE* **2015**, *10*, e0120709. [CrossRef] [PubMed]
42. Koh, T.; Murakami, Y.; Tanaka, S.; Machino, M.; Sakagami, H. Re-evaluation of anti-inflammatory potential of eugenol in IL-1β-stimulated gigngival fibroblast and pulp cells. *In Vivo* **2013**, *27*, 269–274. [PubMed]

43. Ma, Y.; Jiang, J.; Gao, Y.; Shi, T.; Zhu, X.; Zhang, K.; Lu, K.; Xue, B. Research progress of the relationship between pyroptosis and disease. *Am. J. Transl. Res.* **2018**, *10*, 2213–2219. [PubMed]

44. Guamán-Ortiz, L.M.; Orellana, M.I.; Ratovitski, E.A. Natural compounds as modulators of non-apoptotic cell death in cancer cells. *Curr. Genom.* **2017**, *18*, 132–155. [CrossRef] [PubMed]

45. Sakagami, H.; Okudaira, N.; Masuda, Y.; Amano, O.; Yokose, S.; Kanda, Y.; Suguro, M.; Natori, T.; Oizumi, H.; Oizumi, T. Induction of apoptosis in human oral keratinocyte by doxorubicin. *Anticancer Res.* **2017**, *37*, 1023–1029. [PubMed]

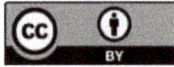

![medicines](medicines logo)   **MDPI**

Review

Recent Progress of Basic Studies of Natural Products and Their Dental Application

Hiroshi Sakagami [1,*], Taihei Watanabe [2], Tomonori Hoshino [2], Naoto Suda [3], Kazumasa Mori [4], Toshikazu Yasui [5], Naoki Yamauchi [6], Harutsugu Kashiwagi [7], Tsuneaki Gomi [8], Takaaki Oizumi [9], Junko Nagai [10], Yoshihiro Uesawa [10], Koichi Takao [11] and Yoshiaki Sugita [11]

1   Meikai University Research Institute of Odontology (M-RIO), 1-1 Keyakidai, Sakado, Saitama 350-0283, Japan
2   Division of Pediatric Dentistry, Meikai University School of Dentistry, 1-1 Keyakidai, Sakado, Saitama 350-0283, Japan; taiheidental10627@gmail.com (T.W.); thoshino1@dent.meikai.ac.jp (T.H.)
3   Division of Orthodontics, Meikai University School of Dentistry, 1-1 Keyakidai, Sakado, Saitama 350-0283, Japan; n-suda@dent.meikai.ac.jp
4   Division of First Oral and Maxillofacial Surgery, Meikai University School of Dentistry, 1-1 Keyakidai, Sakado, Saitama 350-0283, Japan; kazu-mori@dent.meikai.ac.jp
5   Division of Oral Health, Meikai University School of Dentistry, 1-1 Keyakidai, Sakado, Saitama 350-0283, Japan; yasui@dent.meikai.ac.jp
6   Masuko Memorial Hospital, 35-28 Takehashi-cho, Nakamura-ku, Nagoya 453-8566, Japan; yamauchi@masuko.or.jp
7   Ecopale Co., Ltd., 885 Minamiisshiki, Nagaizumi-cho, Suntou-gun, Shizuoka 411-0932, Japan; ecopale@fujibamboogarden.com
8   Gomi clinic, 1-10-12 Hyakunin-cho, Shinjuku-ku, Tokyo 169-0073, Japan; fwkz9633@mb.infoweb.ne.jp
9   Daiwa Biological Research Institute Co., Ltd., 3-2-1 Sakado, Takatsu-ku, Kawasaki, Kanagawa 213-0012, Japan; takaakio@daiwaseibutsu.co.jp
10   Department of Medical Molecular Informatics, Meiji Pharmaceutical University, 2-522-1 Noshio, Kiyose, Tokyo 204-8588, Japan, nagai-j@my-pharm.ac.jp (J.N.); uesawa@my-pharm.ac.jp (Y.U.)
11   Department of Pharmaceutical Sciences, Faculty of Pharmacy and Pharmaceutical Sciences, Josai University, Sakado, Saitama 350-0295, Japan; ktakao@josai.ac.jp (K.T.); sugita@josai.ac.jp (Y.S.)
*   Correspondence: sakagami@dent.meikai.ac.jp; Tel.: +81-49-279-2758

Received: 14 November 2018; Accepted: 19 December 2018; Published: 25 December 2018

Abstract: The present article reviews the research progress of three major polyphenols (tannins, flavonoids and lignin carbohydrate complexes), chromone (backbone structure of flavonoids) and herbal extracts. Chemical modified chromone derivatives showed highly specific toxicity against human oral squamous cell carcinoma cell lines, with much lower toxicity against human oral keratinocytes, as compared with various anticancer drugs. QSAR analysis suggests the possible correlation between their tumor-specificity and three-dimensional molecular shape. Condensed tannins in the tea extracts inactivated the glucosyltransferase enzymes, involved in the biofilm formation. Lignin-carbohydrate complexes (prepared by alkaline extraction and acid-precipitation) and crude alkaline extract of the leaves of *Sasa* species (SE, available as an over-the-counter drug) showed much higher anti-HIV activity, than tannins, flavonoids and Japanese traditional medicine (Kampo). Long-term treatment with SE and several Kampo medicines showed an anti-inflammatory and anti-oxidant effects in small size of clinical trials. Although the anti-periodontitis activity of synthetic angiotensin II blockers has been suggested in many papers, natural angiotensin II blockers has not yet been tested for their possible anti-periodontitis activity. There should be still many unknown substances that are useful for treating the oral diseases in the natural kingdom.

Keywords: polyphenol; chromone; lignin-carbohydrate complex; alkaline extract; Kampo medicine; glucosyltransferase; angiotensin II blocker; QSAR analysis; oral diseases; dental application

1. Introduction

The etiology of stomatitis is largely unclear [1]. However, oral inflammation such as stomatitis are considered to be triggered or aggravated by various factors including bacterial and viral infections, nutritional deficiencies, declined immune functions, allergic reactions, radiotherapy, stress, cigarettes, diseases and genetic backgrounds [1,2]. Applications of topical steroids, transdermal patches, vitamins, throat lozenges, mouth washes and cryotherapy are sometimes not effective for the treatment of stomatitis and therefore exploration of new-type of treatment are necessary [3]. In this sense, natural products having broader spectrum of biological activities are potential candidates as alternative medicine for oral diseases.

Polyphenols in the natural kingdom are defined as substances that possess an aromatic ring bearing one or more hydroxyl substituents and roughly classified into tannins, flavonoids and lignin-carbohydrate complexes (LCC) (Figure 1) [4].

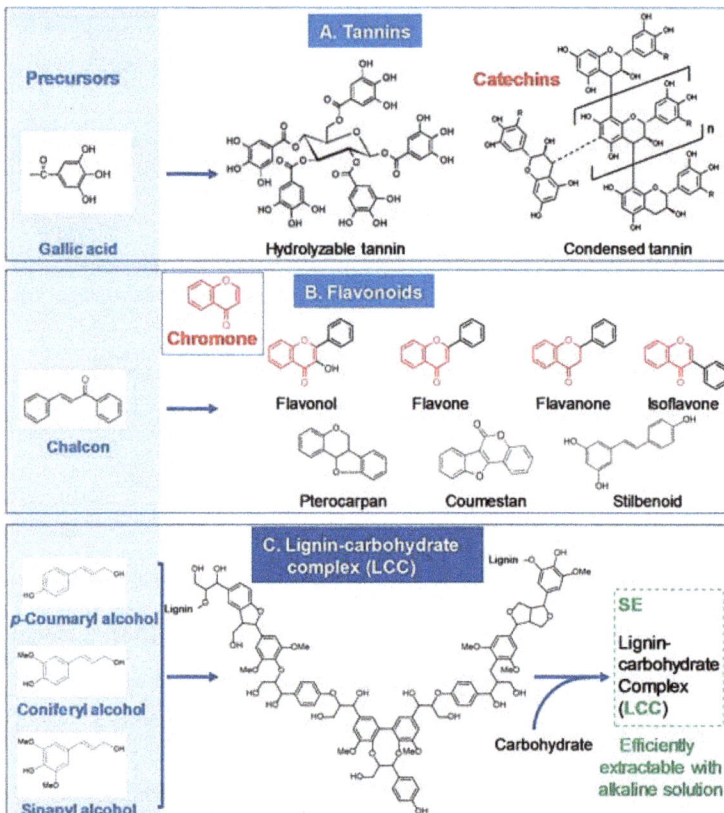

Figure 1. Three major polyphenols, that is tannins (**A**), flavonoids with or with backbone structure of chromone (**B**) and lignin-carbohydrate complex (LCC) (**C**), in the natural kingdom. Cited and modified from Reference [4] with permission.

Tannins are further classified into hydrolysable tannins (in which a polyalcohol is esterified with a galloyl, hexahydroxydiphenoyl, valoneoyl or dehydrohexahydroxydiphenoyl group) and condensed tannins (composed of catechin, epicatechin or their analogs) (Figure 1A) [5].

Flavonoids, synthesized from chalcones [6], are classified into flavonols, flavones, flavanones and isoflavones (that contain the chromone structure in the molecule), pterocarpan and coumestan (Figure 1B). Due to the recent development of separation technology [7,8], chemical structures and biological functions of thousands of tannins and flavonoids have been elucidated.

Lignin is formed by dehydrogenative polymerization of *p*-coumaryl, *p*-conifery and sinapyl alcohols and forms a complex with some polysaccharides (Figure 1C). Lignin-carbohydrate complex (LCC) has amorphous structure with very high molecular weight, thus making it difficult to determine the complete chemical structure, although it shows prominent anti-HIV activity [9]. Since LCC can be prepared by alkaline solution and acid-precipitation, it was not surprising that alkaline extract of the leaves of *Sasa* species (*Sasa* sp.) (SE) described later contains significant amount of LCC and shows several over-lapped biological activities with LCC.

It is generally accepted that improvement of oral functions by periodontal treatment [10], insertion of dentures and implants [11], oral hygiene [12], nutrition [13] and fluoride treatment [14] elevates the general health and quality of life [10,11]. Orally administered products directly contact the oral tissues or cells where they may exert their effects very fast, without being metabolizing and excretion [15], if they have a chance to bind to the target molecules or pattern-recognition receptors such as TLR2 (Toll-like receptor 2), TLR4, Dectin-1 (receptor for glucan) and Dectin-2 (receptor for LCC or mannan) in keratinocytes, macrophages, monocytes and dendritic cells [16]. This article reviews the recent progress of three major polyphenols (tannins, flavonoids and LCCs), chromone (backbone structure of flavonoids) and herbal extracts, glucosyltransferase inhibitor and angiotensin II blocker on dental diseases.

2. Chromone Derivatives as New Type of Anticancer Candidate

2.1. Most of Anticancer Drugs Show Severe Keratinocyte Toxicity

Development of anticancer drugs is shifting from classical anti-cancer drugs to molecular targeted therapeutic agents. However, the incidence of complete response in gastroesophageal cancer patients treated with targeted agents has been reported to be 2.0%, only 0.3 increase from the control arms [17]. ErbB receptor-targeting inhibitors failed to show any significant differences on overall response rate, clinical benefit rate and overall survival, with the increased risk of serious adverse events [18]. Likewise, cyclin-dependent kinase inhibitor combined with chemotherapy slightly increased the mean progression-free survival but also stimulated the senescence-associated (SA) marker expression (assessed by the accumulation of by SA β-galactosidase in the lysosome) by yet unknown mechanism [19]. This points out another unfavorable effect of targeted therapy, the resolution of which we have to find urgently.

Administration of anticancer agents has been reported to induce skin toxicity [20–26]. This prompted us to re-evaluate the cytotoxicity and tumor-specificity of anticancer drugs. We demonstrated for the first time that classical anticancer drugs (doxorubicin, daunorubicin, etoposide, mitomycin C, methotrexate, 5-fluorouracil, melphalan) and molecular targeted therapeutic drug (gefinitib) are highly toxic to epithelial normal cells (keratinocytes) as well as human oral squamous cell carcinoma (OSCC) cell lines. Tumor specificity (TS), determined with human normal oral epithelial cells *vs* OSCC cells (TS_E = 0.1 to 1.5) was usually one to two-orders lower than TS, determined with mesenchymal normal cells *vs* OSCC cells (TS_M = 3.8 to 92.9) [27] (Exp. 1, Table 1).

Also, doxorubicin induced apoptosis characterized by chromatin condensation, nuclear fragmentation and loss of cell surface microvilli) (A) and caspase-3 activation (cleavage of PARP and pro-caspase-3) (B) in human oral keratinocytes [27] (Figure 2). This urged us to survey many natural products which show lower keratinocyte toxicity.

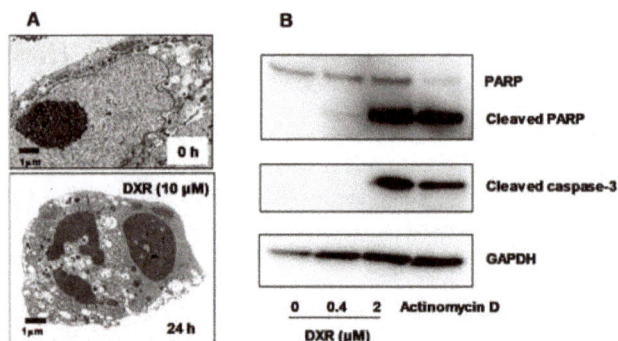

Figure 2. Doxorubicin induced apoptosis in human oral keratinocyte, demonstrated by transmission electron (**A**) and western blot analysis (**B**). Cited from Reference [27] with permission.

2.2. Limitations of Apoptosis-Oriented Research

Many studies have reported the apoptosis-inducing activity of tannins and flavonoids but have not tested for their toxicity to normal cells or tumor selectivity. We reevaluated the antitumor effect of various groups of natural products, based on the TS values determined as shown in the insert of Figure 3. As expected, anticancer drugs showed excellent tumor-specificity (TS_M, determined by the ratio of mean CC_{50} for human normal oral mesenchymal cells to that for human OSCC cell lines, indicated by red color). We found that one among14 poly-herbal formula extracts (supplied by Himalaya drug company) showed excellent tumor-specificity [28]. The active principle (s) are yet to be determined. It was surprising that the tumor selectivity of flavonoids, procyanidins, macrocyclic ellagitannins, hydrolysable tannins, catechins and gallic acid, which has been reported to induce apoptosis, was surprisingly low ($TS_M = 1$ to 5) (green color), as compared with anticancer agents. Similarly, antioxidants (vitamin C, chlorogenic acid, curcumin), ketones (α,β-unsaturated ketones, α-hydroxyketones, β-diketones, trifluoromethylketones, zulenequinones) and amides (pheylpropanoid amides, piperic acid amides, oleoylamides) showed lower TS_M values. On the other hand, the tumor selectivity of eight chromone derivatives (A–H) described later was relatively high (yellow color) (Figure 3).

2.3. Synthesis of Chromone Derivatives Having High Tumor-Specificity and Low Keratinocyte Toxicity

Chromone (4*H*-1-benzopyran-4-one) is a backbone structure of flavonols, flavones, flavanones and isoflavones [29] (Figure 1B). We synthesized eight classes of chromones derivatives (total 134 compounds): 3-styrylchromones (15 compounds) [30,31] (containing compound A), 3-benzylidenechromanones (17 compounds) [32] (containing compound B), 3-styryl-2*H*-chromenes (16 compounds) [33] (containing compound C), 2-azolylchromones (24 compounds) [34] (containing compound D), 3-(*N*-cyclicamino)chromones (15 compounds) [35] (containing compound E), 2-(*N*-cyclicamino)chromones (15 compounds) [36] (containing compound F), furo[2,3-*b*]chromones (12 compounds) [37] (containing compound G) and pyrano[4,3-*b*]chromones (20 compounds) [38] (containing compound H). The eight compounds that produced the highest TS value in each group are listed in Figure 4.

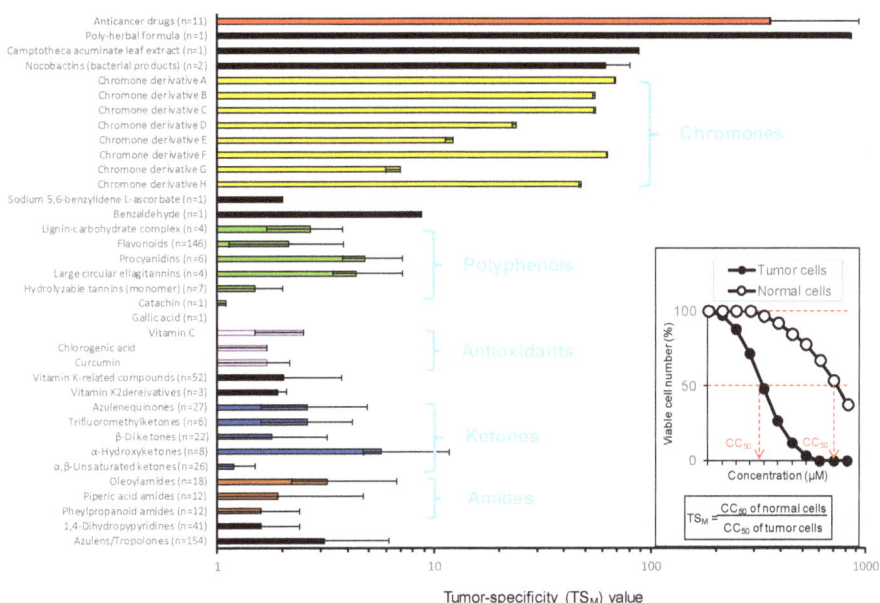

Figure 3. Chromone derivatives showed higher tumor-specificity (TS$_M$) value than most of the polyphenols. TS$_M$ was determined by the following equation: TS$_M$ = (mean CC$_{50}$ for human OSCC cell lines/mean CC$_{50}$ for human normal oral mesenchymal cells. Tumor and normal cells in the insert represent human OSCC cell lines and human normal oral mesenchymal cells. Data of chromones [30,32–38] and other compounds [4] were cited with permission. n, number of compounds tested.

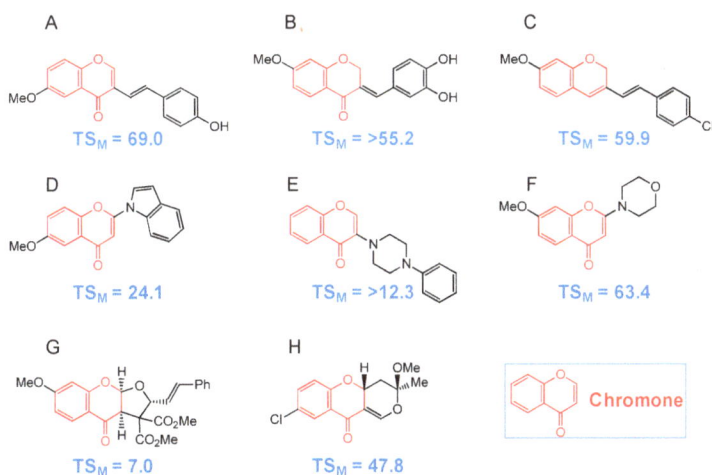

Figure 4. Compounds that showed the highest tumor-specificity (TS$_M$) values (determined with human OSCC and human oral mesenchymal cell) in eight groups of chromone derivatives. Structure and TS$_M$ values of (**A**) that belongs to 3-styrylchromones [30], (**B**) that belongs to 3-benzylidenechromanones [32], (**C**) that belongs to 3-styryl-2*H*-chromenes [33], (**D**) that belongs to 2-azolylchromones [34], (**E**) that belongs to 3-(*N*-cyclicamino)chromones [35], (**F**) that belongs to 2-(*N*-cyclicamino)chromones [36], (**G**) that belongs to furo[2,3-*b*]chromones [37] and (**H**) that belongs to pyrano[4,3-*b*]chromones [38] were cited with permission.

Table 1. Comparison of keratinocyte toxicity between popular anticancer drugs (Exp. 1) and chromone derivatives (Exp. 2).

	CC50 (μM)												TSM	TSE	
	Human Oral Squamous Cell Carcinoma					Human Oral Normal Cells							Mes	Epi	
						Mesenchymal Cells				Epithelial Cells			vs	vs	
Compounds	Ca9-22	HSC-2	HSC-3	HSC-4	mean	HGF	HPLF	HPC	mean	HOK	HGEP	mean	OSCC	OSCC	Ref.
					(A)				(B)			(C)	(B/A)	(C/A)	
Exp. 1 Anticancer drugs:															
CPT	<0.06	<0.06	<0.06	<0.06	<0.06	200	10	146	119	0.3	3.9	2.1	>1853	>33	[27]
SN-38	<0.06	<0.06	<0.06	<0.06	<0.06	143	29	16	63	<0.075	1.5	0.77	>979	<12	[27]
DXR	0.13	0.06	0.09	0.06	0.09	7.3	13	9.3	6.0	0.1	0.2	0.1	69.9	1.7	[27]
DNR	0.27	0.07	0.13	0.09	0.14	4.9	10.0	8.2	7.7	<0.004	0.4	<0.21	54.6	<1.5	[27]
ETP	11.3	3.0	2.7	2.5	4.9	351	500	500	450	1.8	3.2	2.5	92.9	0.5	[27]
MMC	3.97	0.36	0.14	0.78	1.31	22	65	34	40	0.10	0.28	0.19	30.8	0.1	[27]
MTX	9.0	0.2	<0.13	<0.13	<2.35	>400	>400	>400	>400	1000	<0.13	500	>170	>212	[27]
5-FU	15.3	100.3	186.3	92.7	98.7	1000	1000	1000	1000	1000	14.2	500	>10	0.1	[27]
DOC	<0.03	<0.03	<0.03	<0.03	<0.03	70	100	91	87	11.7	0.03	12.9	>2708	>2.4	[27]
MEL	114.0	29.0	18.3	19.0	45.1	153	197	170	173	13.5	18.7	16.1	3.8	0.4	[27]
Gefitinib	18.0	22.3	15.7	13.7	17.4	58	68	83	70	3.5	4.1	3.8	4.0	0.2	[27]
Exp. 2 Chromone derivatives:															
A	2.1	1.0	3.6	1.2	2.0	67	74	272	138	19	>800	>410	69.0	>205	[30]
B	3.2	11.3			7.3	>400	>400		>400	3.8	3.3	3.6	55.2	0.5	[32]
C	3.5	1.5	5.5	8.3	4.7	400	41	400	280	>400	>400	>400	59.9	>85.1	[33]
D	1.6	1.3			1.5	36	35		36				24.1		[34]
E	46.0	20.0	36.7	26.3	32.3	390	>400	>400	>397	>400		>400	>12.3	>12.4	[36]
F	9.1	6.0	3.7	3.1	5.5	244	>400	>400	>348	356		355.7	63.4	65.2	[35]
G	13.8		27.7	70.1	37.2	185	273	324	261				7.0		[37]
H	4.7	5.3			5.0	247	233		240	20		20	47.8	4.1	[38]

The mean of 50% cytotoxic concentration (CC50) of each test compound for human oral squamous cell carcinoma (OSCC) cell lines (Ca9-22, HSC-2, HSC-3, HSC-4) (A) and human normal oral mesenchymal cells (human gingival fibroblast HGF, human periodontal ligament fibroblast HPLF, human pulp cell HPC) (B) and human normal oral epithelial cells (HOK, HGEP) (C) were determined after incubation for 48 h with various concentrations of them. Tumor-specificity (TS) for mesenchymal normal cells *vs* OSCC cells (TSM) and that for epithelial normal cells *vs* OSCC cells (TSE) was determined by the following equation: TSM = B/A, TSE = C/A. Structures of A–H (Exp. 2) that showed the highest tumor-specificity in each group are shown in Figure 4. A, (*E*)-3-(4-hydroxystyryl)-6-methoxy-4*H*-chromen-4-one; B, (3*E*)-2,3-dihydro-3-[(3,4-dihydroxyphenyl)methylene]-7-methoxy-4*H*-1-benzopyran-4-one; C, (*E*)-3-(4-cholorostyryl)-7-methoxy-2*H*-chromene; D, 2-(1*H*-indol-1-yl)-6-methoxy-4*H*-1-benzopyran-4-one; E, 2-(4-phenyl-1-piperazinyl)-4*H*-1-benzopyran-4-one; F, 7-methoxy-2-(4-morpholinyl)-4*H*-1-benzopyran-4-one; G, (2*R*,3a*R*,9a*R*)-rac-3a,9a-dihydro-7-methoxy-4-oxo-2-(2-phenylethenyl)-4*H*-furo[2,3-*b*][1]benzopyran-3,3(2*H*)-dicarboxylic acid 3,3-dimethyl ester; H, 8-chloro-4,4a-dihydro-3-methoxy-3-methyl-3*H*,10*H*-pyrano[4,3-*b*][1]benzopyran-10-one.

All compounds showed much higher cytotoxicity against human oral squamous cell carcinoma (OSCC) cell lines (Ca9-22, HSC-2, HSC-3, HSC-4) than against human normal oral mesenchymal cells (gingival fibroblast HGF, periodontal ligament fibroblast HPLF, pulp cell HPC). These compounds except for 3-benzylidenechromanones were 2.6~2000-fold less cytotoxic to human oral keratinocytes as compared with doxorubicin (Exp. 2, Table 1). We reported that 3-styrylchromones [30] and azolylchromones [34] induced apoptosis (caspase-3 activation) in human OSCC cell line. On the contrary, 7-methoxy-2-(4-morpholinyl)-4*H*-1-benzopyran-4-one, the most active compound among fifteen 2-(*N*-cyclicamino)chromone derivatives (structure depicted in Figure 4F) showed an excellent tumor-specificity (TS = 63.4) (Figure 5A), low keratinocyte toxicity (Table 1, Exp. 2), without induction of apoptosis in human OSCC cell line (HSC-2), as evidenced by the lack of caspase-3 activation (cleavage of PARP and procaspase-3) (Figure 5B) nor of the accumulation of subG$_1$ population (Figure 5C).

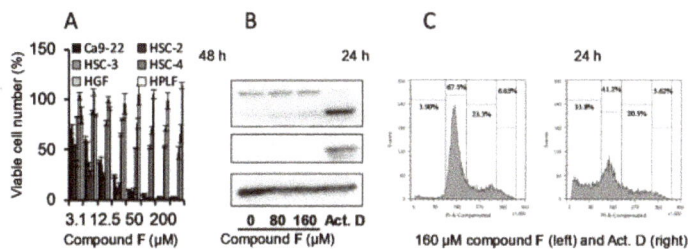

Figure 5. 7-Methoxy-2-(4-morpholinyl)-4*H*-1-benzopyran-4-one (Compound F, Figure 4F) showed higher cytotoxicity against human OSCC cell lines as compared with normal oral mesenchymal cells (**A**), without induction of caspase-3 activation (**B**) nor producing subG$_1$ cell population (**C**). Actinomycin (Act. D) (1 μM) was used as positive control. Cited from Reference [35] with permission.

In order to perform the QSAR analysis with each group of compounds, the 3D structure of each chemical structure was optimized by CORINA Classic (Molecular Networks GmbH, Nürnberg, Germany) with forcefield calculations (amber-10: EHT) in Molecular Operating Environment (MOE) version 2018.0101 (Chemical Computing Group Inc., Quebec, Canada). Approximately 3000 chemical descriptors were analyzed for their correlation with cytotoxicity against tumor cells (**T**) and normal cells (**N**) and tumor-specificity (**T–N**), suggesting that molecular shape is the most important determinant for tumor-specificity (Table 2). For example, we have reported previously that **T–N** of 3-styrylchromones can be estimated by diameter (largest value in the distance matrix defined by the elements Dij), vsurf_DD23 and R3 OH (n = 15, R^2 = 0.764, Q^2 = 0.570, s = 0.308) (right), according to the following equation: **T–N** = 0.607($\pm$ 0.169)diameter − 0.121 ($\pm$0.035)vsurf_DD23 + 1.11 ($\pm$0.235)R3OH − 7.17 ($\pm$ 2.26) [30]. QSAR analysis can be applied to estimate the most potent chemical structures. By repeating the process of synthesis of the estimated structure and reconfirmation of its activity, more active compounds with defied structure will be manufactured.

Table 2. Top six chemical descriptors that showed the highest correlation to cytotoxicity to tumor cells (**T**) or normal cells (**N**) or tumor-specificity (**T–N**). Descriptors are explained in the footnote. Pink, molecular size; yellow, 3D shape; orange, topological shape; blue, electrostatic; green, lipophilicity.

	Category	Number of Descriptors Searched	T	N	T-N	Ref.
A	3-Styrylchromones		OMe at R1 OH at R3	vsurf_DD23 Glu	OH at R3 vsurf_DD23 G2u	[30]
B	3-Benzylidenechromanones	3134	RDF095i RDF095u RDF095e vsurf_IW6 vsurf_ID7 vsurf_ID1	Mor03v Mor03m Mor09m Glu Mor03p R3m+	Mor3m Mor03v SpMAD_AEA(dm) vsurf_HB7 R3m+ Mor25v	[32]

Table 2. *Cont.*

Category		Number of Descriptors Searched	T	N	T-N	Ref.
C	3-Styryl-2*H*-chromenes	330	chi1v	std_dim2	std_dim3	[33]
			KierFlex	E_tor	BCUT_SLOGP_1	
			KierA1	E_oop	vsurf_D4	
			SMR_VSA7	std_dim3	vsurf_R	
			KierA3	vsurf_A	vsurf_D5	
			Weight	BCUT_SMR_1	E-oop	
D	2-Azolylchromones	3062	G3m	SpMin8_Bh(s)	Kp	[34]
			G3e	Q_RPC-	P1p	
			G3v	G3s	Mor32i	
			Gm	G3e	P2p	
			G3p	G3m	Mor32u	
			G3s	Gm	CATS2D_02_LL	
E	3-(*N*-Cyclicamino)chromones	3096	RDF075v	Mor28s	CATS3D_12_LL	[36]
			RDF075p	CATS3D_02_A	VE3sign_G	
			Mor06s	CATS2D_02_A	J_D/Dt	
			SpMAD_AEA(dm	Inflammat-80	FCASA-	
			RDF090p	Depressant-80	CATS3D_11_LL	
			E3m	TDB05i	Chi_G/D	
F	2-(*N*-Cyclicamino)chromones	3089	SpPosA_B(m)	Mor32u	Mor22m	[35]
			SpPosA_B(e)	Mor32e	GCUT_SLOGP_1	
			GCUT_SLOGP	VR2_G/D	Mor17v	
			Mor17v	JGI4	Mor17m	
			Mor17m	VR2_G		
			VE1sign_B(v)	SPH		
G	Furo[2,3-*b*]chromones	2820	b_double	rsynth	b_double	[37]
			SlogP_VSA2	b_double	SlogP_VSA2	
			rsynth	SlogP_VSA2	rsynth	
			std_dim3	std_dim3	std_dim3	
			E_str	E_str	b_rotR	
			dens	dens	E_str	
H	Pyrano[4,3-*b*]chromones	3072	R8s	R6v+	R8s	[38]
			J_G	R1s	HATS7i	
			RDF055s	R4v	HATS3i	
			R7s	J_G	HATS3u	
			HATS7s	R4p	HATS7u	
			R1s	R3v+	Mor10i	

b_double: Number of double bonds. Aromatic bonds are not considered to be double bonds. b_rotR: Fraction of rotatable bonds; CATS2D_02_AL: CATS2D Acceptor-lipophilic at lag 02; CATS2D_02_LL: CATS2D Lipophilic-Lipophilic at lag 02; CATS3D_02_AL: CATS3D Acceptor-lipophilic BIN 02 (2.000-3.000Å); CATS3D_11_LL: CATS3D lipophilic-lipophilic BIN 11 (11.000-12.000Å); CATS3D_12_LL: CATS3D Lipophilic-Lipophilic BIN 12 (12.000-13.000Å); Chi_G/D: Randic-like index from distance/distance matrix; chi1v: atomic valence connectivity index; dens: Mass density: molecular weight divided by van der Waal's volume; Depressant-80: Ghose-Viswanadhan-Wendoloski antidepressant-like index at 80%; E3m: 3rd component accessibility directional WHIM index/weighted by mass; E_oop: out-of-plane potential energy; E_str: Bond stretch potential energy; E_tor: torsion potential energy; FCASA-: Fractional CASA-(negative charge weighted surface area, ASA-times max { qi<0 }) calculated as CASA-/accessible surface area; GCUT_SLOGP_1: The GCUT descriptors using atomic contribution to logP (using the Wildman and Crippen SlogP method); Gm: total symmetry index/weighted by mass; G1u: (the first component symmetry directional WHIM index/unweighted encoding molecular symmetry that extracts the global symmetry information; G2u: (the second component symmetry directional WHIM index/unweighted encoding molecular symmetry that extracts the global symmetry information; G3e: 3rd component symmetry directional WHIM index/weighted by Sanderson electronegativity; G3m: 3rd component symmetry directional WHIM index/weighted by mass; G3p: 3rd component symmetry directional WHIM index/weighted by polarizability; G3s: 3rd component symmetry directional WHIM index/weighted by I-state; G3v: 3rd component symmetry directional WHIM index/weighted by van der Waals volume; HATS3i: Leverage-weighted autocorrelation of lag 3/weighted by ionization potential; HATS3u: Leverage-weighted autocorrelation of lag 3/unweighted; HATS7i: Leverage-weighted autocorrelation of lag 7/weighted by ionization potential; HATS7s: Leverage-weighted autocorrelation of lag 7/weighted by I-state; HATS7u: Leverage-weighted autocorrelation of lag 7/unweighted; Inflammat-80: Ghose-Viswanadhan-Wendoloski anti-inflammatory-like index at 80%; J_D/Dt: Balaban-like index from distance/detour matrix; J_G: Balaban-like index from geometrical matrix; JGI4: Mean topological charge index of order 4; KierA1: First alpha modified shape index; KierA3: Third alpha modified shape index; KierFlex: Kier molecular flexibility index; Kp: K global shape index/weighted by polarizability; Mor03m: signal 03/weighted by mass; Mor03p: signal 03/weighted by polarizability; Mor03v: signal 03/weighted by van der Waals volume; Mor06s: Signal 06/weighted by I-state; Mor09m: signal 09/weighted by mass; Mor10i: Signal 10/weighted by ionization potential; Mor17m: Signal 17/weighted by mass; Mor17v: Signal 17/weighted by van der Waals volume; Mor22m: Signal 22/weighted by mass; Mor25v: signal 25/weighted by van der Waals volume; Mor28s: Signal 28/weighted by I-state; Mor32e: Signal 32/weighted by Sanderson electronegativity; Mor32i: signal 32/weighted by ionization potential in 3D-MoRSE descriptors; Mor32u: signal 32/unweighted in 3D-MoRSE descriptors; OMe at R1: methoxy substitution at the 6-position on the chromone ring group; OH at R3: 4′-hydroxy substitution in the phenyl group of styryl moiety; P1p: 1st component shape directional WHIM index/weighted by polarizability; P2p: 2nd component shape directional WHIM index/weighted by polarizability;Q_RPC-: Relative negative partial charge: the smallest negative partial charge atom i divided by the sum of the negative partial charge atom i; RDF055s: Radial Distribution Function- 055/weighted by I-state; RDF075p: Radial distribution function-075/weighted by polarizability; RDF075v: Radial distribution function-075/weighted by van der Waal's volume RDF; RDF090p: Radial distribution function-090/weighted by polarizability;RDF095i: Radial Distribution Function - 095/weighted by ionization potential;

RDF095u: Radial Distribution Function - 095/unweighted; RDF095e: Radial Distribution Function - 095/weighted by Sanderson electronegativity; rsynth: The synthetic reasonableness or feasibility, of the chemical structure; RTs: R total index/weighted by I-state; R1s: R autocorrelation of lag 1/weighted by I-state; R3m+: R maximal autocorrelation of lag 3/weighted by mass; R3v+: R maximal autocorrelation of lag 3/weighted by van der Waals volume; R4p: R autocorrelation of lag 4/weighted by polarizability; R4v: R autocorrelation of lag 4/weighted by van der Waals volume; R6v+: R maximal autocorrelation of lag 6/weighted by van der Waals volume; R7s: R autocorrelation of lag 7/weighted by I-state; R8s: R autocorrelation of lag 8/weighted by I-state; SCUT_SLOGP_1: using atomic contribution to logP1; SCUt_SMR_1: using atomic contribution to molar refractivity1; SlogP_VSA2: Sum of approximate accessible van der Waal's surface area i such that logP for atom i is from -0.2 to 0; SMR_VSA7: sum of vi such that Ri > 0.56; SPH: Spherosity; SpMAD_AEA: Spectral mean absolute deviation from augmented edge adjacency matrix weighted by dipole moment edge adjacency indices; SpPosA_B(e): Normalized spectral positive sum from Burden matrix weighted by Sanderson electronegativity; SpPosA_B(m): Normalized spectral positive sum from Burden matrix weighted by mass; SpMin8_Bh(s): Smallest eigenvalue n. 8 of Burden matrix weighted by I-state; std_dim2, std_dim3: standard dimension 2 or 3 that depend on the structure connectivity and conformation; TDB05i: 3D Topological distance based descriptors-lag 5 weighted by ionization potential; VE1sign_B(v): Coefficient sum of the last eigenvector from Burden matrix weighted by van der Waals volume; VE3sign_G: logarithmic coefficient sum of the last eigenvector from geometrical matrix; VR2_G: Normalized Randic-like eigenvector-based index from geometrical matrix; VR2_G/D: Normalized Randic-like eigenvector-based index from distance/distance matrix; vsurf_A: amphiphilic moment; vsurf_D4: hydrophobic volume 4; vsurf_D5: hydrophobic volume 5; vsurf_DD23: the interaction with hydrophobic probe assumed surrounding the molecule; vsurf_HB7: H-bond donor capacity 7; vsurf_ID1: Hydrophobic interaction-energy moment 1; vsurf_IW6: Hydrophilic interaction-energy moment 6; vsurf_ID7: Hydrophobic interaction-energy moment 7; vsurf_R: surface rugosity; Weight: molecular weight.

Metabolomic analysis is powerful to determine the early event of cell death induction process. We have reported that compoun. A (which induced apoptosis) increased the intracellular levels of diethanolamine and CDP-choline and reduced that of choline, suggesting the down-regulation of the glycerophospholipid pathway [31]. It remains to be determined which metabolic pathway is first affected at early stages after treatment with compound F (which did not induce apoptosis).

3. Catechins as Inhibitors of Glucosyltransferase

3.1. Classification of Oral Streptococcal GTF Enzymes

Dental plaque is the oral biofilm that consists of bacteria themselves and bacterial metabolites. Glucan, polymer of glucose, is one of the metabolically-produced polysaccharides as the basic structures of the dental plaque and is produced from sucrose by glucosyltransferase enzymes (GTFs). Since dental plaque is a fertile ground of the pathogenic bacteria and virus that cause oral disease such as stomatitis, dental caries, gingivitis and periodontitis, glucan and/or GTFs are the pathogen of those diseases. These GTFs are produced mainly by streptococci in oral cavity [39,40].

Oral streptococcal GTFs (EC: 2.4.1.5) [41] are encoded by *gtf* genes, belong to the glycosyl hydrolase family 70 and basically catalyze the transfer of D-glucopyranosyl units from sucrose to acceptor molecules [42]. Biochemically, GTFs are classified into mainly 2 types according to their products, water-soluble glucan (WSG) and water-insoluble glucan (WIG), main components of oral biofilm. Especially in *Streptococcus mutans (S. mutans)*, GTFB, water-insoluble glucan synthesizing glucosyltransferase enzyme is one of virulence factors for dental caries, because water-insoluble glucan plays an important role in adhesion and establishment of *S. mutans* on tooth surface [43–45].

To clarify the ancestry of streptococcal GTFs, we investigated the distribution of GTFs among bacteria, such as *Lactobacillus*, *Leuconostoc* and *Lactococcus* and phylogenetically analyzed glycosyl hydrolase family 70 enzymes [46]. The sequences of glycosyl hydrolase family 70 proteins used in this study were obtained from GenBank at NCBI (http://www.ncbi.nlm.nih.gov/) with reference to Pfam (http://pfam.sanger.ac.uk/). Sequence alignment was performed using ClustalW software version 1.83 [47] (http://clustalw.ddbj.nig.ac.jp/index.php?, DNA Data Bank of Japan, Mishima, Japan). Multiple alignment files saved by ClustalW in Clustal format were converted to MEGA format with the MEGA version 5 software [48] (http://www.megasoftware.net/). Phylogenetic analysis was performed by the maximum parsimony methods using MEGA version 4.0 software. We analyzed 20 glucosyltransferases from *Streptococcus*; 2 glucosyltransferases, 9 dextran sucrases and 1 alternan sucrase from *Leuconostoc*; 10 glucan sucrases from *Lactobacillus*; and 1 glucosyltransferases from *Lactococcus*. PspA, glucosyltransferases from *Lactococcus* was defined as the convenient ancestor in this analysis (Figure 6) [46].

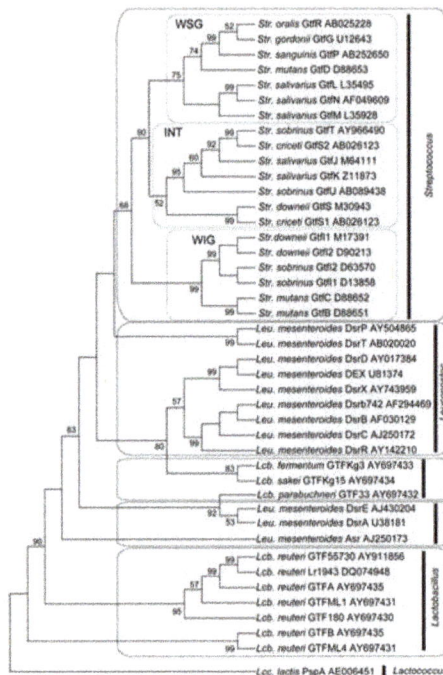

Figure 6. Phylogenetic analysis of glycosyl hydrolase family 70 enzymes by amino acid sequence. Cited from Reference [46] with permission.

The accession numbers in NCBI of these glycosyl hydrolases are provided after species and enzyme name in Figure 6. Here, we have shown that enzymes in the lower part of the phylogenetic tree synthesize glucans with various linkage types such as α-1,3; α-1,6; α-1,2; and α-1,4, while those in the upper part of the tree synthesize only water-soluble α-1,6-linked glucans. The phylogenetic tree would suggest that the streptococcal GTFs were derived from other lactic acid bacteria following their spread through the genera in the order of *Lactococcus, Lactobacillus, Leuconostoc* and *Streptococcus* and that the streptococcal GTF family can be phylogenetically classified into 3 clusters: the water-soluble glucan-synthesizing group (WSG), the water-insoluble glucan synthesizing group (WIG) and the intermediate group (INT).

A phylogenetic tree was constructed using the maximum parsimony (MP) method. The value on each branch is the estimated confidence limit (expressed as a percentage) for the position of the branches, as determined by bootstrap analysis. Only values exceeding 50% are shown. [46]

3.2. Purification of GTF Enzymes

Streptococcal GTFs can be divided into 2 types, WIG- and WIG- synthesizing GTFs by glucan product. Native WIG-synthesizing GTF, for example, GTFB and GTFC was purified from *S. mutans* MT8148, cultured in TTY medium [49,50]. The bacteria were collected by centrifugation and the cell-associated GTF (CA-GTF) was extracted by 8 M urea. The extract was precipitated by 60% saturated ammonium sulfate, applied to a DEAE Sepharose FF and eluted with a linear gradient of 0 to 1.0 M NaCl in the same buffer. Active fractions measured were concentrated by ammonium sulfate precipitation and then applied to a Bio-Scale CHT10-I column and then eluted with a 10 to 500 mM potassium phosphate buffer (KPB) linear gradient [51]. To select the GTFB and GTFC fractions, we carried out glucan synthesis assay [52], ELISA using anti-CA-GTF antibody, SDS-PAGE and Western blot using anti-GTF-I (GTFB) monoclonal antibody and anti-GTF-SI (GTFC) monoclonal antibody (Figure 7) [49].

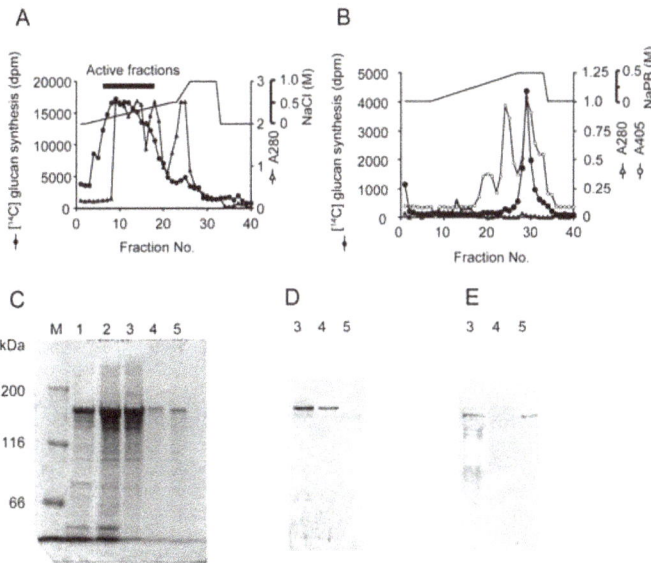

Figure 7. Purification of GTFB and GTFC from *S. mutans* MT8148, by sequential chromatography on. DEAE Sepharose FF column (collecting No. 6 to No. 17 fractions) (**A**) and Bio-Scale CHT10-I column (collecting No.29 and No.24 fraction as purified GTFB and GTFC, respectively) (**B**). The sample in each purification step was separated by SDS-PAGE (**C**) and assessed with Western blot analyses using anti-GTF-I (**D**), anti-GTF-SI (**E**) antiserum. Lane M, molecular weight marker; 1, 8 M-urea extraction; 2, precipitant of 1 by ammonium sulfate; 3, GTF-active fraction eluted with DEAE Sepharose column; 4, No. 29 fraction eluted with CHT10-I column; No. 24 fraction eluted with CHT10-I column. Cited from Reference [49] with permission.

Native WSG-synthesizing GTF, for example, GTFR was purified from *Streptococcus oralis* (*S. oralis*) ATCC 10557 [53], cultured in dialyzed TTY medium [50]. The culture supernatant was precipitated by 60% saturated ammonium sulfate and then applied to a Q Sepharose FF column and eluted with a linear gradient of 0 to 1.0 M NaCl [51]. Active fractions (indicated by bars) were pooled, applied to a Bio-Scale CHT10-I column and then eluted with a 10 to 500 mM KPB linear gradient [51]. To select the GTFR, the glucan synthesis assay and SDS-PAGE were carried out (Figure 8) [53].

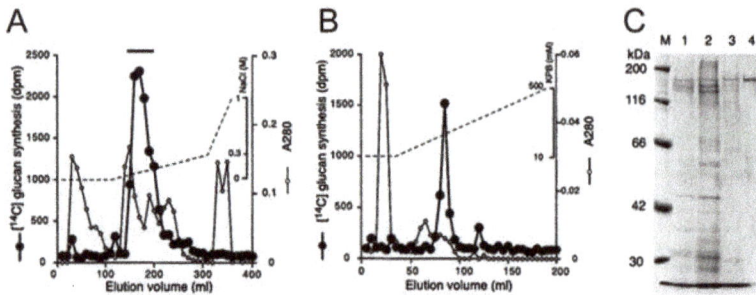

Figure 8. Purification of GTFR from *Streptococcus oralis* (*S. oralis*) ATCC 10557 by sequential chromatography on a Q Sepharose FF column (eluted with a linear gradient of 0 to 0.3 M NaCl) (**A**) and Bio-Scale CHT10-I column (**B**). Elution was done with a 10 to 500 mM KPB linear gradient. (**C**) SDS-PAGE of GTase preparations at different stages of purification. Lanes: 1, culture supernatant; 2, ammonium sulfate precipitate; 3, pooled active fractions from Q-ion-exchange chromatography; 4, pooled active fraction from CHT-10 hydroxylapatite chromatography; M, molecular mass markers. Cited from Reference [53] with permission.

In summary, purification of oral streptococcal GTFs would be commonly carried out by three steps method, ammonium sulfate precipitation, ion-exchange chromatography and hydroxyapatite chromatography [54–58]. Recombinant GTF (rGTF) would be produced as the other approach of GTF preparation using expression vector [59–63]. rGTF would be purified by ammonium sulfate precipitation, chromatography using His-tag and so on. These native and/or recombinant GTFs were used for the suppression analysis of glucan production by inhibitor and the recovery analysis of biofilm formation by addition of GTF. For these reasons, preparation of oral streptococcal GTFs would be important in the study of prevention of oral infectious diseases such as dental caries, periodontitis and so on.

3.3. Inhibitors of Oral Streptococcal GTFs

In GTFR from *S. oralis*, some inorganic salts suppressed the synthesis of water-soluble glucan. The synthesis of water-soluble glucan was reduced especially by divalent cation. Therefore, divalent cation could be inhibitors. However, in water-insoluble GTF from *Streptococcus sobrinus* 6715, high concentrations of monovalent (above 100 mM) and divalent (above 20 mM) cations stimulated the formation of insoluble glucan, whereas lower concentrations of monovalent (below 10 mM) and divalent (below 1 mM) cations reduced the formation of insoluble glucan to a negligible amount [64]. Thus, it would be difficult to adopt inorganic salts an inhibitor of oral streptococcal GTFs, considering their opposing actions between high and low concentrations.

It has been well known that natural products, for example, hydrolysable tannins (gallotannin, ellagitannin), condensed tannins (proanthocyanin, catechins), complex tannins, as from plant origin such as green tea, Oolong tea, cocoa, coffee and traditional Chinese medicine, inhibit glucan synthesis of oral streptococcal GTFs [65–71]. Especially, polyphenol mixtures from Oolong tea or cacao beans among them inhibited glucan-synthesis activity of GTFs from *S. mutans*. For example, OTF6, one of polyphenol fraction extracted from Oolong tea inhibited glucan-synthesis activity of rGTFB, rGTFC and rGTFD (Figure 9) [72]. With the increase of substrate of GTF, the production of glucan reached the plateau (near saturation) level. Even if the substrate concentration is enough, OTF6 effectively inhibited the production of glucan, suggesting its application to the dental plaque and caries. Since they can be inhibitors against other diseases, for example, stomatitis, periodontitis and aspiration pneumonia, they are expected to inhibit the formation of various glucan-biofilm, which contains some pathogenic organisms [73].

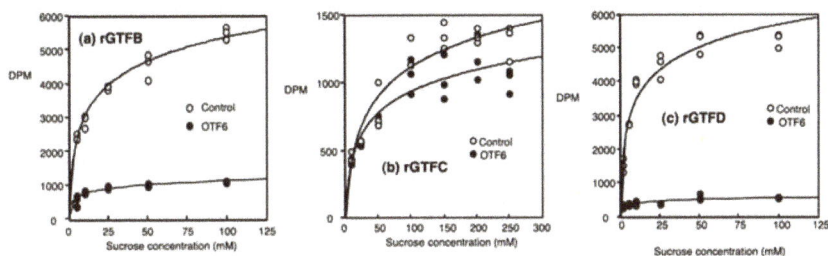

Figure 9. Changes in the quantity of glucan produced by recombinant GTFs. GTF activity was measured with [14C-glucose] sucrose. The OTF6 concentration in all displayed data was 1.0 mg/mL. Data are given in counts per minute. GTFs and sucrose were reacted without (○) and with (●) OTF6. Cited from Reference [72] with permission.

Nearly half of the commensal bacterial population of the human body is present in the oral cavity. An increase in the number of oral microorganisms may produce infective endocarditis, aspiration pneumonia and oral infections. When hydroxypropylcellulose strips containing green tea catechin were applied once a week for 8 weeks in pockets as a slow release local delivery system, the patient's periodontal status was significantly improved [74]. Gel-entrapped catechin (GEC) was manufactured by mixing catechins (epigallocatechin, epigallocatechin gallate, epicatechin, epicatechin gallate, gallocatechin, catechin and gallocatechin gallate) with polysaccharide, dextrin, citric acid, potassium chloride and stevia, to maintain the moistness in the oral cavity of elderly patients. GEC inhibited the growth of the Actinomyces, periodontopathic bacteria and Candida strains, possibly due to the produced hydrogen peroxide [75]. Local treatment of GEC seems to be important, since orally-administered catechin have been reported to increase the blood mitochondrial heme amounts and catalase activity, that may neutralize the antimicrobial activity of GEC [76].

4. Lignin-Carbohydrate Complex (LCC) as Anti-HIV Resources of the Natural Kingdom

We have previously reported anti-HV activity of three major polyphenols, tannins, flavonoids and lignin-carbohydrate complex (LCC), that were purified by our group. The potency of anti-HIV activity (SI) was calculated from the following equation: SI = CC_{50}/EC_{50}, where the CC_{50} is the concentration that reduced the viable cell number of the uninfected cells by 50% and the EC_{50} is the concentration that increased the viable cell number of the HIV-infected cells up to 50% that of the control (mock-infected, untreated) cells. Among them, LCC from pine cones of *Pinus parviflora* Sieb. et Zucc, pine cone of *Pinus elliottii var.* Elliottii, pine seed shell of *Pinus parviflora* Sieb. et Zucc, bark of *Erythroxylum catuaba* Arr. Cam, husk and mass of cacao beans of Theobroma, *Lentinus edodes* mycelia extract (L·E·M) and from precipitating fiber fraction of mulberry juice [77–84] showed the highest value (SI = 14, 28, 12, 43, 311, 46, 94 and 7), although much lower than that of popular anti-IIV agents (dextran sulfate, curdlan sulfate, azidothymidine, 2′,3′-dideoxycytidine) (SI = 2956 to 23261) (Table 3). Lignin but not carbohydrate moiety, seems to be essential to exert the anti-HIV activity, since synthetic lignin, manufactured by dehydrogenation polymerization of phenylpropenoids showed the comparable anti-HIV activity [85], whereas neutral and uronic acid-containing polysaccharides were inactive (SI = 1) [86]. We also found that monomer of phenylpropanoid monomers (*p*-coumaric acid, ferulic acid, caffeic acid) were inactive (SI < 1) [85], suggesting the importance of higher-ordered complicated structures for anti-HIV activity induction.

On the other hand, both hydrolysable and condensed tannins (see Figure 1A for classification) [87] (SI = 1.8 to 7.3 and 1.1) and flavonoids (Figure 1B) [88] (SI = 1.5) showed much lower anti-HIV activity. It is noted that anti-HIV activity of hydrolysable tannins increased with degree of polymerization: monomer (SI = 1.8) < dimer (SI = 2.3) < timer (SI = 3.4) < tetramer (SI = 7.3) [87].

Table 3. Anti-HIV activity of natural products.

Samples		Anti-HIV activity (SI)	Ref.
Lignin-carbohydrate complex			
Pine cone of *Pinus parviflora* Sieb. et Zucc		14	[77]
Pine cone of *Pinus elliottii* var. Elliottii		28	[78]
Pine seed shell of *Pinus parviflora* Sieb. et Zucc		12	[79]
Bark of *Erythroxylum catuaba* Arr. Cam.		43	[80]
Husk of cacao beans of Theobroma		311	[81]
Mass of cacao beans of Theobroma		46	[82]
Lentinus edodes mycelia extract (L·E·M)		94	[83]
Precipitating fiber fraction of mulberry juice		7	[84]
Dehydrogenation polymers of phenylpropenoids (n = 23)		105	[85]
Polysaccharides			
Neutral polysaccharides of pine cone of *P. parviflora* Sieb. et Zucc		1	[86]
Uronic acid-containing polysaccharides of pine cone		1	[86]
Lower molecular weight polyphenols			
Hydrolysable tannins (monomer) (MW: 484–1255) (n = 21)		1.8 ± 2.8	[87]
Hydrolysable tannins (dimer) (MW: 1571–2282) (n = 39)		2.3 ± 3.2	[87]
Hydrolysable tannins (trimer) (MW: 2354–2658) (n = 4)		3.4 ± 3.7	[87]
Hydrolysable tannins (tetramer) (MW: 3138–3745) (n = 3)		7.3 ± 6.5	[87]
Condensed tannins (MW: 290–1764) (n = 8)		1.1 ± 0.4	[87]
Flavonoids (MW: 84–648) (n = 92)		1.5 ± 1.9	[88]
Herb extracts			
Green tea leaves	Hot water extraction		[89]
	Alkaline extraction	3	
Oolong tea leaves	Hot water extraction	<0.033	[89]
	Alkaline extraction	13	
Orange flower	Hot water extraction	<0.5	[89]
	Alkaline extraction	>15	
Licorice root	Hot water extraction	4	[90]
	Alkaline extraction	42	
Alkaline extract of leaves of *Sasa* sp.		86	[86]
Kampo medicines (n = 10)		1.0 ± 0.0	[91]
Constituent plant extracts of Kampo medicines (n = 25)		1.3 ± 0.8	[91]
Chromones			
(*E*)-3-(4-Hydroxystyryl)- 6-methoxy-4*H*-chromen-4-one		<1	[30]
(*E*)-3-(4-Chlorostyryl)-7-methoxy-2*H*-chromene		<1	[30]
Positive Controls			
Dextran sulfate (molecular mass, 5 kDa)		2956	
Curdlan sulfate (molecular mass, 79 kDa)		11718	
Azidothymidine		23261	
2′,3′-Dideoxycytidine (ddC)		2974	

Alkaline extraction of green tea leaves, oolong tea leaves, orange flower, licorice root was more efficient than hot water extraction to recover the anti-HIV substances: SI = 3 *vs* < 0.022; 13 *vs* < 0.033; > 15 *vs* < 0.5; 42 *vs* 4, respectively [89,90]. Likewise, alkaline extract of leaves of *Sasa* sp. showed much higher anti-HIV activity (SI = 86) than Japanese traditional medicines, Kampo (SI = 1.0) and constituent plant extracts (SI = 1.3) [91]. Chromone, such (*E*)-3-(4-hydroxystyryl)-6-methoxy-4*H*-chromen-4-one and (*E*)-3-(4-Chlorostyryl)-7-methoxy-2*H*-chromene were inactive [30] (Table 3).

5. Alkaline Extract of the Leaves of *Sasa* sp. (SE)

5.1. Prominent Anti-HIV, Anti-UV, Anti-Inflammation and Neuroprotective Activities (in vitro)

Although alkaline extracts of plants showed much higher anti-HIV activity than corresponding hot water extracts [86,89–91], only three papers from other groups have reported the anti-angiogenic and neuroprotective activity of alkaline extracts [92–94]. Also, only two papers have been published on the isolation and fractionation of lignin from bamboo, however, they reported no data of biological activity [95,96]. Based on these backgrounds, we reviewed mostly our research topics of SE.

Alkaline extract of the leaves of *Sasa* sp. (SE) is an over-the counter (OTC) drug in Japan, which is available in the drug store without the prescription of doctors. SE (dry weight: 58.8 mg/mL) contains Fe (II)-chlorophyllin, LCC and its degradation products and so forth. SE showed higher anti-HIV [86], anti-UV [97,98], anti-inflammatory [99] and neuroprotection activities [100], as compared with other lower molecular polyphenols (Table 4). SE has many good partners for exerting synergistic actions: anti-HIV activity with azidothymidine, 2′,3′-dideoxycytidine, dextran sulfate or curdlan sulfate [101]; anti-HSV activity with acyclovir [101], anti-bacterial activity with isopropyl methylphenol [102] and anti-UV activity [103] and radical scavenging activity with vitamin C [104]. SE also showed osteogenic activity [105].

Among three SE products, produc. A (100% pure SE that contains Fe(II)-chlorophyllin) showed 1~5-fold higher anti-HIV, anti-UV and hydroxyl radical scavenging activity and 3~7-fold lower CYP3A4 inhibitory activity than product B (contain Cu(II)-chlorophyllin and less LCC) and product C (product B further supplemented with ginseng and *Pinus densiflora* leaf extracts) [106]. Based on this finding, we used produc. A for the following studies and manufacturing the toothpaste.

Table 4. SE shows prominent anti-HIV, anti-UV, anti-inflammation and neuroprotective activities.

Samples	Anti-HIV	Anti-UV	Anti-Inflammation	Neuroprotection
(Target cells)	(T-cell leukemia)	(HSC-2)	(HPLF)	(Differentiated PC12)
Evaluated by	CC_{50}/EC_{50} (+HIV)	CC_{50}/EC_{50}(+UV)	CC_{50}/EC_{50}(+IL-1β)	CC_{50}/EC_{50}(+Aβ_{25-35})
SE	86	38.5	>96.8	56.8
Curcumin		<1.0	1.5	17.3
Gallic acid	<1.0	5.4	0.9	
Ferulic acid	<1.0		>2.9	
p-Coumaric acid	<1.0		>3.1	
EGCG	<1.0	7.7		10.7
Resveratrol		<1.0		<1.0
Rikkosan	<1.0	24.1	>4.3	
Hangesyashinto	<1.0	>4.9	285	
Glycyrrhiza	<1.0	4.3	59	
Ref.	[84]	[97,98]	[99]	[100]

5.2. Improvement of Lichenoid Dysplasia by SE

Oral *lichen planus* is a chronic mucocutaneous disease that affects tongue and oral mucosa, characterized by white lacy streaks on the mucosa or as smaller papules. The cause of lichen planus is not known. A biopsy was taken from a 43-year-old male patient and diagnosed as lichenoid dysplasia in 7 July 7 2003 (physician in charge: Dr. K. Mori). Treatment with vitamin B_1 improved the patient's symptoms but discontinuation of the treatment resulted in the disease recurrence. The patient was subjected to the SE treatment for 11 months (12 April 2011 until 12 March 2012), according to the guideline of Intramural Ethic Committee (no. A0901). The patient was orally administered 13.3 ml SE (diluted two-fold with water, thus containing 33 mg dried materials/mL) three times-a-day, 30 min before each meal. At each administration, the patient swallowed and retained SE in the oral cavity for 1 min before washing it down. The patient did not take any other medications during the treatment period. The patient's oral cavity was photographed with a digital camera and the total saliva was collected just before lunch and then every two weeks, after the start of SE administration.

When a patient had been treated for 12 months with SE, white areas of lacy streaks in the several areas of buccal mucosa progressively reduced (Figure 10A). Oral intake of SE also improved the patient's symptoms of pollen allergy and loose teeth, giving an impression that the oral mucosa became much tighter. Three weeks after treatment, uneven, rough and cut mucosa became much smoother. At four weeks, the rough mucosa was narrowed into a smaller area and the patient could eat without any pungent feeling on the oral mucosa. SE treatment reduced the salivary concentration of IL-6 from 0.052 ± 0.030 ng/mL (n = 5) to 0.01 ng/mL and that of IL-8 from 5.25 ± 1.06 ng/mL (n = 5) to 1.11 ng/mL [107].

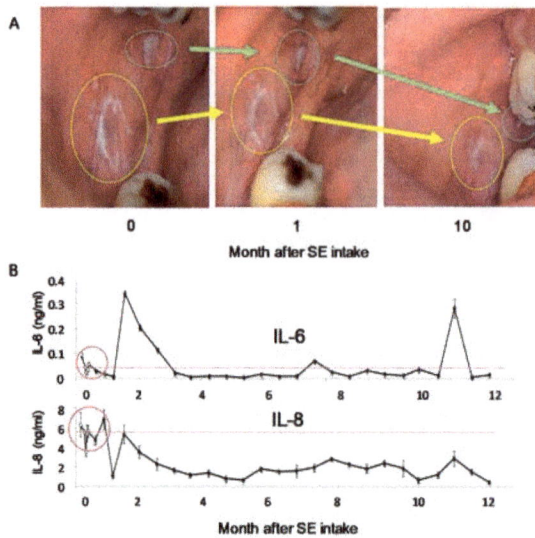

Figure 10. Effect of SE treatment on the oral lichenoid dysplasia. (**A**) Oral inspection with a digital camera, (**B**) salivary IL-6 and IL-8 concentrations. Cited from Reference [107] with permission.

5.3. Anti-Oxidative Stress Effect of SE in Chronic Dialysis Patients

With the cooperation of 10 maintenance dialysis patients in Masuko Memorial Hospital for 2 years from 2000, clinical data of SE were accumulated (Figure 11A–E).

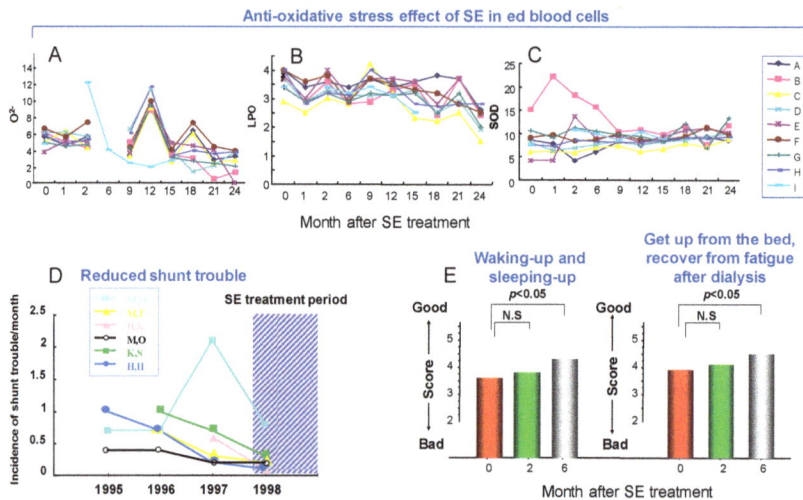

Figure 11. Anti-oxidative stress effects on chronic dialysis patients. (**A**) Superoxide (O^{2-}) (measured by luciferin chemiluminescence method), (**B**) LPO (measured by HPLC), (**C**) SOD activity (xanthine · xanthine oxidase reaction) of red blood cells. (**D**) Incidence of shunt problem from 1996–1998. Patients were treated with SE after 1 November 1997. (**E**) Questionnaire about the clinical effect of SE. Cited from Reference [108] with permission.

By treatment with SE, superoxide (O^{2-}) was gradually declined. Although the drift was seen in the middle of 12 months, possibly due to the measuring problem with instruments and after

24 months, cases exceeding the initial level were not observed (A). Likewise, LPO showed a decreasing tendency, possibly due to the elimination of O^{2-}, although no significant difference was observed (B). In support of this finding, the SOD activity gradually increased (C), suggesting the enhancement of the antioxidant action. Concentration of markers for the impairment of vascular endothelium (thrombomodulin and von Willebrand factor) did not show any significant fluctuation (measured by SRL Inc.), with large variation of the data due to small numbers of patients [108].

A shunt, which is a bypass connecting the artery and vein of the brachium to perform blood maintenance dialysis, is indispensable. However, the pressure due to the dialysis causes expansion, the bending and extension of blood vessel, the thickening of vein wall and the ectopic calcification due to the repeated puncture, leading to the blockage due to the decreased blood pressure, stagnation of blood flow and enhancement of coagulability. All patients frequently repeat the clotting in the part of shunt during dialysis. However, the incidences of such shunt troubles were apparently reduced by SE treatment (D) and questionnaire on the clinical effects of SE showed the good outcome (E) (Figure 11). Although this clinical trial has ended once in 2 years, one patient (84 years old) still receives the clinical trial, with little or no trouble of the shunt, possibly due to the preservation of blood fluidity and maintenance of blood vessel possibly by iron chlorophyllin and antioxidants in SE [108].

5.4. Anti-Halitosis Effect of Toothpaste Supplemented with SE

Considering the potent anti-HIV, anti-inflammatory effects of SE, we have manufactured SE containing toothpaste (SETP) for the first time. The SETP is composed of 26.2% SE, 0.1% isopropylmethylphenol, base materials, cleaning agents, humectants, flavoring substances, sweetening agent, stabilizers, binding agent and washing soap). We have selected the 26.2% SE, since treatment of periodontal ligament fibroblasts for 1 min with 50% of SE did not affect the cell viability and approximately 8 ml of saliva were produced and accumulated in the oral cavity by 5 min of tooth brushing. SETP can be obtained at the drug store. We investigated its anti-halitosis effect with the collaboration of a total of 12 volunteers, according to the guideline of Intramural Ethic Committee (no. A1219). They brushed their teeth immediately after meals three times each day with STEP or placebo toothpaste (omitting only SE). Halitosis in the breath and bacterial number on the tongue were measured by portable apparatuses at 11:00 AM in the morning. We found that SETP significantly reduced halitosis ($p = 0.046$) but not the number of bacterial on the tongue ($p = 0.60$) [109].

5.5. Other Unpublished Case Reports

The female subject (28 years old) was bothered by atopy since her infancy. When her living environment changed by getting a job three years ago, the symptoms worsened further especially in early spring, rainy season and dry winter. She unexpectedly found that pasting the *Sasa* sp. extract-immersed cotton on her skin improved the symptoms. In another when red eczema and skin roughness became apparent (A), she applied just a pearl-size amount of "Moisture Creamy Gel" (containing to 1.8% *Sasa* sp. extract), her skin of cheek and face line three times a day. The creamy gel produced no bleeding, in contrast to other commercially available lotions. After 1 week, area of red eczema began to diminish and rough skin became smooth, thus reducing the application time to twice a day. After 2 weeks, eczema has completely healed (B) (Figure 12).

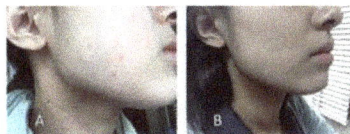

Figure 12. Facial photo before (**A**) and two weeks after application (**B**) of SE Moisture Creamy Gel (taken on 17 April 2018) (unpublished data).

Recently, diacetyl (2,3-butanedione), mostly produced by *Staphylococcus aureus* and *Staphylococcus epidermidis*, has been reported to be a key contributor to unpleasant odors emanating from the axillae, feet and head regions [110]. There was one case report that when male healthy volunteer (69 years old) take daily drink of SE (40 mL, 2.4 g dry weight) mixed with lemon and orange juice after lunch except for Sunday, he experienced the significant reduction in the fecal smell (after 1 week), tongue cloth (after 1 month) and body odor (after three months) and no stress-induced stomatitis for 7 months.

6. Kampo Medicines

Xerostomia is a disease in which a reduction in salivary secretion causes oral dryness and it may also be further complicated with odontonecrosis, periodontal disease, candidiasis, and taste disorders. The exacerbation of these diseases has a substantial effect on the QOL, so it is necessary in such cases to clarify the causes and select the most appropriate treatment. Herbal treatment alleviated thirst and oral dryness in most cases but many cases showed a slower increase in salivary production than the cases administered cevimeline hydrochloride [111] (Figure 13).

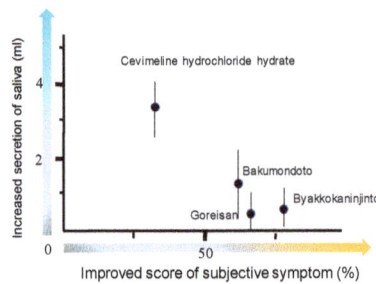

Figure 13. Regarding subjective symptoms, a questionnaire is issued about (i) mouth dryness, (ii) swallowing difficulty and (iii) oral pain, using the VAS method. When the average of these three items is 0, 1~20, 21~40, 41~60, 61~80, 81~100, the score is counted as 1, 2, 3, 4 and 5 points, respectively. The extent of subjective symptom improvement was calculated by dividing the subjective symptom score before the administration by that before starting administration and the multiplied by 100. Cited from Reference [111] with permission.

When the patient with xerostomia-induced glossitis was treated with Byakkokaninjinto (3 g three times a day) for two months, glossitis largely disappeared, and the subjective symptoms decreased (Figure 14).

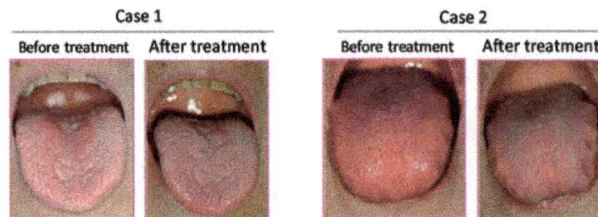

Figure 14. Effect of *Byakkokaninjinto* on glossitis. Cited from Reference [112] with permission.

7. Dental Application of Angiotensin II Receptor Blocker for Severe Periodontitis

7.1. Angiotensin II Receptor Blocker (ARB) in Marfan Syndrome

Marfan syndrome is an autosomal dominant connective tissue disease that affects about one in 5000 individuals [113]. The responsible gene of this syndrome is FBN1 which encodes the extracellular matrix protein fibrillin-1 [113]. FBN1 mutations lead to defects in multiple organs including skeletal, cardiovascular and ocular systems [114]. Among them, the most serious problems are seen in the cardiovascular system, such as, aortic regurgitation, aneurysm and dissection of the aortic root, mitral valve prolapse and mitral regurgitation, causing a short life expectancy in patients [115].

Fibrillin-1 regulates the function of endogenous transforming growth factor (TGF)-β by targeting the respective complexes to the extracellular cell matrix [116]. Studies of animal [117] and human [118] reported that TGF-β signaling drives aneurysm progression in the aorta [119]. Since Marfan syndrome patients have cardiovascular problems, the surgical replacement of aortic and mitral valve and aortic roots is often required [115]. It is known that effects of angiotensin II are mediated by two receptors, type 1 (AT1) and type 2 (AT2) receptor [120]. AT1-receptor signaling can increase the production of TGF-β ligands and receptors [121]. Angiotensin II-receptor blockers (ARBs) selectively block the binding of angiotensin II to its receptor within the renin–angiotensin system [122]. AT1-receptor blockade decreases TGF-β signaling and thus inhibit the phosphorylation of Smad2. Recently, losartan, one of ARBs, have been reported to suppress the progression of aortic root dilation by inhibiting TGF-β signaling [117,123]. Application of ARBs are now providing great benefit to Marfan syndrome patients by improving cardiovascular conditions.

7.2. Periodontal Disease Frequently Seen in Marfan Syndrome

Oral manifestations are not included as diagnostic criteria of Marfan syndrome but this disease is frequently affected with severe periodontitis [124–126]. Periodontitis affects periodontal tissues, including gingiva, periodontal ligament (PDL) and alveolar bone [127]. Approximately 15% of the adult population has an advanced form of periodontitis, making multiple negative impacts on quality of life [128,129]. Consequences of periodontitis include negative esthetics and functional problems in occlusion, chewing and speaking and finally result in tooth loss [130,131]. Periodontitis is initiated by chronic inflammation and immune reactions to bacterial pathogens [132]. Several bacteria play important roles in the pathogenesis of periodontitis but *Porphyromonas gingivalis* plays a central role in pathogenesis of periodontitis [133]. It is reported that 87.5% of Marfan syndrome patients had periodontitis with more than 4 mm of periodontal pocket depth, while only 35.7% of healthy volunteers showed such manifestation [134]. Interestingly, higher percentage of periodontitis with more than 4 mm of periodontal pocket depth was seen in patients with cardiovascular disease than those without cardiovascular disease [135]. Many Marfan syndrome patients have these cardiovascular problems, often necessitating the surgical replacement of aortic and mitral valve and aortic roots [115]. Because of this surgical replacement, it is essential to prevent dental infection, such as infectious endocarditis caused by the periodontitis.

The reason of higher incidence of severe periodontitis in Marfan in not known. However, the lower number of caries has been reported in adult Marfan syndrome patients than in healthy volunteers [124]. This implies that periodontal tissues but not teeth have structural problems making susceptible to severe periodontitis. The abnormal alignment of collagen fibers was observed in one of the model mice of Marfan syndrome (MgR mice). Homozygous MgR mice show the 72% of reduction in Fbn1 (encoding mouse fibrillin-1) expression because of transcriptional interference by insertion of the PGKneo-cassette [136] and resemble the phenotype of Marfan syndrome by showing 10% longer long bones than wild-type (WT) littermates. A comparable level of type I collagen, which is the most major collagen in periodontal ligaments, was expressed in PDL-cells of homozygous MgR mice as in WT mice [137]. However, multi-oriented collagen fiber bundles with a thinner appearance were noted in homozygous mice. These observations were never seen in WT mice showing well-organized definite collagen fiber bundles. This suggests that normal level of fibrillin-1 is essential for the normal architecture of periodontal ligament.

7.3. Progression of Periodontal Disease and Application of ARB

Telmisartan (4'-[[4-methyl-6-(1-methyl-1*H*-benzimidazol-2-yl)-2-propyl-1*H*-benzimidazol-1-yl] methyl]biphenyl-2-carboxylic acid) is a non-peptide ARBs used in the management of hypertension [138,139] and expected as an effective drug for the management of vascular condition in Marfan syndrome [140]. This drug has a binding affinity 3,000 times higher for AT1 than AT2 [141]. Heterozygous MgΔ mice, another mice model of Marfan syndrome, show half level of Fbn1 as WT mice [136]. Six-week-old male heterozygous MgΔ and WT mice were challenged with *P. gingivalis* with and without telmisartan application [142]. Infection of *P. gingivalis* induced alveolar bone resorption in both heterozygous MgΔ and wild-type mice. The amount of alveolar bone resorption was significantly larger in the former than the latter. Interleukin (IL)-17 and tumor necrosis factor (TNF)-α levels were significantly higher in infected MgΔ mice than infected WT mice. Telmisartan treatment significantly suppressed the alveolar bone resorption of infected Mg mice. Telmisartan also significantly reduced the levels of TGF-β, IL-17 and TNF-α in infected MgΔ mice to those seen in infected WT mice. These suggest that ARB can prevent the severe periodontitis frequently seen in Marfan syndrome. Combination with Chinese medicine and angiotensin-converting enzyme inhibitors (ACEI) or ARB showed kidney protection effect [143,144] and tannic acid inhibited AT1 gene expression and cellular response [145]. However, previous studies have not yet investigated whether traditional medicines and dietary polyphenols inhibit the periodontitis through blocking the AT1.

8. Future Direction

The present article demonstrated that chromone derivatives show high tumor-specificity, low keratinocyte toxicity, without or with induction of apoptosis, suggesting that apoptosis induction is not the absolute necessity for exploration of anticancer drugs. Chromone ring is a natural material, distributing into many flavonoids. By introducing an appropriate substituent thereto with the guidance of QSAR analysis, more active derivatives can be manufactured. Synthesis of ^{13}C-labled chromone derivatives is underway to investigate the cellular uptake and binding to the specific acceptor molecules in the cells. Since all data of chromone derivatives are produced in vitro, in vivo study with implanted tumors are necessary to confirm the selective action against tumor cells. Also, possibility of synergistic action with anticancer drugs and effects on CYP-3 enzymes that affect the stability of accompanying drugs should be monitored before the clinical application.

LCC and SE, both are extracted from plants by alkaline extraction showed extremely higher anti-HIV, anti-inflammatory and neuroprotective activity. Our recent study demonstrated that SE stimulated the growth of differentiated neuronal cells and human gingival epithelial progenitor (HGEP) at lower concentration. This hormetic action of SE may explain its ability to protect the cells from amyloid peptides. The pathogenesis of dementia is thought to be due to the collapse of cerebral nerve cells and the reduction of neurotransmitters by the senile plaques produced by the accumulation of amyloid beta (Aβ) and tau protein (Tau) in the brain. It remains to be investigated whether SE prevent the dementia, if so by what mechanism.

We have previously reported that LCC of SE, prepared by repeated acid-precipitation and alkaline solubilization, has greenish color (absorption peak = 655 nm), characteristic to chlorophyllin (absorption peak = 629 nm) and that 68.5% of SE eluted as a single peak at the retention time of 22.175 min in HPLC [146]. This suggests that LCC in SE may easily bind to or entangled with chlorophyllin and other components to make large molecule under physiological condition. Such arge molecule may non-specifically bind to many cell surface receptors including dectin-2, causing its unique biological activity.

This review suggests the efficacy of GTF inhibitors and ARBs to prevent the biofilm formation and periodontitis, respectively. It is crucial to search for these inhibitors and blockers from the natural kingdom and elucidate their action mechanism.

Author Contributions: H.S., T.O. and T.Y. organized the review; T.W. and T.H. wrote the section of GTFs: N.S. wrote section of ARBs; K.M. wrote the section of Kampo; N.Y. wrote the section of anti-oxidative stress effect; H.K. wrote the section of anti-eczema effect; T.G. wrote the section of body odor; J.N. and Y.U. performed the QSAR analysis; K.T. and Y.S. synthesized chromone derivatives.

Funding: This research was funded by Daiwa Biological Research Institute Co., Ltd., Kanagawa, Japan and partially supported by KAKENHI from the Japan Society for the Promotion of Science (JSPS): Sakagami H, 16K11519.

Acknowledgments: The authors acknowledge Daiwa Biological Research Institute Co., Ltd for the supply of SE and Meikai University School of Dentistry for the support for the research.

Conflicts of Interest: One of the authors (H.S.) has been donated from the research fund from Daiwa Biological Research Institute Co., Ltd., Kanagawa, Japan. The authors wish to confirm that such financial support has not influenced the outcome the experimental data.

Abbreviations

ARB	Angiotensin II receptor blocker
AT1	Angiotensin II type 1 receptor
AT2	Angiotensin II type 2 receptor
AZT	Azidothymidine
CC_{50}	50% cytotoxic concentration
CDP-choline	Cytidine diphosphate-choline
CPT	Camptothecin
DNR	Daunorubicin
DOC	Docetaxel
DXR	Doxorubicin
EGCG	Epigallocatechin-3-gallate
ELISA	EnzymelLinked immunoSorbent assay
ETP	Etoposide
FBN1	Gene that codes fibrillin-1 in humans
5-FU	5-Fluorouracil
GTF	Glucosyltransferase GTF
HIV	Human immuno-deficiency virus
HPLC	High-performance liquid chromatography HPLC
HSVV	Herpes simplex virus
IL	Interleukin
LCC	Lignin carbohydrate complex
LPO	Lipid peroxide
MEL	Melphalan
MgR mice	model mice of Marfan syndrome
MMC	Mitomycin C
O_2^{-}	Superoxide
OSCC	Oral squamous cell carcinoma
PDL	Periodontal ligament
QASR	Quantitative structure-activity relationship
Sasa sp.	*Sasa* species
SA	Senescence-associated
SE	Alkaline extract of the leaves of *Sasa* sp.
SN-38	Active metabolite of irinotecan
SOD	Superoxide dismutase
TGF	Transforming growth factor
TNF	Tumor necrosis factor
TRL	Toll-like receptor

TS	Tumor-specificity
TS$_E$	Tumor-specificity determined with human normal oral epithelial cells *vs* OSCC cells
TS$_M$	Tumor-specificity determined with human normal oral mesenchymal cells *vs* OSCC cells
UV	Ultraviolet
WIG	water-insoluble glucan
WSG	water-soluble glucan WSG

References

1. Queiroz, S.I.M.L.; Silva, M.V.A.D.; Medeiros, A.M.; Oliveira, P.T.; Gurgel, B.C.V.; Silveira, É.J.D.D. Recurrent aphthous ulceration. An epidemiological study of etiological factors, treatment and differential diagnosis. *An. Bras. Dermatol.* **2018**, *93*, 341–346. [CrossRef]

2. Chiang, C.P.; Chang, J.; Wang, Y.P.; Wu, Y.H.; Wu, Y.C.; Sun, A. Recurrent aphthous stomatitis—Etiology, serum autoantibodies, anemia, hematinic deficiencies, and management. *J. Formos. Med. Assoc.* **2018**. [CrossRef] [PubMed]

3. Abdel Moneim, A.E.; Guerra-Librero, A.; Florido, J.; Shen, Y.Q.; Fernández-Gil, B.; Acuña-Castroviejo, D.; Escames, G. Oral Mucositis: Melatonin Gel an Effective New Treatment. *Int. J. Mol. Sci.* **2017**, *18*, 1003. [CrossRef] [PubMed]

4. Sakagami, H. Biological activities and possible dental application of three major groups of polyphenols. *J. Pharmacol. Sci.* **2014**, *126*, 92–106. [CrossRef] [PubMed]

5. Okuda, T.; Yoshida, T.; Hatano, T. Hydrolyzable tannins and related polyphenols. In *Fortschritte der Chemie Organischer Naturstoffe/Progressinthe Chemistry of Organic Natural Products*; Springer: Vienna, Austria, 1995; pp. 1–117.

6. Nomura, T.; Hano, Y.; Fukai, T. Chemistry and biosynthesis of isoprenylated flavonoids from Japanese mulberry tree. *Proc. Jpn. Acad. Ser. B Phys. Biol. Sci.* **2009**, *85*, 391–408. [CrossRef] [PubMed]

7. Cendrowski, A.; Ścibisz, I.; Mitek, M.; Kieliszek, M.; Kolniak-Ostek, J. Profile of the Phenolic Compounds of Rosa rugosa Petals. *J. Food Qual.* **2017**, *2017*. [CrossRef]

8. Cendrowski, A.; Ścibisz, I.; Kieliszek, M.; Kolniak-Ostek, J.; Mitek, M. UPLC-PDA-Q/TOF-MS profile of polyphenolic compounds of liqueurs from Rose petals (Rosa rugosa). *Molecules* **2017**, *22*, 1832. [CrossRef] [PubMed]

9. Sakagami, H.; Hashimoto, K.; Suzuki, F.; Ogiwara, T.; Satoh, K.; Ito, H.; Hatano, T.; Takashi, Y.; Fujisawa, S. Molecular requirements of lignin-carbohydrate complexes for expression of unique biological activities. *Phytochemistry* **2005**, *66*, 2108–2120. [CrossRef]

10. Olsen, I.; Singhrao, S.K. Can oral infection be a risk factor for Alzheimer's disease? *J. Oral. Microbiol.* **2015**, *7*, 29143. [CrossRef]

11. Furuta, M.; Yamashita, Y. Oral health and swallowing problems. *Curr. Phys. Med. Rehabil. Rep.* **2013**, *1*, 216–222. [CrossRef]

12. Olmsted, J.L.; Rublee, N.; Zurkawski, E.; Kleber, L. Public health dental hygiene. An option for improved quality of care and quality of life. *J. Dent. Hyg.* **2013**, *87*, 299–308.

13. Hägglund, P.; Olai, L.; Ståhlnacke, K.; Persenius, M.; Hägg, M.; Andersson, M.; Koistinen, S.; Carlsson, E. Study protocol for the SOFIA project: Swallowing function, Oral health, and Food Intake in old Age. A descriptive study with a cluster randomized trial. *BMC Geriatr.* **2017**, *78*. [CrossRef] [PubMed]

14. Bardellini, E.; Amadori, F.; Majorana, A. Oral hygiene grade and quality of life in children with chemotherapy-related oral mucositis. A randomized study on the impact of a fluoride toothpaste with salivary enzymes, essential oils, proteins and colostrum extract versus a fluoride toothpaste without menthol. *Int. J. Dent. Hyg.* **2016**, *14*, 314–319. [CrossRef] [PubMed]

15. Siddiqui, I.A.; Sanna, V. Impact of nanotechnology on the delivery of natural products for cancer prevention and therapy. *Mol. Nutr. Food Res.* **2016**, *60*, 1330–1341. [CrossRef] [PubMed]

16. Feller, L.; Khammissa, R.A.; Chandran, R.; Altini, M.; Lemmer, J. Oral candidosis in relation to oral immunity. *J. Oral. Pathol. Med.* **2014**, *43*, 563–569. [CrossRef]

17. Pang, Y.; Shen, Z.; Sun, J.; Wang, W. Does the use of targeted agents in advanced gastroesophageal cancer increase complete response. A meta-analysis of 18 randomized controlled trials. *Cancer Manag. Res.* **2018**, *10*, 5505–5514. [CrossRef] [PubMed]

18. Zhou, S.; Zuo, L.; He, X.; Pi, J.; Jin, J.; Shi, Y. Efficacy and safety of rh-endostatin (Endostar) combined with pemetrexed/cisplatin followed by rh-endostatin plus pemetrexed maintenance in non-small cell lung cancer. A retrospective comparison with standard chemotherapy. *Thorac. Cancer.* **2018**, *9*, 1354–1360. [CrossRef]

19. Harada, T.; Ijima, A. Pharmacological profile and clinical findings of palbociclib (IBRANCE®capsule 25 mg/125 mg). *Folia Pharmacol. Jpn.* **2018**, *152*, 206–318. (In Japanese) [CrossRef] [PubMed]

20. Lulli, D.; Carbone, M.L.; Pastore, S. Epidermal growth factor receptor inhibitors trigger a type I interferon response in human skin. *Oncotarget* **2016**, *7*, 47777–47793. [CrossRef] [PubMed]

21. Ferrari, D.; Codecà, C.; Bocci, B.; Crepaldi, F.; Violati, M.; Viale, G.; Careri, C.; Caldiera, S.; Bordin, V.; Luciani, A.; et al. Anti-epidermal growth factor receptor skin toxicity. A matter of topical hydration. *Anticancer Drugs* **2016**, *27*, 144–146. [CrossRef]

22. Benjakul, R.; Kongkaneramit, L.; Sarisuta, N.; Moongkarndi, P.; Müller-Goymann, C.C. Cytotoxic effect and mechanism inducing cell death of α-mangostin liposomes in various human carcinoma and normal cells. *Anticancer Drugs* **2015**, *26*, 824–834. [CrossRef] [PubMed]

23. Do, N.; Weindl, G.; Grohmann, L.; Salwiczek, M.; Koksch, B.; Korting, H.C.; Schäfer-Korting, M. Cationic membrane-active peptides–anticancer and antifungal activity as well as penetration into human skin. *Exp. Dermatol.* **2014**, *23*, 326–331. [CrossRef] [PubMed]

24. Moreno Garcia, V.; Thavasu, P.; Blanco Codesido, M.; Molife, L.R.; Vitfell Pedersen, J.; Puglisi, M.; Basu, B.; Shah, K.; Iqbal, J.; de Bono, J.S.; et al. Association of creatine kinase and skin toxicity in phase I trials of anticancer agents. *Br. J. Cancer* **2012**, *107*, 1797–1800. [CrossRef] [PubMed]

25. Benedict, A.L.; Knatko, E.V.; Dinkova-Kostova, A.T. The indirect antioxidant sulforaphane protects against thiopurine-mediated photo-oxidative stress. *Carcinogenesis* **2012**, *33*, 2457–2466. [CrossRef] [PubMed]

26. Fischel, J.L.; Formento, P.; Ciccolini, J.; Etienne-Grimaldi, M.C.; Milano, G. Lack of contribution of dihydrofluorouracil and Alpha-fluoro-beta-alanine to the cytotoxicity of 5′-deoxy-5-fluorouridine on human keratinocytes. *Anticancer Drugs* **2004**, *15*, 969–974. [CrossRef] [PubMed]

27. Sakagami, H.; Okudaira, N.; Masuda, Y.; Amano, O.; Yokose, S.; Kanda, Y.; Suguro, M.; Natori, T.; Oizumi, H.; Oizumi, T. Induction of apoptosis in human oral keratinocyte by doxorubicin. *Anticancer Res.* **2017**, *37*, 1023–1029.

28. Miyamoto, M.; Sakagami, H.; Minagawa, K.; Kikuchi, H.; Nishikawa, H.; Satoh, K.; Komatsu, N.; Fujimaki, M.; Nakashima, H.; Gupta, M.; et al. Tumor-specificity and radical scavenging activity of poly-herbal formula. *Anticancer Res.* **2002**, *22*, 1217–1224.

29. Gaspar, A.; Matos, M.J.; Garrido, J.; Uriarte, E.; Borges, F. Chromone. A valid scaffold in medicinal chemistry. *Chem Rev.* **2014**, *114*, 4960–4992. [CrossRef]

30. Shimada, C.; Uesawa, Y.; Ishii-Nozawa, R.; Ishihara, M.; Kagaya, H.; Kanamto, T.; Terakubo, S.; Nakashima, H.; Takao, K.; Sugita, Y.; et al. Quantitative structure–cytotoxicity relationship of 3-styrylchromones. *Anticancer Res.* **2014**, *34*, 5405–5412.

31. Sakagami, H.; Shimada, C.; Kanda, Y.; Amano, O.; Sugimoto, M.; Ota, S.; Soga, T.; Tomita, M.; Sato, A.; Tanuma, S.; et al. Effects of 3-styrylchromones on metabolic profiles and cell death in oral squamous cell carcinoma cells. *Toxicol. Rep.* **2015**, *2*, 1281–1290. [CrossRef]

32. Uesawa, Y.; Sakagami, H.; Kagaya, H.; Yamashita, M.; Takao, K.; Sugita, Y. Quantitative structure-cytotoxicity relationship of 3-benzylidenechromanones. *Anticancer Res.* **2016**, *36*, 5803–5812. [CrossRef] [PubMed]

33. Uesawa, Y.; Ishihara, M.; Kagaya, H.; Kanamoto, T.; Terakubo, S.; Nakashima, H.; Yahagi, H.; Takao, K.; Sugita, Y. Quantitative structure–cytotoxicity relationship of 3-styryl-2*H*-chromenes. *Anticancer Res.* **2015**, *35*, 5299–5308. [PubMed]

34. Sakagami, H.; Okudaira, N.; Uesawa, Y.; Takao, K.; Kagaya, H.; Sugita, Y. Quantitative structure-cytotoxicity relationship of 2-azolylchromones. *Anticancer Res.* **2018**, *38*, 763–770. [PubMed]

35. Shi, H.; Nagai, J.; Sakatsume, T.; Bandow, K.; Okudaira, N.; Sakagami, H.; Tomomura, M.; Tomomura, A.; Uesawa, Y.; Takao, K.; et al. Quantitative structure–cytotoxicity relationship of 2-(*N*-cyclicamino)chromone derivatives. *Anticancer Res.* **2018**, *38*, 3897–3906. [CrossRef] [PubMed]

36. Shi, H.; Nagai, J.; Sakatsume, T.; Bandow, K.; Okudaira, N.; Uesawa, Y.; Sakagami, H.; Tomomura, M.; Tomomura, A.; Takao, K.; et al. Quantitative structure–cytotoxicity relationship of 3-(*N*-cyclicamino)chromone derivatives. *Anticancer Res.* **2018**, *38*, 4459–4467. [CrossRef]

37. Uesawa, Y.; Sakagami, H.; Shi, H.; Hirose, M.; Takao, K.; Sugita, Y. Quantitative structure-cytotoxicity relationship of furo[2,3-*b*]chromones. *Anticancer Res.* **2018**, *38*, 3283–3290. [CrossRef]

38. Nagai, J.; Shi, H.; Kubota, Y.; Bandow, K.; Okudaira, N.; Uesawa, Y.; Sakagami, H.; Tomomura, M.; Tomomura, A.; Takao, K.; et al. Quantitative structure–cytotoxicity relationship of pyrano[4,3-*b*]chromones. *Anticancer Res.* **2018**, *38*, 4449–4457. [CrossRef]

39. Pleszczyńska, M.; Wiater, A.; Bachanek, T.; Szczodrak, J. Enzymes in therapy of biofilm-related oral diseases. *Biotechnol. Appl. Biochem.* **2017**, *64*, 337–346. [CrossRef]

40. Kalesinskas, P.; Kačergius, T.; Ambrozaitis, A.; Pečiulienė, V.; Ericson, D. Reducing dental plaque formation and caries development. A review of current methods and implications for novel pharmaceuticals. *Stomatologija* **2014**, *16*, 44–52.

41. Hehre, E. Enzymic synthesis of polysaccharides. A biological type of polymerization. *Adv. Enzymol. Relat. Subj. Biochem.* **1951**, *11*, 297–337.

42. Kuramitsu, H.K. Virulence factors of mutans streptococci: Role of molecular genetics. *Crit. Rev. Oral Biol. Med.* **1993**, *4*, 159–176. [CrossRef]

43. Caufield, P.W. Dental caries. An infectious and transmissible disease. *Compend. Contin. Educ. Dent.* **2005**, *26*, 10–16. [PubMed]

44. Miller, W.D. *The Microorganisms of the Human Mouth; Ko"nig KG*; Karger: Basel, Switzerland, 1973.

45. Touger-Decker, R.; van Loveren, C. Sugars and dental caries. *Am. J. Clin. Nutr.* **2003**, *78*, 881S–892S. [CrossRef] [PubMed]

46. Hoshino, T.; Fujiwara, T.; Kawabata, T. Evolution of Cariogenic Character in Streptococcus Mutans: Horizontal Transmission of Glycosyl Hydrase Family 70 Genes. *Sci. Rep.* **2012**, *2*, 518. [CrossRef] [PubMed]

47. Jeanmougin, F.; Thompson, J.D.; Gouy, M.; Higgins, D.G.; Gibson, T.J. Multiple sequence alignment with Clustal, X. *Trends. Biochem. Sci.* **1998**, *23*, 403–405. [CrossRef]

48. Tamura, K.; Dudley, J.; Nei, M.; Kumar, S. MEGA4: Molecular evolutionary genetics analysis (MEGA) software version 4.0. *Mol. Biol. Evol.* **2007**, *24*, 1596–1599. [CrossRef] [PubMed]

49. Hoshino, T.; Kondo, Y.; Saito, K.; Terao, Y.; Okahashi, N.; Kawabata, S.; Fujiwara, T. Novel epitopic region of glucosyltransferase B from Streptococcus mutans. *Clin. Vaccine Immunol.* **2011**, *18*, 1552–1561. [CrossRef] [PubMed]

50. Hamada, S.; Torii, M. Effect of sucrose in culture media on the location of glucosyltransferase of Streptococcus mutans and cell adherence to glass surfaces. *Infect. Immun.* **1978**, *20*, 592–599. [PubMed]

51. Hamada, S.; Horikoshi, T.; Minami, T.; Okahashi, N.; Koga, T. Purification and characterization of cell-associated glucosyltransferase synthesizing water-insoluble glucan from serotype c *Streptococcus mutans*. *J. Gen. Microbiol.* **1989**, *135*, 335–344. [CrossRef]

52. Tomita, Y.; Zhu, X.; Ochiai, K.; Namiki, Y.; Okada, T.; Ikemi, T.; Fukushima, K. Evaluation of three individual glucosyltransferases produced by Streptococcus mutans using monoclonal antibodies. *FEMS Microbiol. Lett.* **1996**, *145*, 427–432. [CrossRef]

53. Fujiwara, T.; Hoshino, T.; Ooshima, T.; Sobue, S.; Hamada, S. Purification, characterization, and molecular analysis of the gene encoding glucosyltransferase from *Streptococcus oralis*. *Infect. Immun.* **2000**, *68*, 2475–2483. [CrossRef] [PubMed]

54. Mukasa, H.; Tsumori, H.; Shimamura, A. Isolation and characterization of an extracellular glucosyltransferase synthesizing insoluble glucan from *Streptococcus mutans* serotype c. *Infect. Immun.* **1985**, *49*, 790–796. [PubMed]

55. Shimamura, A.; Tsumori, H.; Mukasa, H. Purification and properties of *Streptococcus mutans* extracellular glucosyltransferase. *Biochim. Biophys. Acta* **1982**, *702*, 72–80. [CrossRef]

56. Mukasa, H.; Shimamura, A.; Tsumori, H. Purification and characterization of basic glucosyltransferase from Streptococcus mutans serotype c. *Biochim. Biophys. Acta* **1982**, *719*, 81–89. [CrossRef]

57. Grahame, D.; Mayer, R. Purification, and comparison, of two forms of dextransucrase from *Streptococcus sanguis. Carbohydr. Res.* **1985**, *142*, 285–298. [CrossRef]

58. Kobs, S.; Husman, D.; Cawthern, K. Mayer R Affinity purification of dextransucrase from *Streptococcus sanguis* ATCC 10558. *Carbohydr. Res.* **1990**, *203*, 156–161. [CrossRef]

59. Aoki, H.; Shiroza, T.; Hayakawa, M.; Sato, S.; Kuramitsu, H. Cloning of a *Streptococcus mutans* glucosyltransferase gene coding for insoluble glucan synthesis. *Infect. Immun.* **1986**, *53*, 587–594. [PubMed]

60. Shiroza, T.; Ueda, S.; Kuramitsu, H. Sequence analysis of the gtfB gene from *Streptococcus mutans. J. Bacteriol.* **1987**, *169*, 4263–4270. [CrossRef] [PubMed]

61. Hanada, N.; Kuramitsu, H. Isolation and characterization of the *Streptococcus mutans* gtfC gene, coding for synthesis of both soluble and insoluble glucans. *Infect. Immun.* **1988**, *56*, 1999–2005. [PubMed]

62. Fukushima, K.; Ikeda, T.; Kuramitsu, H. Expression of *Streptococcus mutans* gtf genes in Streptococcus milleri. *Infect. Immun.* **1992**, *60*, 2815–2822. [PubMed]

63. Honda, O.; Kato, C.; Kuramitsu, H. Nucleotide sequence of the *Streptococcus mutans* gtfD gene encoding the glucosyltransferase-S enzyme. *J. Gen. Microbiol.* **1990**, *136*, 2099–2105. [CrossRef] [PubMed]

64. Mukasa, H.; Shimamura, A.; Tsumori, H. Effect of salts on water-insoluble glucan formation by glucosyltransferase of *Streptococcus mutans*. *Infect. Immun.* **1979**, *23*, 564–570. [PubMed]

65. Sakanaka, S.; Kim, M.; Taniguchi, M.; Yamamoto, T. Antibacterial substances in Japanese green tea extract against *Streptococcus mutans*, a cariogenic bacterium. *Agric. Biol. Chem.* **1989**, *53*, 2307–2311. [CrossRef]

66. Hattori, M.; Kusumoto, I.; Namba, T.; Ishigami, T.; Hara, Y. Effect of tea polyphenols on glucan synthesis by glucosyltransferase from *Streptococcus mutans*. *Chem. Pharm. Bull.* **1990**, *38*, 717–720. [CrossRef] [PubMed]

67. Nakahara, K.; Kawabata, S.; Ono, H.; Ogura, K.; Tanaka, T.; Ooshima, T.; Hamada, S. Inhibitory effect of oolong tea polyphenols on glycosyltransferases of *mutans Streptococci*. *Appl. Environ. Microbiol.* **1993**, *59*, 968–973. [PubMed]

68. Ooshima, T.; Minami, T.; Aono, W.; Izumitani, A.; Sobue, S.; Fujiwara, T.; Kawabata, S.; Hamada, S. Oolong tea polyphenols inhibit experimental dental caries in SPF rats infected with *mutans streptococci*. *Caries Res.* **1993**, *27*, 124–129. [CrossRef] [PubMed]

69. Otake, S.; Makimura, M.; Kuroki, T.; Nishihara, Y.; Hirasawa, M. Anticaries effects of polyphenolic compounds from Japanese green tea. *Caries Res.* **1991**, *25*, 438–443. [CrossRef] [PubMed]

70. Kakiuchi, N.; Hattori, M.; Nishizawa, M.; Yamagishi, T.; Okuda, T.; Namba, T. Studies on dental caries prevention by traditional medicines. VIII. Inhibitory effect of various tannins on glucan synthesis by glucosyltransferase from *Streptococcus mutans*. *Chem. Pharm. Bull.* **1986**, *34*, 720–725. [CrossRef] [PubMed]

71. Wu-Yuan, C.; Chen, C.; Wu, R. Gallotannins inhibit growth, water-insoluble glucan synthesis, and aggregation of *mutans streptococci*. *J. Dent. Res.* **1988**, *67*, 51–55. [CrossRef]

72. Matsumoto, M.; Hamada, S.; Ooshima, T. Molecular analysis of the inhibitory effects of oolong tea polyphenols on glucan-binding domain of recombinant glucosyltransferases from *Streptococcus mutans* MT8148. *FEMS Microbiol. Lett.* **2003**, *228*, 73–80. [CrossRef]

73. Karygianni, L.; Al-Ahmad, A.; Argyropoulou, A.; Hellwig, E.; Anderson, A.C.; Skaltsounis, A.L. Natural Antimicrobials and Oral Microorganisms. A Systematic Review on Herbal Interventions for the Eradication of Multispecies Oral Biofilms. *Front. Microbiol.* **2015**, *6*, 1529. [CrossRef] [PubMed]

74. Hirasawa, M.; Takada, K.; Makimura, M.; Otake, S. Improvement of periodontal status by green tea catechin using a local delivery system. A clinical pilot study. *J. Period. Res.* **2002**, *37*, 433–438. [CrossRef]

75. Tamura, M.; Saito, H.; Kikuchi, K.; Ishigami, T.; Toyama, Y.; Takami, M.; Ochiai, K. Antimicrobial activity of Gel-entrapped catechins toward oral microorganisms. *Biol. Pharm Bull.* **2011**, *34*, 638–643. [CrossRef] [PubMed]

76. Cueno, M.E.; Tamura, M.; Imai, K.; Ochiai, K. Orally supplemented catechin increases heme amounts and catalase activities in rat heart blood mitochondria. A comparison between middle-aged and young rats. *Exp Gerontol.* **2013**, *48*, 1319–1322. [CrossRef] [PubMed]

77. Lai, P.K.; Donovan, J.; Takayama, H.; Sakagami, H.; Tanaka, A.; Konno, K.; Nonoyama, M. Modification of human immunodeficiency viral replication by pine cone extracts. *AIDS Res. Hum. Retrovirus.* **1990**, *6*, 205–217. [CrossRef] [PubMed]

78. Satoh, K.; Kihara, T.; Ida, Y.; Sakagami, H.; Koyama, N.; Premanathan, M.; Arakaki, R.; Nakashima, H.; Komatsu, N.; Fujimaki, M.; et al. Radical modulation activity of pine cone extracts of *Pinus elliottii* var. Elliottii. *Anticancer Res.* **1999**, *19*, 357–364. [PubMed]

79. Sakagami, H.; Yoshihara, M.; Fujimaki, M.; Wada, C.; Komatsu, N.; Nakashima, H.; Murakami, T.; Yamamoto, N. Effect of pine seed shell extract on microbial and viral infection. *Lett. Appl. Microbiol.* **1992**, *6*, 13–16.

80. Manabe, H.; Sakagami, H.; Ishizone, H.; Kusano, H.; Fujimaki, M.; Wada, C.; Komatsu, N.; Nakashima, H.; Murakami, T.; Yamamoto, N. Effects of Catuaba extracts on microbial and HIV infection. *In Vivo* **1992**, *6*, 161–165. [PubMed]

81. Sakagami, H.; Satoh, K.; Fukamachi, H.; Ikarashi, T.; Shimizu, A.; Yano, K.; Kanamoto, T.; Terakubo, S.; Nakashima, H.; Hasegawa, H.; et al. Anti-HIV and vitamin C-synergized radical scavenging activity of cacao husk lignin fractions. *In Vivo* **2008**, *22*, 327–332. [PubMed]

82. Sakagami, H.; Kawano, M.; Thet, M.M.; Hashimoto, K.; Satoh, K.; Kanamoto, T.; Terakubo, S.; Nakashima, H.; Haishima, Y.; Maeda, Y.; Sakurai, K. Anti-HIV and immunomodulation activities of cacao mass lignin carbohydrate complex. *In Vivo* **2011**, *25*, 229–236. [PubMed]

83. Kawano, M.; Sakagami, H.; Satoh, K.; Shioda, S.; Kanamoto, T.; Terakubu, S.; Nakashima, H.; Makino, T. Lignin-like activity of *Lentinus edodes* mycelia extract (LEM). *In Vivo* **2010**, *24*, 543–551. [PubMed]

84. Sakagami, H.; Asano, K.; Satoh, K.; Takahashi, K.; Kobayashi, M.; Koga, N.; Takahashi, H.; Tachikawa, R.; Tashiro, T.; Hasegawa, A.; et al. Anti-stress, anti-HIV and vitamin C-synergized radical scavenging activity of mulberry juice fractions. *In Vivo* **2007**, *21*, 499–505. [PubMed]

85. Nakashima, H.; Murakami, T.; Yamamoto, N.; Naoe, T.; Kawazoe, Y.; Konno, K.; Sakagami, H. Lignified materials as medicinal resources. V. Anti-HIV (human immunodeficiency virus) activity of some synthetic lignins. *Chem. Pharm. Bull.* **1992**, *40*, 2102–2105. [CrossRef] [PubMed]

86. Sakagami, H.; Kushida, T.; Oizumi, T.; Nakashima, H.; Makino, T. Distribution of lignin carbohydrate complex in plant kingdom and its functionality as alternative medicine. *Pharmacol. Ther.* **2010**, *128*, 91–105. [CrossRef] [PubMed]

87. Nakashima, H.; Murakami, T.; Yamamoto, N.; Sakagami, H.; Tanuma, S.; Hatano, T.; Yoshida, T.; Okuda, T. Inhibition of human immunodeficiency viral replication by tannins and related compounds. *Antivir. Res.* **1992**, *18*, 91–103. [CrossRef]

88. Fukai, T.; Sakagami, H.; Toguchi, M.; Takayama, F.; Iwakura, I.; Atsumi, T.; Ueha, T.; Nakashima, H.; Nomura, T. Cytotoxic activity of low molecular weight polyphenols against human oral tumor cell lines. *Anticancer Res.* **2000**, *20*, 2525–2536. [PubMed]

89. Sakagami, H.; Ohkoshi, E.; Amano, S.; Satoh, K.; Kanamoto, T.; Terakubo, S.; Nakashima, H.; Sunaga, K.; Otsuki, T.; Ikeda, H.; et al. Efficient utilization of plant resources by alkaline extraction. *Altern. Integr. Med.* **2013**, *2*, 2013.

90. Ohno, H.; Miyoshi, S.; Araho, D.; Kanamoato, T.; Terakubo, S.; Nakashima, H.; Tsuda, T.; Sunaga, K.; Amano, S.; Ohkoshi, E.; et al. Efficient utilization of licorice root by alkaline extraction. *In Vivo* **2014**, *28*, 785–794. [PubMed]

91. Kato, T.; Horie, N.; Matsuta, T.; Umemura, N.; Shimoyama, T.; Kaneko, T.; Kanamoto, T.; Terakubo, S.; Nakashima, H.; Kusama, K.; et al. Anti-UV/HIV activity of Kampo medicines and constituent plant extracts. *In Vivo* **2012**, *26*, 1007–1013. [PubMed]

92. Huang, W.; Yu, X.; Liang, N.; Ge, W.; Kwok, H.F.; Lau, C.B.; Li, Y.; Chung, H.Y. Anti-angiogenic Activity and Mechanism of Sesquiterpene Lactones from Centipeda minima. *Nat. Prod. Commun.* **2016**, *11*, 435–438.

93. Huang, W.; Wang, J.; Liang, Y.; Ge, W.; Wang, G.; Li, Y.; Chung, H.Y. Potent anti-angiogenic component in Croton crassifolius and its mechanism of action. *J. Ethnopharmacol.* **2015**, *175*, 185–191. [CrossRef] [PubMed]

94. Ho, Y.S.; Yu, M.S.; Lai, C.S.; So, K.F.; Yuen, W.H.; Chang, R.C. Characterizing the neuroprotective effects of alkaline extract of Lycium barbarum on beta-amyloid peptide neurotoxicity. *Brain Res.* **2007**, *16*, 123–134. [CrossRef] [PubMed]

95. Yuan, Z.; Wen, Y.; Kapu, N.S.; Beatson, R.; Mark Martinez, D. A biorefinery scheme to fractionate bamboo into high-grade dissolving pulp and ethanol. *Biotechnol. Biofuels* **2017**, *10*, 38. [CrossRef] [PubMed]

96. Xie, J.; Hse, C.Y.; De Hoop, C.F.; Hu, T.; Qi, J.; Shupe, T.F. Isolation and characterization of cellulose nanofibers from bamboo using microwave liquefaction combined with chemical treatment and ultrasonication. *Carbohydr. Polym.* **2016**, *151*, 725–734. [CrossRef] [PubMed]

97. Sakagami, H.; Sheng, H.; Okudaira, N.; Yasui, T.; Wakabayashi, H.; Jia, J.; Natori, T.; Suguro-Kitajima, M.; Oizumi, H.; Oizumi, T. Prominent Anti-UV activity and possible cosmetic potential of lignin-carbohydrate complex. *In Vivo* **2016**, *30*, 331–339. [PubMed]

98. Nanbu, T.; Shimada, J.; Kobayashi, M.; Hirano, K.; Koh, T.; Machino, M.; Ohno, H.; Yamamoto, M.; Sakagami, H. Anti-UV activity of lignin-carbohydrate complex and related compounds. *In Vivo* **2013**, *27*, 133–140.

99. Kato, T.; Segami, N.; Sakagami, H. Anti-inflammatory activity of hangeshashinto in IL-1β -stimulated gingival and periodontal ligament fibroblasts. *In Vivo* **2016**, *30*, 257–264. [PubMed]

100. Sakagami, H.; Shi, H.; Bandow, K.; Tomomura, M.; Tomomura, A.; Horiuchi, M.; Fujisawa, T.; Oizumi, T. Search of neuroprotective polyphenols using the "overlay" isolated method. *Molecules* **2018**, *23*, 1840. [CrossRef]

101. Sakagami, H.; Fukuchi, K.; Kanamoto, T.; Terakubo, S.; Nakashima, H.; Natori, T.; Suguro-Kitajima, M.; Oizumi, H.; Yasui, T.; Oizumi, T. Synergism of alkaline extract of the leaves of *Sasa senanensis* Rehder and antiviral agents. *In Vivo* **2016**, *30*, 421–426.

102. Sakagami, H.; Amano, S.; Yasui, T.; Satoh, K.; Shioda, S.; Kanamoto, T.; Terakubo, S.; Nakashima, H.; Watanabe, K.; Sugiura, T.; et al. Biological interaction between *Sasa senanensis* Rehder leaf extract and toothpaste ingredients. *In Vivo* **2013**, *27*, 275–284.

103. Matsuta, T.; Sakagami, H.; Kitajima, M.; Oizumi, H.; Oizumi, T. Anti-UV activity of alkaline extracts of the leaves of *Sasa senanensis* Rehder. *In Vivo* **2011**, *25*, 751–755. [PubMed]

104. Sakagami, H.; Amano, S.; Kikuchi, H.; Nakamura, Y.; Kuroshita, R.; Watanabe, S.; Satoh, K.; Hasegawa, H.; Nomura, A.; Kanamoto, T.; et al. Antiviral, antibacterial and vitamin C-synergized radical scavenging activity of *Sasa senanensis* Rehder extract. *In Vivo* **2008**, *22*, 471–476. [PubMed]

105. Tomomura, M.; Tomomura, A.; Oizumi, T.; Yasui, T.; Sakagami, H. Extract of *Sasa senanensis* Rehder leaf promotes osteoblast differentiation in MC3T3-E1 cells. *J. Meikai Dent. Med.* **2017**, *46*, 111–116.

106. Sakagami, H.; Iwamoto, S.; Matsuta, T.; Satoh, K.; Shimada, C.; Kanamoto, T.; Terakubo, S.; Nakashima, H.; Morita, Y.; Ohkubo, A.; et al. Comparative study of biological activity of three commercial products of *Sasa senanensis* Rehder leaf extract. *In Vivo* **2012**, *26*, 259–264. [PubMed]

107. Matsuta, T.; Sakagami, H.; Tanaka, S.; Machino, M.; Tomomura, M.; Tomomura, A.; Yasui, T.; Itoh, K.; Sugiura, T.; Kitajima, M.; et al. Pilot clinical study of *Sasa senanensis* Rehder leaf extract treatment on lichenoid dysplasia. *In Vivo* **2012**, *26*, 957–962. [PubMed]

108. Yamauchi, N.; Nakagawa, R.; Namiki, K.; Hayashi, T.; Iguchi, A.; Kubota, I.; Oizumi, T.; Ito, A. *Effect of Fe Chlorophyllin on Shunt Clot*; Kidney and Free Radical Series 4; Tokyo Igakusha: Tokyo, Japan, 1998; pp. 66–70.

109. Sakagami, H.; Sheng, H.; Ono, K.; Komine, Y.; Miyadai, T.; Terada, Y.; Nakada, D.; Tanaka, S.; Matsumoto, M.; Yasui, T.; et al. Anti-halitosis effect of toothpaste supplemented with alkaline extract of the leaves of *Sasa senanensis* Rehder. *In Vivo* **2016**, *30*, 107–111. [PubMed]

110. Hara, T.; Matsui, H.; Shimizu, H. Suppression of microbial metabolic pathways inhibits the generation of the human body odor component diacetyl by *Staphylococcus* spp. *PLoS ONE* **2014**, *9*, e111833. [CrossRef] [PubMed]

111. Mori, K.; Shoda, H.; Tanura, N.; Takeshima, H.; Shimada, J. Comparisons between the effects of herb treatments and cases in which cevimeline hydrochloride (Saligren®) is administered for xerostomia. *Jpn. J. Oral Diagnos. Oral Med.* **2008**, *21*, 205–211. (In Japanese)

112. Mori, K.; Onuki, H.; Yoshida, A.; Tamura, N.; Maekawa, Y.; Konno, C.; Iida, S.; Shimada, J. Two cases of Xerostomia that showed an improvement after being treated with Chinese herbal medicine. *J. Meikai Dent. Med.* **2008**, *37*, 153–158. (In Japanese)

113. Dietz, H.C. Marfan syndrome caused by a recurrent de novo missense mutation in the fibrillin gene. *Nature* **1991**, *352*, 337–339. [CrossRef]

114. McKusick, V.A. The defect in Marfan syndrome. *Nature* **1991**, *352*, 279–281. [CrossRef] [PubMed]

115. Judge, D.P.; Dietz, H.C. Marfan's syndrome. *Lancet* **2005**, *366*, 1965–1976. [CrossRef]

116. Ramirez, F.; Dietz, H.C. Extracellular microfibrils in vertebrate development and disease processes. *J. Biol. Chem.* **2009**, *284*, 14677–14681. [CrossRef] [PubMed]

117. Habashi, J.P.; Judge, D.P.; Holm, T.M.; Cohn, R.D.; Loeys, B.L.; Cooper, T.K.; Myers, L.; Klein, E.C.; Liu, G.; Calvi, C.; et al. Losartan, an AT1 antagonist, prevents aortic aneurysm in a mouse model of Marfan syndrome. *Science* **2006**, *312*, 117–121. [CrossRef] [PubMed]

118. Brooke, B.S. Angiotensin II blockade and aortic-root dilation in Marfan's syndrome. *N. Engl. J. Med.* **2008**, *358*, 2787–2795. [CrossRef] [PubMed]

119. Neptune, E.R.; Frischmeyer, P.A.; Arking, D.E.; Myers, L.; Bunton, T.E.; Gayraud, B.; Ramirez, F.; Sakai, L.Y.; Dietz, H.C. Dysregulation of TGF-β activation contributes to pathogenesis in Marfan syndrome. *Nat. Genet.* **2003**, *33*, 407–411. [CrossRef]

120. Sumners, C.; Tang, W.; Zelezna, B.; Raizada, M.K. Angiotensin II receptor subtypes are coupled with distinct signal-transduction mechanisms in neurons and astrocytes from rat brain. *Proc. Natl. Acad. Sci. USA* **1991**, *88*, 7567–7571. [CrossRef]

121. Habashi, J.P.; Doyle, J.J.; Holm, T.M.; Aziz, H.; Schoenhoff, F.; Bedja, D.; Chen, Y.; Modiri, A.N.; Judge, D.P.; Dietz, H.C. Angiotensin II type 2 receptor signaling attenuates aortic aneurysm in mice through ERK antagonism. *Science* **2011**, *332*, 361–365. [CrossRef]

122. Holm, T.M.; Habashi, J.P.; Doyle, J.J.; Bedja, D.; Chen, Y.; van Erp, C.; Lindsay, M.E.; Kim, D.; Schoenhoff, F.; Cohn, R.D.; et al. Noncanonical TGFβ signaling contributes to aortic aneurysm progression in Marfan syndrome mice. *Science* **2011**, *332*, 358–361. [CrossRef]

123. Takagi, H.; Yamamoto, H.; Iwata, K.; Goto, S.N.; Umemoto, T.; ALICE (All-Literature Investigation of Cardiovascular Evidence) Group. An evidence-based hypothesis for beneficial effects of telmisartan on Marfan syndrome. *Int. J. Cardiol.* **2012**, *158*, 101–102. [CrossRef]

124. De Coster, P.J.; Martens, L.C.; De Paepe, A. Oral manifestations of patients with Marfan syndrome. A case-control study. *Oral Surg. Oral Med. Oral Pathol. Oral Radiol. Endod.* **2002**, *93*, 564–572. [CrossRef] [PubMed]

125. Shiga, M.; Saito, M.; Hattori, M.; Torii, C.; Kosaki, K.; Kiyono, T.; Suda, N. Characteristic phenotype of immortalized periodontal cells isolated from a Marfan syndrome type I patient. *Cell Tissue Res.* **2008**, *331*, 461–472. [CrossRef] [PubMed]

126. Suda, N.; Shiga, M.; Ganburged, G.; Moriyama, K. Marfan syndrome and its disorder in periodontal tissues. *J. Exp. Zool. B. Mol. Dev. Evol.* **2009**, *312B*, 503–509. [CrossRef] [PubMed]

127. Hujoel, P.; Zina, L.G.; Cunha-Cruz, J.; Lopez, R. Historical perspectives on theories of periodontal disease etiology. *Periodontology* **2012**, *58*, 153–160. [CrossRef] [PubMed]

128. Fox, C.H. New considerations in the prevalence of periodontal disease. *Curr. Opin. Dent.* **1992**, *2*, 5–11. [PubMed]

129. Fox, C.; Jette, A.M.; McGuire, S.M.; Feldman, H.A.; Douglass, C.W. Periodontal disease among New England elders. *J. Periodontol.* **1994**, *65*, 676–684. [CrossRef] [PubMed]

130. O'Dowd, L.K.; Durham, J.; McCracken, G.I.; Preshaw, P.M. Patients' experiences of the impact of periodontal disease. *J. Clin. Periodontol.* **2010**, *37*, 334–339. [CrossRef]

131. Pihlstrom, B.L. Periodontal risk assessment, diagnosis and treatment planning. *Periodontology* **2000**, *2001*, 37–58. [CrossRef]

132. Page, R.C.; Schroeder, H.E. *Periodontitis in Man and Other Animals. A Comparative Review*; Karger Medical and Scientific: Basel, Switzerland, 1982; pp. 5–41.

133. Christersson, L.A.; Zambon, J.J.; Genco, R.J. Dental bacterial plaques. Nature and role in periodontal disease. *J. Clin. Periodontol.* **1991**, *18*, 441–446. [CrossRef]

134. Suzuki, J.; Imai, Y.; Aoki, M.; Fujita, D.; Aoyama, N.; Tada, Y.; Akazawa, H.; Izumi, Y.; Isobe, M.; Komuro, I.; et al. High incidence and severity of periodontitis in patients with Marfan syndrome in Japan. *Heart Vessels* **2015**, *30*, 692–695. [CrossRef]

135. Suzuki, J.; Imai, Y.; Aoki, M.; Fujita, D.; Aoyama, N.; Tada, Y.; Wakayama, K.; Akazawa, H.; Izumi, Y.; Isobe, M.; et al. Periodontitis in cardiovascular disease patients with or without Marfan syndrome—A possible role of Prevotella intermedia. *PLoS ONE* **2014**, *9*, e95521. [CrossRef] [PubMed]

136. Pereira, L.; Lee, S.Y.; Gayraud, B.; Andrikopoulos, K.; Shapiro, S.D.; Bunton, T.; Biery, N.J.; Dietz, H.C.; Sakai, L.Y.; Ramirez, F. Pathogenetic sequence for aneurysm revealed in mice underexpressing fibrillin-1. *Proc. Natl. Acad. Sci. USA* **1999**, *96*, 3819–3823. [CrossRef] [PubMed]

137. Ganburged, G.; Suda, N.; Saito, M.; Yamazaki, Y.; Isokawa, K.; Moriyama, K. Dilated capillaries, disorganized collagen fibers and differential gene expression in periodontal ligaments of hypomorphic fibrillin-1 mice. *Cell Tissue Res.* **2010**, *341*, 381–395. [CrossRef] [PubMed]

138. Karlberg, B.E.; Lins, L.E.; Hermansson, K. Efficacy and safety of telmisartan, a selective AT1 receptor antagonist, compared with enalapril in elderly patients with primary hypertension. TEES Study Group. *J. Hypertens.* **1999**, *17*, 293–302. [CrossRef] [PubMed]

139. Benson, S.C.; Pershadsingh, H.A.; Ho, C.I.; Chittiboyina, A.; Desai, P.; Pravenec, M.; Qi, N.; Wang, J.; Avery, M.A.; Kurtz, T.W. Identification of telmisartan as a unique angiotensin II receptor antagonist with selective PPARgamma-modulating activity. *Hypertension* **2004**, *43*, 993–1002. [CrossRef]

140. Kaschina, E.; Schrader, F.; Sommerfeld, M.; Kemnitz, U.R.; Grzesiak, A.; Krikov, M.; Unger, T. Telmisartan prevents aneurysm progression in the rat by inhibiting proteolysis, apoptosis and inflammation. *J. Hypertens.* **2008**, *26*, 2361–2373. [CrossRef]

141. Ohno, K.; Amano, Y.; Kakuta, H.; Niimi, T.; Takakura, S.; Orita, M.; Miyata, K.; Sakashita, H.; Takeuchi, M.; Komuro, I.; et al. Unique "delta lock" structure of telmisartan is involved in its strongest binding affinity to angiotensin II type 1 receptor. *Biochem. Biophys. Res. Commun.* **2011**, *404*, 434–437. [CrossRef]

142. Suda, N.; Moriyama, K.; Ganburged, G. Effect of angiotensin II receptor blocker on experimental periodontitis in a mouse model of Marfan syndrome. *Infect. Immun.* **2013**, *81*, 182–188. [CrossRef]

143. Mao, W.; Zhang, L.; Zou, C.; Li, C.; Wu, Y.; Su, G.; Guo, X.; Wu, Y.; Lu, F.; Lin, Q.; et al. Rationale and design of the Helping Ease Renal failure with Bupi Yishen compared with the Angiotensin II Antagonist Losartan (HERBAAL) trial. A randomized controlled trial in non-diabetes stage 4 chronic kidney disease. *BMC Complement. Altern. Med.* **2015**, *15*, 316. [CrossRef]

144. Tu, X.; Ye, X.; Xie, C.; Chen, J.; Wang, F.; Zhong, S. Combination Therapy with Chinese Medicine and ACEI/ARB for the Management of Diabetic Nephropathy: The Promise in Research Fragments. *Curr. Vasc. Pharmacol.* **2015**, *13*, 526–539. [CrossRef]

145. Yesudas, R.; Gumaste, U.; Snyder, R.; Thekkumkara, T. Tannic acid down-regulates the angiotensin type 1 receptor through a MAPK-dependent mechanism. *Mol. Endocrinol.* **2012**, *26*, 458–470. [CrossRef] [PubMed]

146. Sakagami, H.; Zhou, L.; Kawano, M.; Thet, M.M.; Tanaka, S.; Machino, M.; Amano, S.; Kuroshita, R.; Watanabe, S.; Chu, Q.; et al. Multiple biological complex of alkaline extract of the leaves of *Sasa senanensis* Rehder. *In Vivo* **2010**, *24*, 735–743. [PubMed]

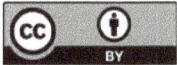

medicines

MDPI

Article

QSAR Prediction Model to Search for Compounds with Selective Cytotoxicity Against Oral Cell Cancer

Junko Nagai [1], **Mai Imamura** [1], **Hiroshi Sakagami** [2] and **Yoshihiro Uesawa** [1,*]

[1]   Department of Medical Molecular Informatics, Meiji Pharmaceutical University, 2-522-1 Noshio, Kiyose, Tokyo 204-8588, Japan; nagai-j@my-pharm.ac.jp (J.N.); y151038@std.my-pharm.ac.jp (M.I.)
[2]   Meikai University Research Institute of Odontology (M-RIO), 1-1 Keyakidai, Sakado, Saitama 350-0283, Japan; sakagami@dent.meikai.ac.jp
*   Correspondence: uesawa@my-pharm.ac.jp; Tel.: +81-42-495-8983

Received: 28 February 2019; Accepted: 26 March 2019; Published: 1 April 2019

Abstract: Background: Anticancer drugs often have strong toxicity against tumours and normal cells. Some natural products demonstrate high tumour specificity. We have previously reported the cytotoxic activity and tumour specificity of various chemical compounds. In this study, we constructed a database of previously reported compound data and predictive models to screen a new anticancer drug. **Methods**: We collected compound data from our previous studies and built a database for analysis. Using this database, we constructed models that could predict cytotoxicity and tumour specificity using random forest method. The prediction performance was evaluated using an external validation set. **Results**: A total of 494 compounds were collected, and these activities and chemical structure data were merged as database for analysis. The structure-toxicity relationship prediction model showed higher prediction accuracy than the tumour selectivity prediction model. Descriptors with high contribution differed for tumour and normal cells. **Conclusions**: Further study is required to construct a tumour selective toxicity prediction model with higher predictive accuracy. Such a model is expected to contribute to the screening of candidate compounds for new anticancer drugs.

Keywords: quantitative structure-activity relationship; machine learning; random forest; natural products; tumour-specificity

---

1. Introduction

Various anticancer drugs are used to treat oral cancer; however, most of these drugs also affect normal cells. Damage to normal cell induces several adverse effects, one of these is oral mucositis (OM). OM of patients who receiving cancer therapy makes difficult to eat and to deprive volition of treatment. OM is an inflammation induced by various factors such as trauma, viruses and bacterial infections, genetic factors, stress, vitamin deficiency, and chemotherapy [1,2]. The mechanism of detail is still not well known; however, toxicity to normal cells is one of the causes. In addition, many anticancer drugs are toxic to normal cells and have low selectivity for tumour cells. For these reasons, anticancer drugs which have low toxicity on normal cells are urgently needed.

Compounds which are highly tumour-specific exist in natural products. Previously, we reported cytotoxic activity against human oral squamous cell carcinoma (OSCC) cell lines and human oral normal cells using a variety of natural and synthesized organic compounds with chromone and azulene, which are present in various natural products, as the mother nucleus [3]. We have recently reported that many anticancer drugs induce keratinocyte toxicity by inducing apoptosis [4]. However, very few reports have been published [5] about the exploration of new synthetic substances that show low keratinocyte toxicity except of our studies (Table 1).

Table 1. Urgency of manufacturing new anticancer drugs with low keratinocyte toxicity (data obtained from SciFinder® [5] on 5 February 2019)

Search Terms	Number of Total Reports (A)	Number of Our Reports (B)	% (B/A) × 100
OSCC	8951 (100)	141	1.6
OSCC + Anticancer Drug	335 (3.70)	60	17.9
OSCC + Anticancer Drug + Tumour-Specificity	50 (0.56)	40	80.0
OSCC + Anticancer Drug + Tumour-Specificity + Newly Synthesized	2 (0.02)	2	100.0
OSCC + Anticancer Drug + Keratinocyte Toxicity	5 (0.06)	4	80.0
OSCC + anticancer drug + QSAR	27 (0.30)	25	92.6
OSCC + Anticancer Drug + QSAR+ Newly Synthesized	3 (0.03)	3	100.0

Based on the notion that similar structures have similar activity, the relationship between chemical structure and activity is referred to as the structure-activity relationship (SAR). Currently, using information about chemical structure which called "descriptor" that is structural, physicochemical and quantum chemical variety of characteristics, data were calculated and used for relation analysis. Conventionally, multiple regression analysis, which is a standard statistical approach, has been employed to analyse the relationship between the characteristic amount and activity of such drugs. Recently, machine-learning methods have been applied to such analyses due to their high prediction performance, and the quantitative structure activity relationship (QSAR) model is used to screen lead compounds in drug discovery research [6–8].

We have also studied the properties of compounds relative to cytotoxicity activity using QSAR analysis of compound and cytotoxic activity reported in the literature [3]. However, we could not employ high performance analysis methods due to the limited number of compounds evaluated in each study.

Thus, in this study, we gathered compound data from our previous reports and developed a database with a sufficient number of compounds to facilitate the use of a more advanced prediction method than single regression analysis. We attempted to construct a prediction model to search for compounds with high cytotoxic activity and tumour specificity score, using the collected data of cytotoxic activity of various compounds against tumour and normal cells.

To construct the prediction model, random forest (RF; one of the machine learning method) [9,10], was adopted, expecting the collection of sufficient numbers of compounds for QSAR analysis.

2. Materials and Methods

2.1. Data Collection and Preparation

We collected our original articles published up to May 2018 (with the exception of literature reviews), and compound and cytotoxicity data were extracted from the collected articles. All OSCC and normal human oral cells were incubated at 2×10^3/96-microwell and incubated for 48 h to produce near confluent cells (approximately half of the plate covered by cells) so that cells can further grow. Cells were then treated with various conditions of samples for 48 h. Controls contains the same concentration of DMSO, and subtracted from the experimental values to correct for DMSO cytotoxicity. Relative viable cell numbers were determined by MTT method. The conditions of cytotoxic assays were the same for all experiments we have done in our previous publications [11–49].

Cytotoxicity data were used as a ratio of mean 50% cytotoxic concentration (CC_{50}) against OSCC cell lines (HSC-2, HSC-3, and HSC-4) and human oral normal cells (human gingival fibroblast, HGF; human pulp cells, HPC; human periodontal ligament fibroblast, and HPLF), and these CC_{50} were converted to $-logCC_{50}$ (pCC_{50}), which is a negative common logarithm.

The tumour cell selective toxic index (selectivity index; SI) was defined as the ratio of the mean CC_{50} of OSCC cell lines to the mean CC_{50} of the human oral normal cells, and the SI was calculated for all individual compounds.

2.2. Chemical Structure Data Acquisition and Descriptor Calculation

The collected compounds were drawn using MarvinSketch 18.10.0 (ChemAxon, Budapest, Hungary) [50] and then converted to SMILES that is a form of a line notation based on graph theory, to obtain numerical data from the chemical structure.

The compound data were dealt with using the integrated computational chemistry system Molecular Operating Environment (MOE) version 2018.0101 (Chemical Computing Group Inc., Quebec, Canada) [51] as follows; salts were removed, structure optimization was calculated, and load partial charges were obtained. The structural data were converted to a 3D format by MOE using "Rebuild 3D" and structural optimization was realized by force field calculation (amber-10: EHT).

From this compound data, we calculated 2D and 3D descriptors using MOE and Dragon (version 7.0.2, Kode srl., Pisa, Italy) [52], respectively. Descriptors were treated independently by the software. Standard deviations were calculated with each descriptor; in cases where the value was zero, the descriptor was excluded. These descriptor data calculated by MOE and Dragon were merged for each compound.

2.3. Preparation of Data Table

The cytotoxic activity and descriptor data were merged to a data table for analysis. The compounds in this data table were checked for duplication by using SMILES. Compounds that had one SMILES to several cytotoxic activity data from different articles adopted the mean pCC_{50}.

2.4. Construction of Prediction Models by RF

The data table was randomly split (2:1 ratio) into a training set and an external validation set [53].

Eight structure-toxicity relationship prediction models were constructed by RF using the training set. The response variables of eight prediction models were three pCC_{50} against each OSCC cell line, three pCC_{50} against each human oral normal cell, the mean pCC_{50} against OSCC cell lines (mean tumour cell), and the mean pCC_{50} against human oral normal cells (i.e., the mean normal cell).

In the same manner, a tumour cell selective toxicity prediction model in which the response variable was the SI was constructed by using RF. Construction of prediction models by RF was performed "Bootstrap Forest" [54] in statistical software JMP® Pro. 13.1.0 (SAS Institute Inc., Cary, NC, USA) [55].

To construct the prediction model, changing parameter settings and largest coefficient of determination prediction model that was selected. Figure 1 shows the procedures from Sections 2.1–2.4.

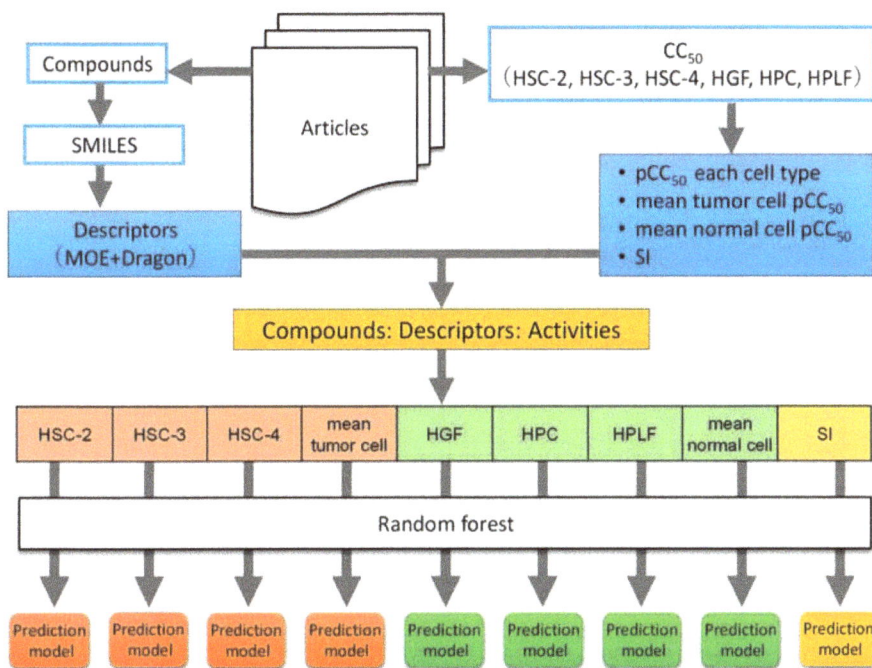

Figure 1. Schematic diagram of data collection and analysis.

3. Results

3.1. Data Collection

We obtained 498 compounds from 39 articles [11–49]. After eliminating duplicate compounds by SMILES, 494 compounds were analysed. Table 2 shows the articles and number of extracted compounds. These 494 compounds belong to the compound groups developed from various natural products, having skeletons shown in Table 2. SMILES data of these compounds are provided in Supplementary Materials (Table S1).

Table 2. Number of compounds and basic skeleton extracted from articles.

No.	Number of Compounds	Basic Skeleton	Ref.
1	9	Isoflavones and Isoflavanones	[9]
2	3	Three β-Diketones	[10]
3	6	Styrylchromones	[11]
4	3	Nocobactins NA-a, NA-b and Their Ferric Complexes	[12]
5	5	Betulinic Acid and Its Derivatives	[13]
6	2	Berberines	[14]
7	20	Coumarin and Its Derivatives	[15]
8	1	Mitomycin C, Bleomycin and Peplomycin	[16]
9	13	4-Trifluoromethylimidazole Derivatives	[17]
10	15	Phenoxazine Derivatives	[18]

Table 2. *Cont.*

No.	Number of Compounds	Basic Skeleton	Ref.
11	7	Vitamin K$_2$ Derivatives	[19]
12	2	4-Trifluoromethylimidazoles	[20]
13	10	Phenoxazines	[21]
14	18	Vitamin K$_2$ Derivatives and Prenylalcohols	[22]
15	10	3-Formylchromone Derivatives	[23]
16	12	5-Trifluoromethyloxazole Derivatives	[24]
17	19	1,2,3,4-Tetrahydroisoquinoline Derivatives	[25]
18	19	1,2,3,4Tetrahydroisoquinoline Derivatives	[26]
19	12	Dihydroimidazoles	[27]
20	24	Tropolones	[28]
21	24	Trihaloacetylazulenes	[29]
22	22	Trihaloacetylazulene Derivatives	[30]
23	10	Licorice Flavonoids	[31]
24	4	1,2,3,4-Tetrahydroisoquinoline Derivatives	[32]
25	19	2-Aminotropones	[33]
26	12	Phenylpropanoid Amides	[34]
27	12	Piperic Acid Amides	[35]
28	15	3-Styrylchromones	[36]
29	16	3-Styryl-2H-chromenes	[37]
30	18	Oleoylamides	[38]
31	17	3-Benzylidenechromanones	[39]
32	18	Licorice Root Extracts	[40]
33	15	Chalcones	[41]
34	11	Piperic Acid Esters	[42]
35	17	Aurones	[43]
36	24	2-Azolylchromones	[44]
37	10	Cinnamic Acid Phenetyl Esters	[45]
38	10	Azulene Amide Derivatives	[46]
39	10	Alkylaminoguaiazulenes	[47]

Descriptors were calculated from each software MOE and Dragon, subsequently excluded in case of the value is constant. After cleaning, 3750 descriptors were remained and used for analyses (319 descriptors calculated by MOE and 3431 descriptors calculated by Dragon).

Figure 2a shows applicability domain (AD). AD is the range of molecular properties or structures for which the model is considered to be applicable [56]. This scatter plot shows the result of principal component analysis using descriptors. The horizontal axis is the first principal component, and the vertical axis is the second principal component. Training set and test set compounds distribute as well balanced.

Moreover, to indicate detailed properties of these compounds, scatter plot of molecular weight (MW) and octanol-water partitioning coefficient (logP) is shown in Figure 2b. These compounds showed characteristic distribution of MW from 114.2 to 1125.8 (median 297.9); and logP from −1.53 to 13.9 (median 3.46).

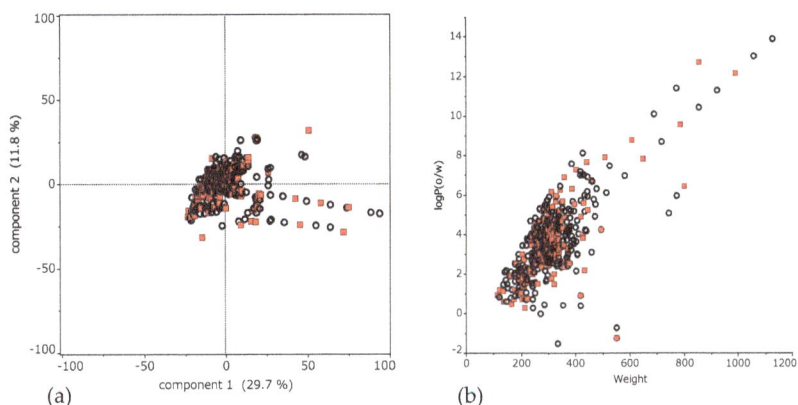

Figure 2. Chemical space of 494 compounds. (**a**) Applicability domain (AD) of 494 compounds. Scatter plot of principal component analysis using descriptors. The horizontal axis is the first principal component, and the vertical axis is the second principal component. These percentage are eigenvalue that represent a partition of the total variation in the multivariate sample. Each dot represents a compound; black circle is the training set and red square is the external validation set. (**b**) The horizontal axis is molecular weight (MW) and the vertical axis is octanol-water partitioning coefficient (logP). Here, each dot represents a compound; black is the training set and red is the external validation set.

3.2. Construction of Prediction Models by RF

Several prediction models were built by parameter turning. Here, the model that demonstrated the largest value was selected. The prediction accuracy and parameters of each model are shown in Table 3. These models were evaluated by using parameters as follows; R^2, root-mean-square error (RMSE), out of bag (OOB) RMSE, maximum absolute value of the residue, mean absolute error (MAE). The OOB RMSE is computed as the square root of the sum of squared errors divided by the number of OOB observations. OOB observations are training observations that are not used to construct a tree in RF. MAE is a mean of error at a model which the value is the closer to zero indicates the model is the higher accuracy.

Table 3. Parameters of each model by random forest

Parameters	Tumour Cells				Normal Cells				SI
	HSC-2	HSC-3	HSC-4	Mean	HGF	HPC	HPLF	Mean	
Number of Tree	100	300	100	100	100	100	100	100	300
Number of Term	952	1000	952	952	952	952	952	952	1000
Number of Maximum Split at Tree	100	1000	2000	2000	2000	2000	2000	2000	2000
Minimum Node Size	3	5	5	5	5	5	3	5	5
Seed Value	29	36	44	77	93	91	730	9045	124
Number of Tree	23	8	21	20	9	4	34	12	8
Number of Term at a Split	1000	1000	952	952	952	952	952	952	1000
R^2 (Training Set)	0.904	0.847	0.868	0.876	0.862	0.815	0.908	0.858	0.817
R^2 (External Validation Set)	0.564	0.568	0.631	0.563	0.554	0.659	0.515	0.576	0.404

Table 3. *Cont.*

Parameters	Tumour Cells				Normal Cells				SI
	HSC-2	HSC-3	HSC-4	Mean	HGF	HPC	HPLF	Mean	
RMSE (External Validation Set)	0.480	0.496	0.496	0.473	0.435	0.372	0.442	0.397	0.340
OOB RMSE	0.808	0.778	0.742	0.760	0.593	0.587	0.618	0.573	0.579
Maximum Absolute Value of the Residue	2.052	1.875	1.424	1.408	1.347	1.758	1.331	1.582	1.188
Mean Absolute Error	0.236	0.255	0.232	0.216	0.216	0.199	0.240	0.198	0.191

Figure 3 shows scatter plots of each RF model obtained using the training and external validation sets, the measured pCC_{50}, the predicted pCC_{50}, the predicted SI, and the observed SI.

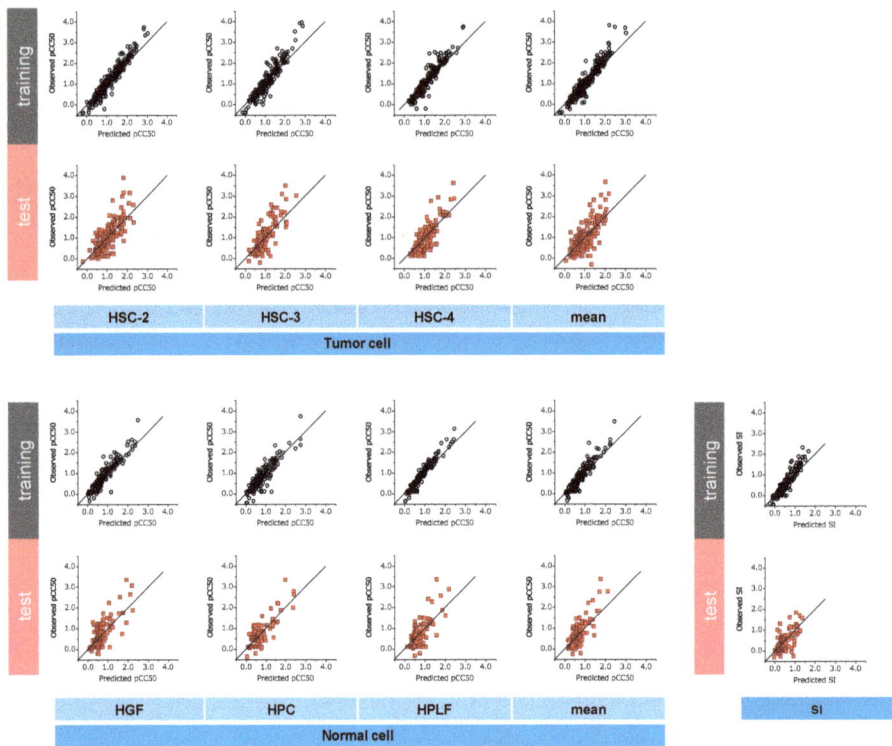

Figure 3. Scatter plot of training set and external validation set. In scatter plots of tumour and normal cell, the horizontal axis is the predicted pCC_{50}, and the vertical axis is the observed pCC_{50} of tumour and normal cell. In scatter plot of SI, the horizontal axis is the predicted SI, and the vertical axis is the observed SI. Each dot represents a compound; black circle is the training set and red square is the external validation set.

The model that demonstrated the greatest R^2 value with the external validation set was the normal cell HPC model ($R^2 = 0.659$, RMSE = 0.372), and the SI model ($R^2 = 0.404$, RMSE = 0.340) demonstrated the smallest R^2 value.

3.3. Large Contribution Descriptor for Prediction Model

Table 4 shows the top five contributing descriptors for the RF prediction model. Importance of descriptor were evaluated "LogWorth" in JMP® Pro software. "LogWorth" is calculated as negative common logarithm of p-value. This p-value is calculated in a complex manner that takes into account the number of different ways splits can occur. This calculation is very fair compared to the unadjusted p-value [57]. In the structure-toxicity relationship prediction model, most descriptors were classified into groups representing the topological shape. Note that descriptors meaning lipophilicity were observed in the tumour cell model, and electric charge descriptors were observed in the normal cell model. Topological or 3D shape descriptors were selected in the tumour cell selective toxicity prediction model.

Table 4. Top five contributing descriptors for random forest prediction model.

Cell Type		Descriptor	Meaning
Tumour Cells	HSC-2	vsurf_D7	Lipophilicity
		vsurf_D2	Lipophilicity
		GCUT_SMR_0	Topological shape
		CATS2D_07_LL	Lipophilicity
		SpMin2_Bh(e)	Topological shape and electric state
	HSC-3	SssNH	Topological shape and electric state
		b_max1len	Topological shape
		Mor13s	3D shape and electric state
		Mor15s	3D shape and electric state
		F01[C-C]	Topological shape
	HSC-4	SpMax_L	Topological shape
		SpAD_EA(dm)	Topological shape and dipole moment
		ATSC2s	Topological shape and electric state
		vsurf_D7	Lipophilicity
		ATSC5s	Topological shape and electric state
	Mean	logP(o/w)	Lipophilicity
		vsurf_D2	Lipophilicity
		vsurf_D6	Lipophilicity
		P_VSA_ppp_L	Topological shape and lipophilicity
		SssNH	Topological shape and electric state
Normal Cells	HGF	GCUT_SLOGP_0	Topological shape
		F10[C-N]	Topological shape
		SssNH	Topological shape and electric state
		SpMin2_Bh(s)	Topological shape
		GCUT_SMR_0	Topological shape
	HPC	VE1_B(p)	Topological shape and polarizability
		b_max1len	Topological shape
		CATS3D_10_PL	3D shape and electric state
		h_pKb	Topological shape and electric state
		SpMin1_Bh(p)	Topological shape and polarizability

Table 4. *Cont.*

Cell Type		Descriptor	Meaning
Normal Cells	HPLF	P_VSA_e_3	Topological shape and electric state
		GCUT_SLOGP_0	Topological shape
		F10[C-N]	Topological shape
		SssNH	Topological shape and electric state
	Mean	h_pavgQ	Topological shape and electric state
		h_pstrain	Topological shape and electric state
		h_pavgQ	Topological shape and electric state
		b_max1len	Topological shape
		SssNH	Topological shape and electric state
		F10[C-N]	Topological shape
SI		TDB08p	3D shape and polarizability
		F06[C-N]	Topological shape
		PEOE_VSA+1	Topological shape and electric state
		R5u+	3D shape and size
		RDF035m	3D shape and size

4. Discussion

From our previous articles, 494 compounds and activity data were obtained. As reported in previous studies, compounds with higher tumour specificity than existing anticancer drugs are present among these 494 compounds. For example, in a study of 3-Styryl-2*H*-chromenes, several compounds showed higher tumour specificity than doxorubicin (at most approximately 4.8 times higher specificity) [39].

In this study, we constructed a database of seed compounds for anticancer drugs, including a sufficient number of compounds for analysis.

Regarding cell type, the structure-toxicity relationship prediction models demonstrated the maximum R^2 value for cytotoxic activity against normal cells. If toxicity against normal cells can be predicted accurately, it is hoped that such prediction models can be applied to the estimation of side effects caused by cytotoxicity against normal cells, such as OM, hematotoxicity alopecia and so on. In contrast, with the training set, the R^2 values were greater than 0.9. In addition, the R^2 values of all structure-toxicity relationship prediction models obtained with the external validation set were greater 0.5.

We consider that the structure responsible for lipophilicity or a combination of lipophilicity and another characteristic descriptors may contribute to cytotoxic activity prediction because lipophilicity was tend to observed in the tumour cell models and not in the normal cell models. Relationship of between lipophilicity and cytotoxicity against tumour cell might be considered that penetration mechanism of compounds into tumour cell is one of the reason, however, further study is needed.

We expect that these findings will be useful relative to examining prediction models in future. In construct to structure-toxicity relationship prediction model, the R^2 results of the tumour cell selective toxicity prediction models were less than 0.5.

In light of these results, further study is required to construct a tumour cell selective toxicity prediction model. With the RF method, the meaning of the top five contributing descriptors tended to differ from the structure-toxicity relationship and tumour cell selective toxicity prediction models.

These results indicate that tumour cell selective toxicity prediction is difficult to realize using the methods employed in the cytotoxic activity prediction model.

Thus, further study involving other methods, parameter tuning, and so on is required to construct a tumour cell selective toxicity prediction model with high prediction accuracy. Superior anticancer drugs require both strong cytotoxicity against tumour cells and selectivity to tumour cells, therefore cytotoxic activity prediction model is needed.

In this study, we constructed prediction models that can estimate cytotoxicity and tumour selective toxicity based on cytotoxic activity data derived from various compounds. The RF machine learning method constructed models with higher prediction accuracy.

In future, using our findings as reference, we would like to construct a high-performance prediction model that can be used to search for candidate compounds for a new anticancer drug.

5. Conclusions

In this study, we constructed a database of different compounds with structure and cytotoxic activity data derived from various compounds reported in previous studies. With this database, cytotoxicity and tumour cell selective toxicity prediction models were constructed by RF method. It was found that the structure-toxicity relationship prediction model tended to demonstrate greater R^2 values.

In future, we expect that collecting addition compound data and investigating various model construction methods will help realize a prediction model with good prediction accuracy, which would facilitate the search for candidate compounds for anticancer drugs.

Supplementary Materials: The following are available online at http://www.mdpi.com/2305-6320/6/2/45/s1, Table S1: SMILES of 494 compounds.

Author Contributions: J.N., M.I. performed QSAR analysis; H.S. performed cytotoxicity assay; Y.U. organized the review.

Funding: This work was partially supported by KAKENHI from the Japan Society for the Promotion of Science (JSPS): 15K08111(Y.U.) and 16K11519(S.H.).

Acknowledgments: The authors acknowledge Yoshiaki Sugita and Koichi Takao for the supply of chromones, and Meikai University School of Dentistry for the support for the research.

Conflicts of Interest: The authors declare no conflict of interest.

Abbreviations

HGF	Human gingival fibroblast
HPC	Human pulp cell
HPLF	Human periodontal fibroblast
Log P	Octanol-water partitioning coefficient
MOE	Molecular Operating Environment
OM	Oral mucositis
OOB	Out-of-bag
OSCC	Oral squamous cell carcinoma
pCC$_{50}$	$-$logCC$_{50}$, a negative common logarithm
QASR	Quantitative structure-activity relationship
R^2	Coefficient of determination
RF	Random forest
RMSE	Root-mean-square error
SAR	Structure-activity relationship

References

1. Sonis, S.T. Mucositis: The impact, biology and therapeutic opportunities of oral mucositis. *Oral Oncol.* **2009**, *45*, 1015–1020. [CrossRef] [PubMed]
2. Yoshino, F.; Yoshida, A.; Nakajima, A.; Wada-Takahashi, S.; Takahashi, S.S.; Lee, M.C. Alteration of the redox state with reactive oxygen species for 5-fluorouracil-induced oral mucositis in hamsters. *PLoS ONE* **2013**, *8*, e82834. [CrossRef] [PubMed]

3.   Sugita, Y.; Takao, K.; Uesawa, Y.; Sakagami, H. Search for New Type of Anticancer Drugs with High Tumor Specificity and Less Keratinocyte Toxicity. *Anticancer Res.* **2017**, *37*, 5919–5924. [PubMed]

4.   Sakagami, H.; Okudaira, N.; Masuda, Y.; Amano, O.; Yokose, S.; Kanda, Y.; Suguro, M.; Natori, T.; Oizumi, H.; Oizumi, T. Induction of apoptosis in human oral keratinocyte by doxorubicin. *Anticancer Res.* **2017**, *37*, 1023–1029.

5.   SciFinder®. Available online: https://www.cas.org/products/scifinder (accessed on 5 February 2019).

6.   Wolfgang, S.; Dina, R. QSAR/QSPR. In *Applied Chemoinformatics*; Thomas, E., Johann, G., Eds.; Wiley-VCH: Weinheim, Germany; Berlin, Germany, 2018; pp. 9–13.

7.   Guohui, S.; Tengjiao, F.; Xiaodong, S.; Yuxing, H.; Xin, C.; Lijiao, Z.; Ting, R.; Yue, Z.; Rugang, Z.; Yongzhen, P. In Silico Prediction of O^6-Methylguanine-DNA Methyltransferase Inhibitory Potency of Base Analogs with QSAR and Machine Learning Methods. *Molecules* **2018**, *23*, 2892.

8.   Tengjiao, F.; Guohui, S.; Lijiao, Z.; Xin, C.; Rugang, Z. QSAR and Classification Study on Prediction of Acute Oral Toxicity of N-Nitroso Compounds. *Int. J. Mol. Sci.* **2018**, *19*, 3015.

9.   Breiman, L. Random forests. *Mach. Learn.* **2001**, *45*, 5–32. [CrossRef]

10.   Svetnik, V.; Liaw, A.; Tong, C.; Culberson, J.C.; Sheridan, R.P.; Feuston, B.P. Random forest: A classification and regression tool for compound classification and QSAR modeling. *J. Chem. Inf. Comput. Sci.* **2003**, *43*, 1947–1958. [CrossRef]

11.   Shirataki, Y.; Wakae, M.; Yamamoto, Y.; Hashimoto, K.; Satoh, K.; Ishihara, M.; Kikuchi, H.; Nishikawa, H.; Minagawa, K.; Motohashi, N.; et al. Cytotoxicity and radical modulating activity of isoflavones and isoflavanones from sophora species. *Anticancer Res.* **2004**, *24*, 1481–1488.

12.   Ishihara, M.; Sakagami, H. Re-evaluation of cytotoxicity and iron chelation activity of three β-diketones by semiempirical molecular orbital method. *In Vivo* **2005**, *19*, 119–124.

13.   Momoi, K.; Sugita, Y.; Ishihara, M.; Satoh, K.; Kikuchi, H.; Hashimoto, K.; Yokoe, I.; Nishikawa, H.; Fujisawa, S.; Sakagami, H. Cytotoxic activity of styrylchromones against human tumor cell lines. *In Vivo* **2005**, *19*, 157–164. [PubMed]

14.   Sakagami, H.; Ishihara, M.; Hoshino, Y.; Ishikawa, J.; Mikami, Y.; Fukai, T. Cytotoxicity of nocobactins NA-a, NA-b and their ferric complexes assessed by semiempirical molecular orbital method. *In Vivo* **2005**, *19*, 277–282. [PubMed]

15.   Ishihara, M.; Sakagami, H.; Liu, W.K. Quantitative structure-cytotoxicity relationship analysis of betulinic acid and its derivatives by semi-empirical molecular-orbital method. *Anticancer Res.* **2005**, *25*, 3951–3956. [PubMed]

16.   Inoue, K.; Kulsum, U.; Chowdhury, SA.; Fujisawa, S.; Ishihara, M.; Yokoe, I.; Sakagami, H. Tumor-specific cytotoxicity and apoptosis-inducing activity of berberines. *Anticancer Res.* **2005**, *25*, 4053–4060. [PubMed]

17.   Ishihara, M.; Yokote, Y.; Sakagami, H. Quantitative structure-cytotoxicity relationship analysis of coumarin and its derivatives by semiempirical molecular orbital method. *Anticancer Res.* **2006**, *26*, 2883–2886. [PubMed]

18.   Sasaki, M.; Okamura, M.; Ideo, A.; Shimada, J.; Suzuki, F.; Ishihara, M.; Kikuchi, H.; Kanda, Y.; Kunii, S.; Sakagami, H. Re-evaluation of tumor-specific cytotoxicity of mitomycin c, bleomycin and peplomycin. *Anticancer Res.* **2006**, *26*, 3373–3380.

19.   Ishihara, M.; Kawase, M.; Sakagami, H. Quantitative structure-activity relationship analysis of 4-trifluoromethylimidazole derivatives with the concept of absolute hardness. *Anticancer Res.* **2007**, *27*, 4047–4052.

20.   Ishihara, M.; Kawase, M.; Westman, G.; Samuelsson, K.; Motohashi, N.; Sakagami, H. Quantitative structure-cytotoxicity relationship analysis of phenoxazine derivatives by semiempirical molecular-orbital method. *Anticancer Res.* **2007**, *27*, 4053–4058. [PubMed]

21.   Ishihara, M.; Sakagami, H. QSAR of molecular structure and cytotoxic activity of vitamin K_2 derivatives with concept of absolute hardness. *Anticancer Res.* **2007**, *27*, 4059–4064.

22.   Takekawa, F.; Nagumo, T.; Shintani, S.; Hashimoto, K.; Kikuchi, H.; Katayama, T.; Ishihara, M.; Amano, O.; Kawase, M.; Sakagami, H. Tumor-specific cytotoxic activity and type of cell death induced by 4-trifluoromethylimidazoles in human oral squamous cell carcinoma cell lines. *Anticancer Res.* **2007**, *27*, 4065–4070.

23.   Suzuki, F.; Hashimoto, K.; Ishihara, M.; Westman, G.; Samuelsson, K.; Kawase, M.; Motohashi, N.; Sakagami, H. Tumor-specificity and type of cell death induced by phenoxazines. *Anticancer Res.* **2007**, *27*, 4233–4238. [PubMed]

Medicines **2019**, 6, 45

24. Sakagami, H.; Hashimoto, K.; Suzuki, F.; Ishihara, M.; Kikuchi, H.; Katayama, T.; Satoh, K. Tumor-specificity and type of cell death induced by vitamin K_2 derivatives and prenylalcohols. *Anticancer Res.* **2008**, *28*, 151–158. [PubMed]

25. Ishihara, M.; Sakagami, H. Quantitative structure-cytotoxicity relationship analysis of 3-formylchromone derivatives by a semiempirical molecularorbital method with the concept of absolute hardness. *Anticancer Res.* **2008**, *28*, 277–282.

26. Ishihara, M.; Kawase, M.; Sakagami, H. Quantitative structure-cytotoxicity relationship analysis of 5-trifluoromethyloxazole derivatives by a semiempirical molecular-orbital method with the concept of absolute hardness. *Anticancer Res.* **2008**, *28*, 997–1004.

27. Ishihara, M.; Hatano, H.; Kawase, M.; Sakagami, H. Estimation of relationship between the structure of 1, 2, 3, 4-tetrahydroisoquinoline derivatives determined by a semiempirical molecular-orbital method and their cytotoxicity. *Anticancer Res.* **2009**, *29*, 2265–2272.

28. Hatano, H.; Takekawa, F.; Hashimoto, K.; Ishihara, M.; Kawase, M.; Qing, C.; Qin-Tao, W.; Sakagami, H. Tumor-specific cytotoxic activity of 1, 2, 3, 4-tetrahydroisoquinoline derivatives against human oral squamous cell carcinoma cell lines. *Anticancer Res.* **2009**, *29*, 3079–3086.

29. Takekawa, F.; Sakagami, H.; Ishihara, M. Estimation of relationship between structure of newly synthesized dihydroimidazoles determined by a semiempirical molecular-orbital method and their cytotoxicity. *Anticancer Res.* **2009**, *29*, 5019–5022. [PubMed]

30. Ishihara, M.; Wakabayashi, H.; Motohashi, N.; Sakagami, H. Quantitative structure-cytotoxicity relationship of newly synthesized tropolones determined by a semiempirical molecular-orbital method (PM5). *Anticancer Res.* **2010**, *30*, 129–134.

31. Ishihara, M.; Wakabayashi, H.; Motohashi, N.; Sakagami, H. Quantitative structure–cytotoxicity relationship of newly synthesized trihaloacetylazulenes determined by a semi-empirical molecular-orbital method (PM5). *Anticancer Res.* **2011**, *31*, 515–520.

32. Ishihara, M.; Wakabayashi, H.; Motohashi, N.; Sakagami, H. Estimation of relationship between the structure of trihaloacetylazulene derivatives determined by a semiempirical molecular–orbital method (PM5) and their cytotoxicity. *Anticancer Res.* **2010**, *30*, 837–842. [PubMed]

33. Ohno, H.; Araho, D.; Uesawa, Y.; Kagaya, H.; Ishihara, M.; Sakagami, H.; Yamamoto, M. Evaluation of cytotoxicity and tumor-specificity of licorice flavonoids based on chemical structure. *Anticancer Res.* **2013**, *33*, 3061–3068.

34. Uesawa, Y.; Mohri, K.; Kawase, M.; Ishihara, M.; Sakagami, H. Quantitative structure–activity relationship (QSAR) analysis of tumor-specificity of 1, 2, 3, 4-tetrahydroisoquinoline derivatives. *Anticancer Res.* **2011**, *31*, 4231–4238. [PubMed]

35. Sekine, S.; Shimodaira, C.; Uesawa, Y.; Kagaya, H.; Kanda, Y.; Ishihara, M.; Amano, O.; Sakagami, H.; Wakabayashi, H. Quantitative structure–activity relationship analysis of cytotoxicity and anti-uv activity of 2-aminotropones. *Anticancer Res.* **2014**, *34*, 1743–1750.

36. Shimada, C.; Uesawa, Y.; Ishihara, M.; Kagaya, H.; Kanamoto, T.; Terakubo, S.; Nakashima, H.; Takao, K.; Saito, T.; Sugita, Y.; et al. Quantitative structure–cytotoxicity relationship of phenylpropanoid amides. *Anticancer Res.* **2014**, *34*, 3543–3548.

37. Shimada, C.; Uesawa, Y.; Ishihara, M.; Kagaya, H.; Kanamoto, T.; Terakubo, S.; Nakashima, H.; Takao, K.; Miyashiro, T.; Sugita, Y.; et al. Quantitative structure–cytotoxicity relationship of piperic acid amides. *Anticancer Res.* **2014**, *34*, 4877–4884.

38. Shimada, C.; Uesawa, Y.; Ishii-Nozawa, R.; Ishihara, M.; Kagaya, H.; Kanamoto, T.; Terakubo, S.; Nakashima, H.; Takao, K.; Sugita, Y.; et al. Quantitative structure–cytotoxicity relationship of 3-styrylchromones. *Anticancer Res.* **2014**, *34*, 5405–5412.

39. Uesawa, Y.; Sakagami, H.; Ishihara, M.; Kagaya, H.; Kanamoto, T.; Terakubo, S.; Nakashima, H.; Yahagi, H.; Takao, K.; Sugita, Y. Quantitative structure–cytotoxicity relationship of 3-styryl-2*H*-chromenes. *Anticancer Res.* **2015**, *35*, 5299–5308. [PubMed]

40. Sakagami, H.; Uesawa, Y.; Ishihara, M.; Kagaya, H.; Kanamoto, T.; Terakubo, S.; Nakashima, H.; Takao, K.; Sugita, Y. Quantitative structure–cytotoxicity relationship of oleoylamides. *Anticancer Res.* **2015**, *35*, 5341–5355. [PubMed]

41. Uesawa, Y.; Sakagami, H.; Kagaya, H.; Yamashita, M.; Takao, K.; Sugita, Y. Quantitative structure-cytotoxicity relationship of 3-benzylidenechromanones. *Anticancer Res.* **2016**, *36*, 5803–5812. [CrossRef]

42. Fukuchi, K.; Okudaira, N.; Adachi, K.; Odai-Ide, R.; Watanabe, S.; Ohno, H.; Yamamoto, M.; Kanamoto, T.; Terakubo, S.; Nakashima, H.; et al. Antiviral and antitumor activity of licorice root extracts. *In Vivo* **2016**, *30*, 777–786. [CrossRef]

43. Sakagami, H.; Masuda, Y.; Tomomura, M.; Yokose, S.; Uesawa, Y.; Ikezoe, N.; Asahara, D.; Takao, K.; Kanamoto, T.; Terakubo, S.; et al. Quantitative structure–cytotoxicity relationship of chalcones. *Anticancer Res.* **2017**, *37*, 1091–1098.

44. Sakagami, H.; Uesawa, Y.; Masuda, Y.; Tomomura, M.; Yokose, S.; Miyashiro, T.; Murai, J.; Takao, K.; Kanamoto, T.; Terakubo, S.; et al. Quantitative structure–cytotoxicity relationship of newly synthesized piperic acid esters. *Anticancer Res.* **2017**, *37*, 6161–6168.

45. Uesawa, Y.; Sakagami, H.; Ikezoe, N.; Takao, K.; Kagaya, H.; Sugita, Y. Quantitative structure–cytotoxicity relationship of aurones. *Anticancer Res.* **2017**, *37*, 6169–6176.

46. Sakagami, H.; Okudaira, N.; Uesawa, Y.; Takao, K.; Kagaya, H.; Sugita, Y. Quantitative structure–cytotoxicity relationship of 2-azolylchromones. *Anticancer Res.* **2018**, *38*, 763–770.

47. Uesawa, Y.; Sakagami, H.; Okudaira, N.; Toda, K.; Takao, K.; Kagaya, H.; Sugita, Y. Quantitative structure–cytotoxicity relationship of cinnamic acid phenetyl esters. *Anticancer Res.* **2018**, *38*, 817–823. [CrossRef] [PubMed]

48. Wada, T.; Maruyama, R.; Irie, Y.; Hashimoto, M.; Wakabayashi, H.; Okudaira, N.; Uesawa, Y.; Kagaya, H.; Sakagami, H. In vitro anti-tumor activity of azulene amide derivatives. *In Vivo* **2018**, *32*, 479–486. [PubMed]

49. Uehara, M.; Minemura, H.; Ohno, T.; Hashimoto, M.; Wakabayashi, H.; Okudaira, N.; Sakagami, H. In vitro antitumor activity of alkylaminoguaiazulenes. *In Vivo* **2018**, *32*, 541–547. [PubMed]

50. Marvin. Available online: https://chemaxon.com/products/marvin (accessed on 15 November 2018).

51. MOE. Available online: http://www.chemcomp.com/MOE-Molecular_Operating_Environment.htm (accessed on 15 November 2018).

52. Dragon. Available online: https://chm.kode-solutions.net/products_dragon.php (accessed on 15 November 2018).

53. Paola, G. Principles of QSAR models validation: Internal and external. *QSAR Comb. Sci.* **2007**, *26*, 694–701.

54. SAS Institute Inc. Chapter 6 Bootstrap Forest. In *JMP® 13 Predictive and Specialized Modeling*, 2nd ed.; SAS Institute Inc.: Cary, NC, USA, 2017; pp. 107–122.

55. JMP®. Available online: https://www.jmp.com/en_us/home.html (accessed on 15 November 2018).

56. Wolfgang, S.; Dina, R. Applicability domain and model acceptability critera. In *Applied Chemoinformatics*; Thomas, E., Johann, G., Eds.; Wiley-VCH: Weinheim, Germany; Berlin, Germany, 2018; pp. 41–43.

57. SAS Institute Inc. Chapter 5 Partition Models. In *JMP® 13 Predictive and Specialized Modeling*, 2nd ed.; SAS Institute Inc.: Cary, NC, USA, 2017; pp. 104–106.

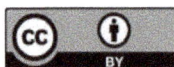

MDPI

St. Alban-Anlage 66

4052 Basel

Switzerland

Tel. +41 61 683 77 34

Fax +41 61 302 89 18

www.mdpi.com

Medicines Editorial Office

E-mail: medicines@mdpi.com

www.mdpi.com/journal/medicines

www.ingramcontent.com/pod-product-compliance
Lightning Source LLC
Chambersburg PA
CBHW051847210326
41597CB00033B/5802